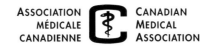

ASSOCIATION
MÉDICALE
CANADIENNE

CANADIAN
MEDICAL
ASSOCIATION

CANADIAN MEDICAL
ASSOCIATION

COMPLETE BOOK OF
MOTHER &
BABY CARE

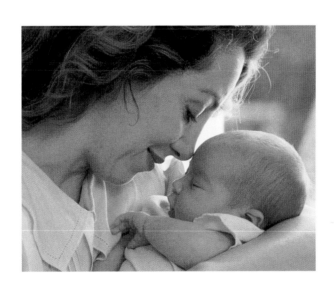

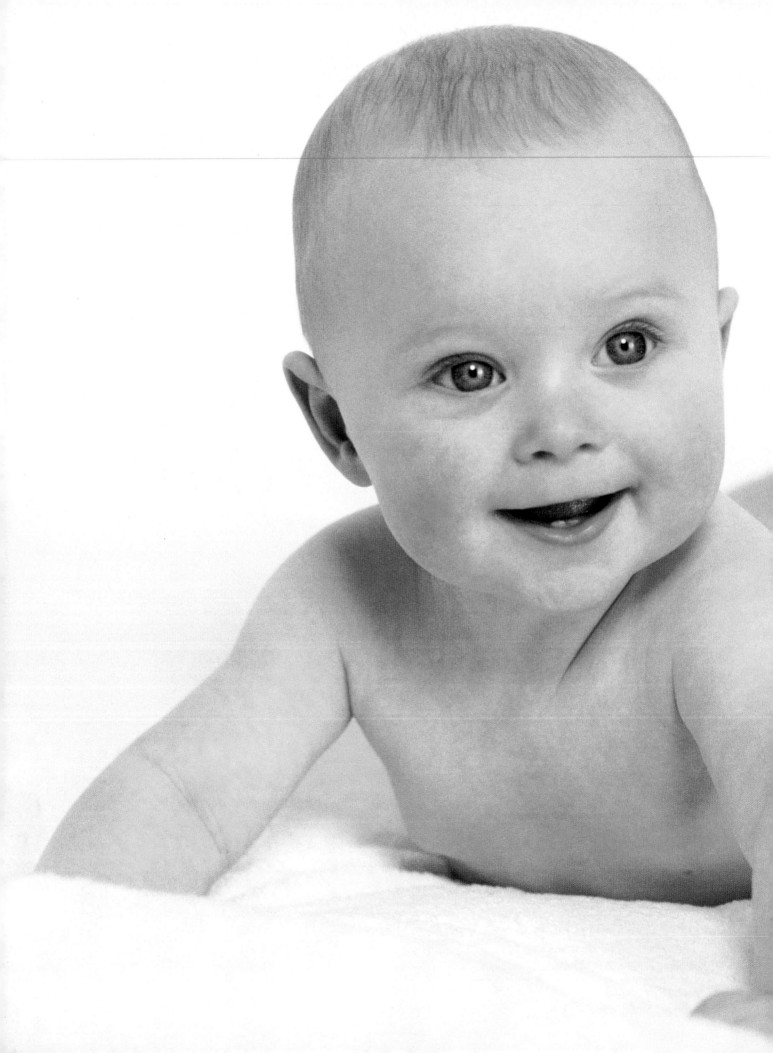

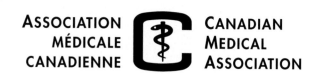

ASSOCIATION MÉDICALE CANADIENNE

CANADIAN MEDICAL ASSOCIATION

CANADIAN MEDICAL ASSOCIATION

COMPLETE BOOK OF MOTHER & BABY CARE

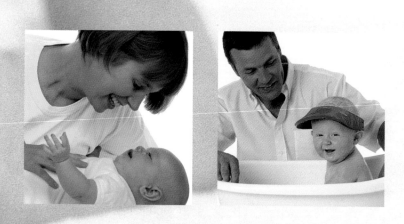

Medical Editor

CATHERINE YOUNGER-LEWIS MD, MJ

www.dk.com

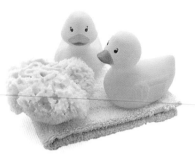

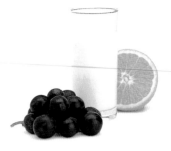

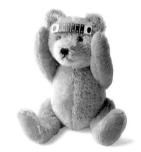

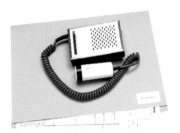

MEDICAL CONSULTANTS

M. Shirley Gross MDCM, CCFP; Sidney Kardash MD, FRCPC
Mary Krywulak DMD, MS; Charmaine Roye MDCM, FRCSC

The CMA acknowledges the valuable contribution of
Health Canada (Consumer Product Safety),
the City of Ottawa Public Health and St. John Ambulance.

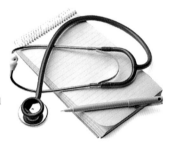

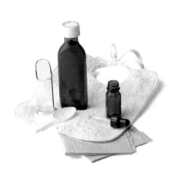

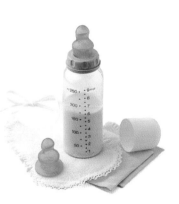

Canadian Cataloguing in Publication Data
Main entry under title:
Canadian Medical Association Complete Mother & Baby Care/
Catherine Younger-Lewis MD, MJ, medical editor.
Includes index.
ISBN 978-1-55363-086-9

III. Infants—Care. 2. Child care. 3. Pregnancy. I. Younger-
Lewis, Catherine II. Canadian Medical Association.
III. Title: Complete Mother & Baby Care. IV. Title: Complete
Mother and Baby Care.

RG525.C34 2002   649'.122   C2002-901558-8

Colour reproduction by Colourscan, Singapore
Printed and bound by Neografia, Slovakia

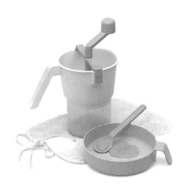

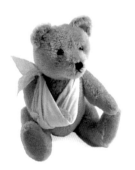

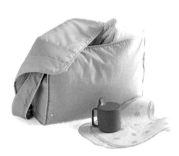

Having a baby opens up a new, joyful and exciting world for the mother, the father, other children in the family, and the grandparents-to-be. But it's also full of challenges. There's a lot to learn and unforeseen events can take place. Although parents may handle these challenges in different ways, there's often an "easiest" or "best" way. That's what the *Complete Book of Mother & Baby Care* is about.

This updated version features hundreds of beautiful illustrations and clearly written text covering the entire period from the beginning of pregnancy to early childhood. It offers sensible, easy-to-understand pointers on nutrition, exercise, self-care, baby care, and on getting the most out of medical and obstetric care (including important questions to ask your physician). It also reflects the emerging complexities of the Canadian family. And it includes online resources, updated information on immunization and prenatal tests, and a revised section on breast-feeding with an emphasis on preventing problems.

The *Complete Book of Mother & Baby Care* is more than a self-help or "how-to" book; it was written and reviewed by health professionals who are experts in the field. The book tells parents what they need to know about the way physicians are currently practicing obstetrics and pediatrics, about what to do in an emergency before medical help arrives, about when to call the doctor.

The *Complete Book of Mother & Baby Care* reflects the Canadian health care system and Canadian medical practice. It is a welcome companion to the Canadian Medical Association's series of health guides for the general public, notably the *Complete Home Medical Guide*.

I hope this practical book will help you both in every stage of your pregnancy, delivery, and care of your young child and will allow you to more fully enjoy, as I have, the greatest gift of life — your child.

Dana W. Hanson MD, FRCPC
President, Canadian Medical Association

CONTENTS

PREGNANCY AND BIRTH
8–73

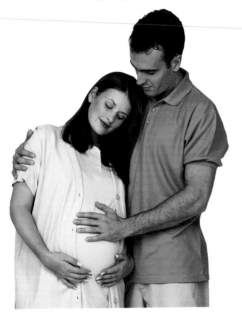

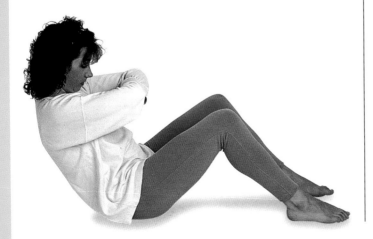

CARING FOR YOUR BABY
74–177

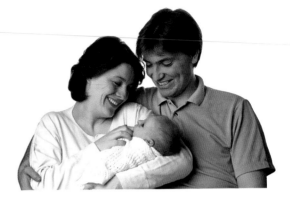

YOUR CHILD'S HEALTH
178–253

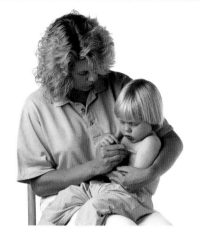

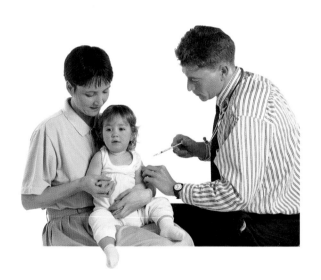

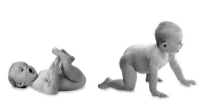
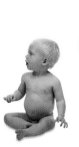
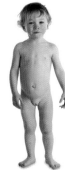

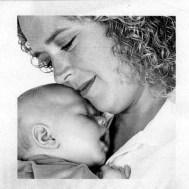

PREGNANCY
AND BIRTH

An illustrated guide to a healthy and happy pregnancy, incorporating practical self-help advice for labor and birth.

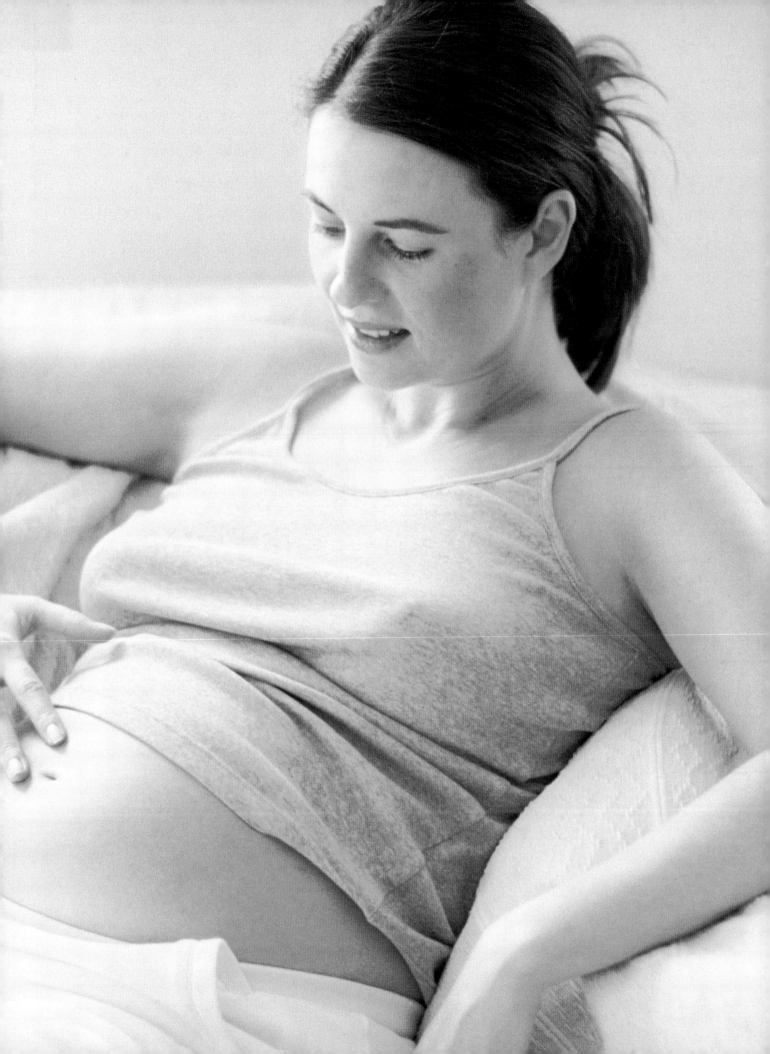

THINKING ABOUT PREGNANCY

There are a number of steps you can take to increase your chances of conceiving and giving birth to a normal, healthy baby. Ideally, you and your partner should plan for pregnancy at least three months before you conceive. It is in the first few weeks, when you may not even know you are pregnant, that a baby's development can be most easily affected. Keeping 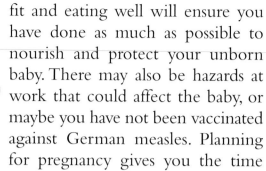 fit and eating well will ensure you have done as much as possible to nourish and protect your unborn baby. There may also be hazards at work that could affect the baby, or maybe you have not been vaccinated against German measles. Planning for pregnancy gives you the time you need to consider these kinds of risks and, if necessary, to do something positive about them.

CHECKLIST FOR PREGNANCY

Use these questions as a checklist if you want to have a baby or have just discovered that you are pregnant. A few may not apply to you, but it is important to ask yourself all of them. Talk to your partner too, because some of the questions relate directly to him. If any frighten you, consult your doctor.

Are you immune to German measles?
German measles (often referred to as rubella) can cause serious defects in the baby if you develop it in pregnancy, especially early pregnancy, when the baby's internal organs are forming. So before you become pregnant, ask your doctor for a blood test to make sure that you are immune to the disease. If you are not, your doctor can vaccinate you. Arrange to have the test done right away because you shouldn't try to become pregnant for a minimum of three months after you have had a rubella vaccination.

Do you or your partner have a family history of inherited disease?
Some medical conditions, such as hemophilia and cystic fibrosis, are inherited. If either you or your partner have a close relative with an inherited disease, there is a chance that it might be passed on to your baby. See your doctor before you start trying to become pregnant, and if necessary he or she may refer you to a genetic counselor who can assess the level of risk that you will be taking if you have a baby and advise you accordingly.

Do you have a long-standing medical condition?
If you have a medical disorder, such as diabetes or epilepsy, you should talk to your doctor before trying to become pregnant. Your doctor may want to change your drug treatment, either because the drugs you are on might affect the baby, or because they might make it more difficult for you to conceive.

> ### "How important is folic acid in pregnancy?"
>
> Folic acid is a vitamin that has been shown to be *very* important in the formation of the fetus's spine and spinal cord. This formation takes place in the first four weeks of pregnancy, so it is strongly recommended that all women of childbearing potential ensure adequate folic acid in their diets. It is very important to do this before becoming pregnant and to continue until you have completed the first three months of pregnancy. Ask your doctor for guidelines.

If you're on the pill, when should you stop taking it?
It is best to stop taking the pill several months before you plan to conceive, to allow your body time to return to its normal cycle. Wait until you have had three menstrual periods before trying to become pregnant. (Find alternative means of birth control during this time.) If you conceive before the regular rhythm of your periods has been re-established, it may be difficult to predict your due date with reasonable accuracy.

Does your work bring you into contact with any risks?
If you or your partner has a job that involves working with chemicals, lead, anesthesia, or X-rays, this may affect your chances of conceiving, or involve a risk to the baby, so talk to your doctor. If possible, consider changing to a safer job before you become pregnant, or at least avoid the risk as much as possible. Once you are pregnant, you should take further steps to protect yourself. Your doctor may also advise you to change jobs if yours involves heavy lifting. Computer VDTs (video display terminals) are now believed to cause no harm to the developing baby.

How much do you weigh?

Ideally, your weight should be normal for your height for at least six months before conceiving, so if you are seriously over- or underweight, see your doctor for advice on attaining the right weight. Unless you have a serious weight problem, never diet in pregnancy, lest you deprive your body or baby of vital nutrients.

Are you eating a balanced diet?

You will increase your chances of having a healthy baby if you eat a properly balanced diet throughout your pregnancy.

Do you smoke or drink?

Both you and your partner should stop smoking and drinking alcohol as soon as you decide to become pregnant, because tobacco and alcohol can affect fertility in men as well as women. Smoking and drinking can also harm the growing baby (see page 13).

Are you exercising regularly?

To keep fit, aim for at least 20 minutes of exercise each day. Walking and swimming are great before and during pregnancy.

FOLIC ACID

Take a folic acid supplement for at least three months prior to conception, and for the first three months of pregnancy. Folic acid, also called folate or folacin, is one of the B vitamins. It is one of the few nutrients that is known to prevent neural tube defects (NTDs) such as spina bifida or anencephaly. The neural tube, which goes on to form the baby's spine, develops very soon after conception—probably even before you realize that you are pregnant. Without sufficient folic acid, the neural tube may fail to fuse completely along its length, exposing the spinal cord and resulting in the condition known as spina bifida. Infants with anencephaly die shortly after birth because most or all of the brain is absent.

SOURCES OF FOLIC ACID

Research has shown that an increased intake of folic acid can prevent up to 70 percent of cases of spina bifida.

Good natural food sources of folic acid include spinach and broccoli, orange juice, kidney beans, Brussels sprouts, canteloupe, and egg yolks. Try to eat vegetables lightly steamed or raw to preserve the nutritional content. Some foods have also been fortified with folic acid. These include white flour, enriched pasta and enriched cornmeal.

However, you must not depend on food sources alone to supply you with this vital nutrient. You should start to take a folic acid supplement as soon as you decide to stop using contraception. To reduce the risk of your baby having spina bifida you need to take a multivitamin tablet that contains 0.4mg of folic acid every day. These tablets can be bought over the counter without a prescription, from any pharmacy. If you have had one child with a neural tube defect, you have an increased risk of having another child with the same defect. If this is the case for you, your doctor will advise you to take a tablet containing a higher dose of folic acid each day.

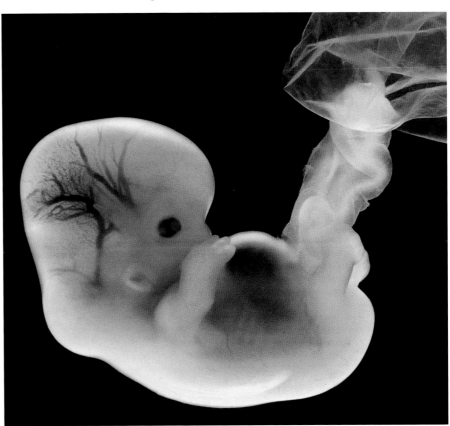

The developing embryo
Your unborn baby will stand a better chance of developing normally if you take a folic acid supplement. This should be taken before conception and during the first 12 weeks of pregnancy.

A PREGNANCY CALENDAR

This month-by-month calendar will show the changes in your body and emotions as it follows the baby's development from conception to the last days in the womb. There is advice on each stage, as well as reassuring answers to questions and worries you might have. Each month explains at least one additional aspect, such as options for prenatal classes or measuring yourself for a nursing bra. Every pregnancy varies, so don't be surprised if some changes don't happen to you exactly as they are described here. The calendar counts day one of pregnancy as the first day of your last menstrual period, so two weeks after conception (according to the calendar), you are four weeks pregnant.

BECOMING PREGNANT

If you are thinking of becoming pregnant, make sure your lifestyle involves nothing that might harm the baby. All the major organs are formed during the first three months, and it is then that his development can be harmed most easily. Once you have conceived, you may suspect that you are pregnant because of signs such as heavy breasts or nausea. Most changes are set off by the increase in hormone levels, as your body prepares to nurture the baby. The discomforts often lessen or disappear around week 12.

EARLY SIGNS OF PREGNANCY

One or more of these changes can indicate that you are pregnant. You may not notice any of them at first, however, you might still instinctively know you are pregnant because you "feel" different.

★ A missed period—but if your periods are normally irregular, or you are anxious, busy, or ill, this may not be a reliable guide to whether you have conceived. It is also possible after you have become pregnant to experience slight bleeding around the time you would normally expect your period.

★ Enlarged, tender breasts, which may tingle a little.

★ A strange metallic taste in your mouth.

★ Tiredness, not just in the evening, but during the day.

★ Feeling faint, and perhaps dizzy.

★ An increase in normal vaginal discharge.

★ Nausea and perhaps vomiting; this may happen at any time of day.

★ A strong dislike of some things, such as alcohol, coffee, and cigarette smoke, and a craving for others.

★ Feeling unusually emotional (because of hormone changes).

★ A frequent need to urinate.

CONFIRMING THE PREGNANCY

Have the pregnancy confirmed as soon as possible. Your doctor or a family planning clinic can test a urine sample. About two weeks after conception, a hormone will appear in your urine, and this confirms the pregnancy. Alternatively, buy a home pregnancy testing kit from a drugstore and do the test yourself. Your physician may examine you internally to confirm the age of the pregnancy.

HOME PREGNANCY TESTING KITS

All pregnancy-testing kits contain a chemical solution that you mix with a few drops of urine to detect the presence of Human Chorionic Gonadotropin (βHCG), the pregnancy hormone. Some suggest that you do the test immediately after rising in the morning, when the concentration of hormones is highest; check the manufacturer's instructions. Various indicators, such as a color change, will suggest whether or not you are pregnant. These tests are accurate if you follow the instructions carefully.

CALCULATING YOUR DELIVERY DATE

Pregnancy lasts about 266 days from conception to birth. The most likely time of conception is when you ovulate. In a normal 28-day cycle, this happens about 14 days before the next period is due, so to calculate your approximate delivery date, count 280 days (266 plus 14) from the first day of your last period. Remember, this is only a guide. While the average pregnancy is 40 weeks, a normal pregnancy can be anywhere from 37 to 42 weeks long.

A healthy pregnancy
From conception onward, it is important to avoid ingesting any substance that could harm your unborn baby.

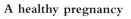

WHAT TO AVOID

Avoid smoking, alcohol, and any form of medication, unless confirmed as safe by your doctor, throughout pregnancy. This is especially important during the first three months, when the baby's organs are forming.

Smoking

This deprives the baby of oxygen. Babies of mothers who smoke are more likely to be premature and have a low birthweight. Smoking also increases the chances of having a miscarriage, a stillbirth, a malformed baby, or a baby that dies directly after birth. The more you smoke, the greater the risk, so stop smoking completely. If you really can't give it up entirely, switch to a low-tar brand, ration the number of cigarettes you smoke, don't inhale, and stub out your cigarette when you've smoked half of it. Doctors now believe that the smoke you breathe in from other people's cigarettes could be a factor in crib death, so avoid smoky atmospheres when pregnant.

Alcohol

Drinking heavily in pregnancy can seriously affect the developing baby. No one knows what a "safe" level of drinking is, so it's best not to drink at all while pregnant.

Medication

Many drugs can have harmful or unknown effects on the baby, so avoid taking medication in pregnancy, unless it is prescribed by a doctor who knows you are pregnant. This includes many of the remedies you would normally take for minor complaints. Medications to control a condition such as thyroid disease may have to be adjusted.

Other risks

Cats' feces, and raw or undercooked meat, may contain a parasite called toxoplasma, which can seriously harm the unborn baby. Don't eat undercooked meat and wash your hands after handling raw meat. Avoid emptying cat litter trays (if you must, wear gloves and then wash your hands). Wear gloves for gardening. Wash all fruit and vegetables well before eating to remove any soil.

THE START OF LIFE

During the first eight weeks of pregnancy, the baby develops from a single cell at conception to a fetus that is starting to look human.

CONCEPTION TO WEEK FOUR

1 Ovulation

Around day 14 of your menstrual cycle, a ripe egg is released from one of your ovaries, and fertilization becomes possible. The egg is caught by the "fingers" at the end of the fallopian tube, and drawn into it. The egg can survive for up to 24 hours; if it isn't fertilized, it passes out of the vagina with the lining of the womb in your next monthly period.

The swim of the sperm

During orgasm, a man may ejaculate between 200 and 400 million sperm into a woman's vagina. Many spill out again, or are lost along the way, but some swim through the mucus secreted by the cervix (the neck of the womb), which becomes thin and soft around ovulation, and cross the womb into the fallopian tube. If an egg hasn't been released, the sperm can survive in the tube for up to 48 hours.

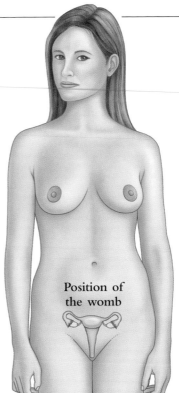

Position of the womb

5 Implantation

The fertilized egg begins to embed itself in the soft, thick lining of the womb at about the end of week three. This is called implantation. When the egg is securely attached to the lining of the womb, conception is complete.

Sponge-like fingers from the outer cells of the embryo start to burrow into the lining, to link up with the mother's blood vessels. These later form the placenta. Some of the cells also develop into the umbilical cord and the membranes that protect the baby. The inner cells divide into three layers, which develop into the different parts of your baby's body.

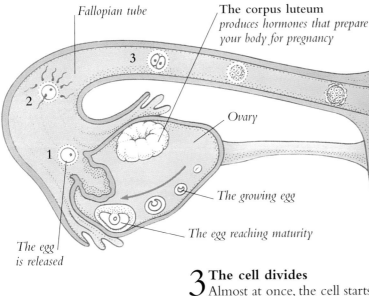

Fallopian tube

The corpus luteum
produces hormones that prepare your body for pregnancy

Ovary

The growing egg

The egg reaching maturity

The egg is released

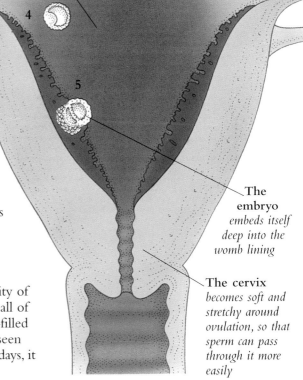

Womb

The embryo *embeds itself deep into the womb lining*

The cervix *becomes soft and stretchy around ovulation, so that sperm can pass through it more easily*

2 Fertilization

Sperm carry a substance that can dissolve the outer covering of the egg, so that one of them can penetrate it. As soon as the successful sperm enters the egg, no other sperm can get through. The sperm loses its tail and its head begins to swell. It fuses with the egg, forming a single cell.

3 The cell divides

Almost at once, the cell starts to divide. It continues to divide into more and more cells as it travels down the fallopian tube.

4 Reaching the womb

On about the fourth day after fertilization, the egg reaches the cavity of the womb. It has developed into a ball of about 100 cells with a hollow, fluid-filled center, but it is still too small to be seen by the naked eye. For the next few days, it floats around in the womb cavity.

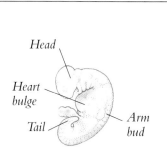

Head
Heart bulge
Tail
Arm bud

About week six

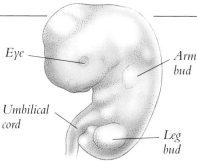

Eye
Arm bud
Umbilical cord
Leg bud

About week seven

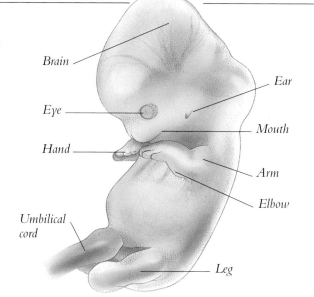

Brain
Ear
Eye
Mouth
Hand
Arm
Elbow
Umbilical cord
Leg

About week eight

WEEKS FIVE TO SIX

★ The embryo is floating in a fluid-filled sac.
★ It has a simple brain, spine, and central nervous system.
★ Four shallow pits have appeared on the head, which will later become the baby's eyes and ears.
★ The embryo has the beginnings of a digestive system, a mouth, and a jaw.
★ The stomach and chest are developing. The heart can be seen as a large bulge at the front of the chest; by the end of the week it will start beating.
★ A system of blood vessels is forming.
★ Four tiny limb buds have developed.

Length: The embryo is now 6mm (¼ in), about the size of an apple seed.

WEEK SEVEN

★ The head looks large and is bent onto the chest. A face is forming, though the eyes are on the sides of the head and still sealed. Black pigment can be seen under the skin overlying the eyes.
★ The arms and legs are clearly visible, with clefts at the end, which become fingers and toes.
★ The heart starts to circulate blood around the embryo's body.
★ The outline of the baby's nervous system is already nearly complete.
★ Bone cells are beginning to develop.
★ The embryo has lungs, an intestine, a liver, kidneys and internal sex organs, but all are not yet fully formed.

Length: The embryo is now 1.3cm (½in), about the size of a small grape.

WEEK EIGHT

★ The embryo can now be called a fetus, which means "young one."
★ All the major internal organs have developed, although they are still in a simple form, and may not be in their final position.
★ A face is recognizable: the nose seems to have a tip, the nostrils have formed, and the two sides of the jaw have joined to make a mouth. A tongue has already formed.

★ The inner parts of the ears, responsible for balance and hearing, are forming.
★ The fingers and toes are becoming more distinct, although they are joined by webs of skin.
★ The arms and legs have grown longer, and shoulders, elbows, hips, and knees are detectable.
★ The baby moves around a lot, although you can't actually feel him yet.

Length: The fetus is now 2.5cm (1in), about the size of a strawberry.

TWINS

About one in 80 pregnancies results in twins. If twins run in your family, your chances of having them are greater.
Fraternal twins occur when two separate eggs are fertilized by two separate sperm. They are three times as common as identical twins. The twins each have their own placenta, may or may not be the same sex, and are no more alike than any other brothers or sisters.
Identical twins are produced when the egg that is fertilized divides into two separate halves, each of which develops into an identical baby. The twins share a placenta, are always of the same sex, and have the same physical characteristics and genetic makeup.

"What is a trimester?"

Q&A

Trimesters are simply a convenient way of subdividing the nine months of your pregnancy (see Calculating Your Delivery Date, page 13) into three somewhat uneven periods of about three months each. The first trimester covers weeks 1 to 12; the second trimester runs from the 13th to the 28th week; and the third, the most variable, is measured from the 29th week to the end of the pregnancy.

WEEK
12

The baby looks much more human, although his head is still large in proportion to his body, and his limbs, although fully formed, are small. You should find that the discomforts of early pregnancy are beginning to wear off. Make sure you have your first visit with a doctor around now.

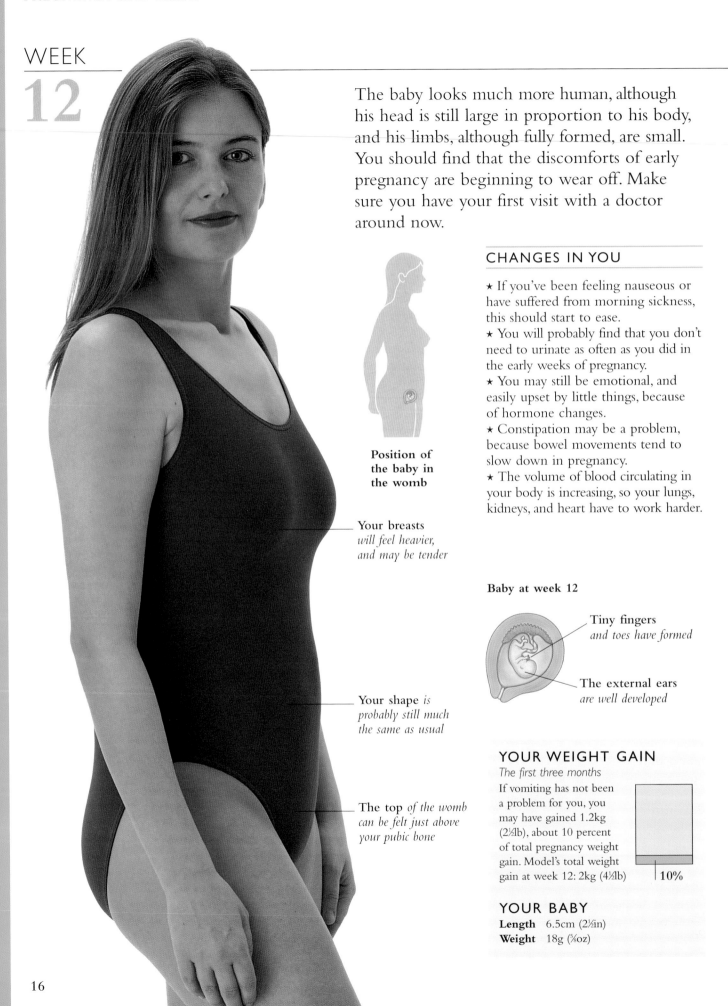

Position of the baby in the womb

Your breasts *will feel heavier, and may be tender*

Your shape *is probably still much the same as usual*

The top *of the womb can be felt just above your pubic bone*

CHANGES IN YOU

★ If you've been feeling nauseous or have suffered from morning sickness, this should start to ease.
★ You will probably find that you don't need to urinate as often as you did in the early weeks of pregnancy.
★ You may still be emotional, and easily upset by little things, because of hormone changes.
★ Constipation may be a problem, because bowel movements tend to slow down in pregnancy.
★ The volume of blood circulating in your body is increasing, so your lungs, kidneys, and heart have to work harder.

Baby at week 12

Tiny fingers *and toes have formed*

The external ears *are well developed*

YOUR WEIGHT GAIN
The first three months
If vomiting has not been a problem for you, you may have gained 1.2kg (2½lb), about 10 percent of total pregnancy weight gain. Model's total weight gain at week 12: 2kg (4½lb)

10%

YOUR BABY
Length 6.5cm (2½in)
Weight 18g (⅝oz)

WHAT TO DO

★ Buy a bra that will support your breasts well.
★ Check that you are eating a varied diet of fresh foods.
★ Guard against constipation by drinking plenty of water and including high-fiber foods in your diet.
★ Make an appointment with your dentist for a check-up.
★ Tell your employer that you are pregnant, so that you can adjust your work schedule.
★ Visit the doctor for your first prenatal check-up.
★ Find out about insurance benefits and parental leave policies.
★ Practice prenatal exercises regularly. Go swimming.
★ Enrol for prenatal exercise classes if you want to.
★ Find out about other prenatal classes in your area.

YOUR GROWING BABY

★ All of the internal organs are formed, and most are working, so the baby is far less likely to be harmed by infections or drugs.
★ The eyelids have developed, and are closed over the eyes.
★ The baby has earlobes.
★ The limbs are formed, with fingers and toes. Miniature fingernails and toenails are growing.
★ Muscles are developing, so the baby moves much more. He can curl and fan his toes. He can make a fist.
★ He can move the muscles of his mouth to frown, purse his lips, and open and close his mouth.
★ He can suck. He swallows the fluid that surrounds him and he passes urine.

see also:
Prenatal clinic *pages 34–36*
Prenatal exercises *pages 45–47*
Eating healthily *pages 50–53*
Frequent urination *page 41*
Morning sickness *page 41*
Pregnancy bra *page 23*
Protecting your back *page 44*

PRENATAL CLASSES

Start thinking about the type of class that will best suit you and your partner. Often you can go to introductory classes now—on ways to keep healthy in pregnancy, for example—and the classes themselves start eight to ten weeks before the baby is due. Prenatal exercise classes can continue throughout your pregnancy.

CHOOSING A CLASS

Prepared childbirth classes are run by hospitals, individual instructors, as well as various organizations and local groups such as the YWCA, the community health center, or (in Quebec) the CLSC. To find one, start by checking the professional adverstising section of community newspapers and bulletin boards. Ask your doctor or friends for recommendations. Make sure that you reserve a spot early, even if classes won't begin until you are 28 to 32 weeks pregnant. Most feature a weekly two-hour session, scheduled over a six- to eight-week period. To find the one that suits your feelings about pregnancy, labor, and delivery best, you might want to observe a session before you sign up.

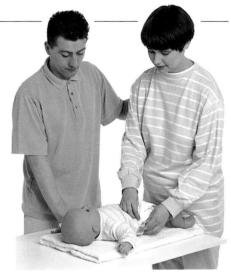

Basics of babycare
It's fun and helpful to learn how to look after your baby at the classes.

What will you learn

Though the course content may vary according to the philosophy of the instructor, all childbirth classes teach couples basic information about pregnancy, the stages and pain of labor and delivery, relaxation techniques, physical exercises, medication and anesthesia, and everything you might need to know about different hospital procedures and policies. A tour of the hospital is often included. Classes can be invaluable for first-time mothers and fathers, and even in a second or third pregnancy the review is almost always worthwhile. Most emphasize the close working relationship a woman will want to have with the person she chooses to have by her side during the birth, her labor partner. If your baby's father isn't going to be there, a relative or close friend can join in the preparation. Some classes cover the postnatal period and include tips on caring for a newborn, breast-feeding, postpartum depression, and exercises for getting back into shape.

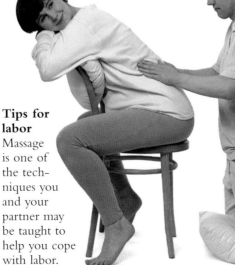

Tips for labor
Massage is one of the techniques you and your partner may be taught to help you cope with labor.

WEEK 16

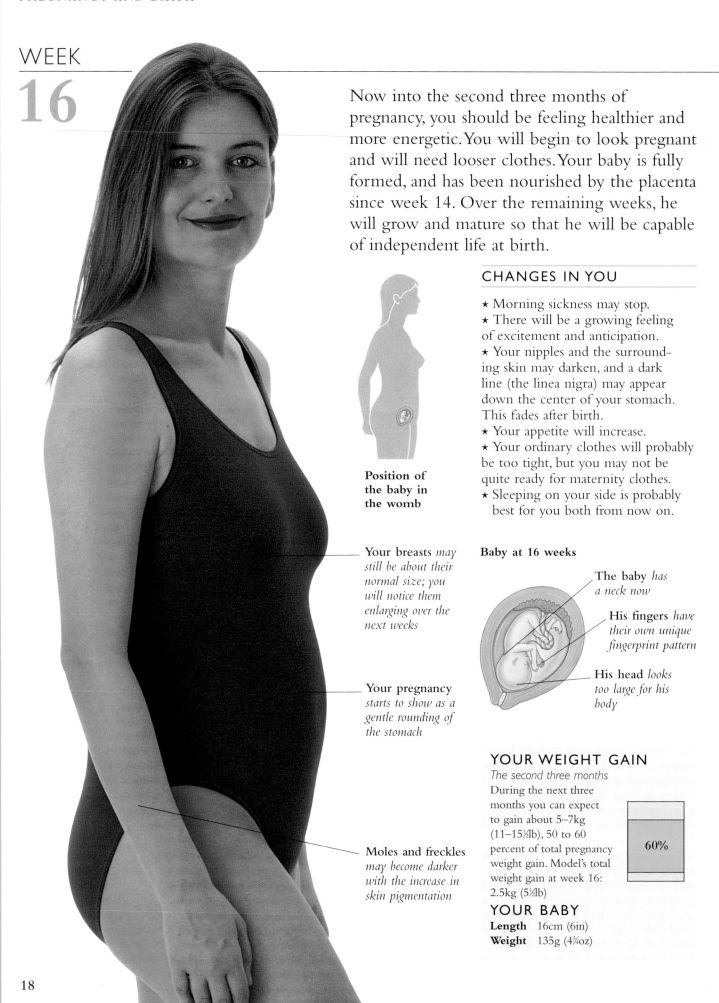

Now into the second three months of pregnancy, you should be feeling healthier and more energetic. You will begin to look pregnant and will need looser clothes. Your baby is fully formed, and has been nourished by the placenta since week 14. Over the remaining weeks, he will grow and mature so that he will be capable of independent life at birth.

Position of the baby in the womb

CHANGES IN YOU

★ Morning sickness may stop.
★ There will be a growing feeling of excitement and anticipation.
★ Your nipples and the surrounding skin may darken, and a dark line (the linea nigra) may appear down the center of your stomach. This fades after birth.
★ Your appetite will increase.
★ Your ordinary clothes will probably be too tight, but you may not be quite ready for maternity clothes.
★ Sleeping on your side is probably best for you both from now on.

Your breasts *may still be about their normal size; you will notice them enlarging over the next weeks*

Your pregnancy *starts to show as a gentle rounding of the stomach*

Moles and freckles *may become darker with the increase in skin pigmentation*

Baby at 16 weeks

The baby *has a neck now*

His fingers *have their own unique fingerprint pattern*

His head *looks too large for his body*

YOUR WEIGHT GAIN

The second three months
During the next three months you can expect to gain about 5–7kg (11–15½lb), 50 to 60 percent of total pregnancy weight gain. Model's total weight gain at week 16: 2.5kg (5½lb)

60%

YOUR BABY
Length 16cm (6in)
Weight 135g (4¾oz)

WHAT TO DO

★ Give up smoking if you have not already done so. Encourage your partner to do the same.
★ Eat nutritiously and watch weight gain.
★ Continue to take iron and folic acid supplements as prescribed by your doctor. Take supplements on a full stomach.
★ Obstetrical visits are scheduled once a month now. An ultrasound scan may be done to confirm your due date. A maternal serum screen (MSS), a blood test for possible fetal abnormalities, may be offered. Amniocentesis is also done now if there is any chance of the baby being abnormal.

YOUR GROWING BABY

★ Eyebrows and eyelashes are growing, and he has fine downy hair on his face and body (known as lanugo).
★ His skin is so thin that it is transparent; networks of blood vessels can be seen underneath.
★ Arm and leg joints have formed and hard bones are beginning to develop.
★ His sex organs are sufficiently mature for his sex to be evident, but this is not always detectable by an ultrasound scan.
★ The baby makes breathing movements with his chest.
★ He can suck his thumb.
★ He moves around vigorously, but you probably won't be able to feel him yet.
★ His heart is beating about twice as fast as your own; the doctor can hear it with a special device after week 14.
★ He grows rapidly during this month.

see also:
MSS test *page 37*
Amniocentesis *page 37*
Healthy eating *pages 50–53*
Relaxation and breathing *pages 48–49*
Skin color *page 21*
Smoking *page 13*
Supplements *page 52*
Ultrasound *page 37*

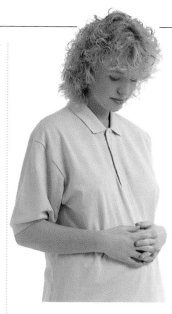

You
It's only natural for your feelings of excitement and anticipation to be clouded sometimes by negative thoughts. You may worry about loving the baby, but once he's born and you get to know each other, love will grow. You may also feel depressed about your changing shape, and even resent the baby for putting your body through such strains. But most major bodily changes disappear after birth, and with some gentle exercising your shape will return.

Your partner
The baby may become a reality for the first time when you see him on an ultrasound screen. Up to now you may have felt left out, and perhaps jealous of all the attention your mate and the baby have been receiving. If you're worried about money and having enough to support your new family, try to plan and budget.

Both of you
It's normal to feel excited about the new baby, yet to worry that you're not yet ready for parenthood. If you're anxious about labor and birth, learn all about them, and practice techniques, such as deep breathing, so you can feel more confident and in control when the time comes.

MIXED FEELINGS

You and your partner are bound to have mixed emotions about the pregnancy, so don't be surprised if as well as feeling elated and excited, you sometimes feel anxious or sad. Try to tolerate and understand any negative feelings; they are normal emotions.

COMMON WORRIES
The best way to dispel any worries you may have about the baby or parenthood is to talk about them frankly with each other. It also helps to find out as much as you can about pregnancy, so you understand the changes taking place.

Q&A
"How can I be sure the baby will be all right?"

The chances of the baby being abnormal are very small. Most abnormalities occur in the first weeks, and end in an early miscarriage. By week 13 the baby is fully formed and very little can go wrong. Make sure that your lifestyle involves nothing that could harm him, and you can reduce the risk even further.

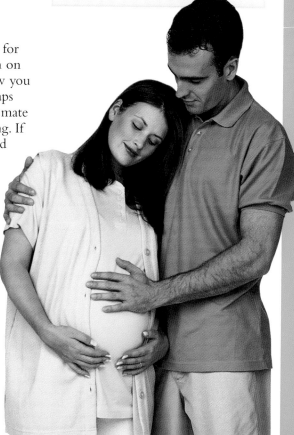

WEEK
20

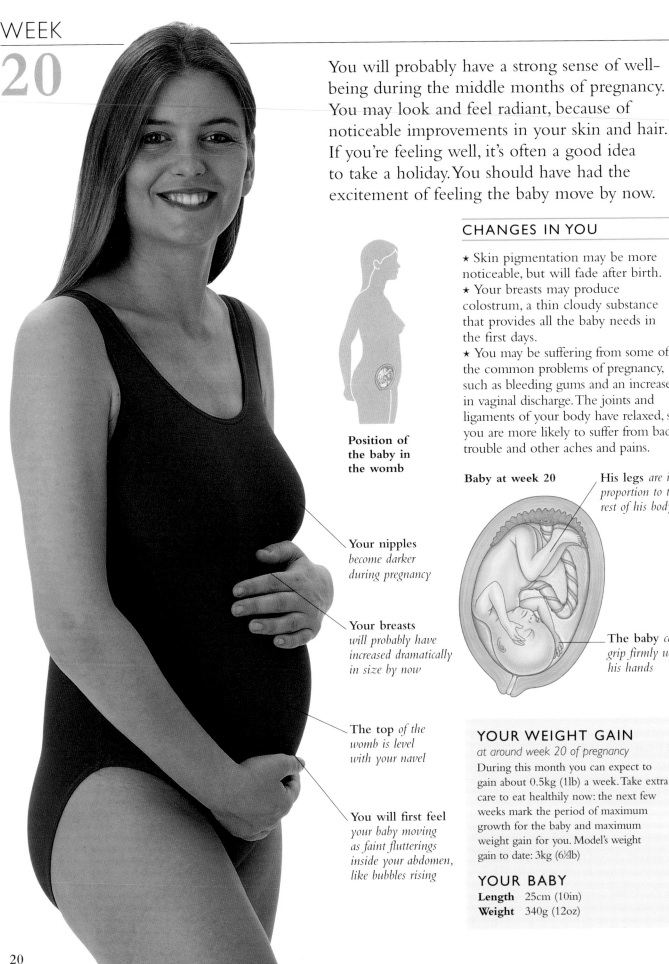

You will probably have a strong sense of well-being during the middle months of pregnancy. You may look and feel radiant, because of noticeable improvements in your skin and hair. If you're feeling well, it's often a good idea to take a holiday. You should have had the excitement of feeling the baby move by now.

CHANGES IN YOU

★ Skin pigmentation may be more noticeable, but will fade after birth.
★ Your breasts may produce colostrum, a thin cloudy substance that provides all the baby needs in the first days.
★ You may be suffering from some of the common problems of pregnancy, such as bleeding gums and an increase in vaginal discharge. The joints and ligaments of your body have relaxed, so you are more likely to suffer from back trouble and other aches and pains.

Position of the baby in the womb

Baby at week 20

His legs *are in proportion to the rest of his body*

The baby *can grip firmly with his hands*

Your nipples *become darker during pregnancy*

Your breasts *will probably have increased dramatically in size by now*

The top *of the womb is level with your navel*

You will first feel *your baby moving as faint flutterings inside your abdomen, like bubbles rising*

YOUR WEIGHT GAIN
at around week 20 of pregnancy
During this month you can expect to gain about 0.5kg (1lb) a week. Take extra care to eat healthily now: the next few weeks mark the period of maximum growth for the baby and maximum weight gain for you. Model's weight gain to date: 3kg (6¼lb)

YOUR BABY
Length 25cm (10in)
Weight 340g (12oz)

WHAT TO DO

★ Make sure you are holding yourself well, and that you avoid straining your back. Wear low-heeled shoes.
★ Take the practical steps suggested on pages 40–42 to relieve any other discomforts that you may have.
★ Start to think about essential clothes and equipment for the baby, such as an infant seat.

Q&A "Is a long journey advisable?"

There's usually no reason why you shouldn't travel in pregnancy, but preferably not on your own, especially on a long car journey. Wear loose, comfortable clothes, and break the journey up by walking around for a few minutes at least every two hours, to help your circulation. Always remember to take your pregnancy record with you.

YOUR GROWING BABY

★ Hair appears on the baby's head.
★ Teeth are developing.
★ Vernix, the white greasy substance that protects the baby's skin in the womb, forms.
★ The baby's arms and legs are well developed.
★ Protective substances may be transferred to the baby through your blood to help him resist disease in the first weeks.
★ The baby is very active; you should have felt his movements for the first time as a faint fluttering. He may even react to noises outside the womb, but don't worry if he doesn't move around much; it's fairly common for babies to have a quiet period now.

see also:
Common complaints pages 40–42
Eating healthily pages 50–53
Essentials for the baby page 27
Protecting your back page 44

LOOKING GOOD

You may look and feel your best during the middle months of pregnancy, with lustrous hair, rosy cheeks, and healthy skin. But not everyone blooms; the high hormone levels can have less flattering effects on your skin, nails, and hair, though any adverse changes usually disappear after birth.

HAIR
Thick, shiny hair is often a bonus of pregnancy. However, not all hair improves, and greasy hair may become more oily, and dry hair, drier and more brittle, so that you may seem to lose more hair than usual. Facial and body hair also tends to darken.

Have your hair cut *into a style that is easy to look after*

What to do
If your hair is dry and splits easily, use a mild shampoo and conditioner, and don't brush it too often or too vigorously. Wash greasy hair frequently to keep it shiny. As hair is so unpredictable during pregnancy, avoid perms or having your hair colored.

Your skin *may become smooth and blemish-free*

SKIN TEXTURE
Your skin will probably improve in pregnancy: blemishes disappear, and skin texture becomes smooth and silky. However, you may find that your skin becomes very dry, or greasy, and perhaps spotty.
What to do Cleanse your skin thoroughly. If it is dry, gently rub moisturizer over the dry areas, and add bath oil to your bath water. Use as little soap as possible.

NAILS
You may notice that your nails split and break more easily than usual.
What to do Wear gloves for household chores and gardening.

SKIN COLOR
An increase in skin pigmentation is normal during pregnancy. Moles, birthmarks, scars, and especially freckles usually darken and grow in size, and a brown line often appears on the stomach. You may also notice a brownish patch, or "butterfly mask", across your face and neck. Don't worry, since this disappears soon after the birth.
What to do Avoid strong sunlight since this makes pigmentation worse, but if you have to go out in the sun, use sun-cream with a strong filter. Don't try to bleach the mask; if you want to disguise it, you can use a skin-blemish covering stick.

WEEK
24

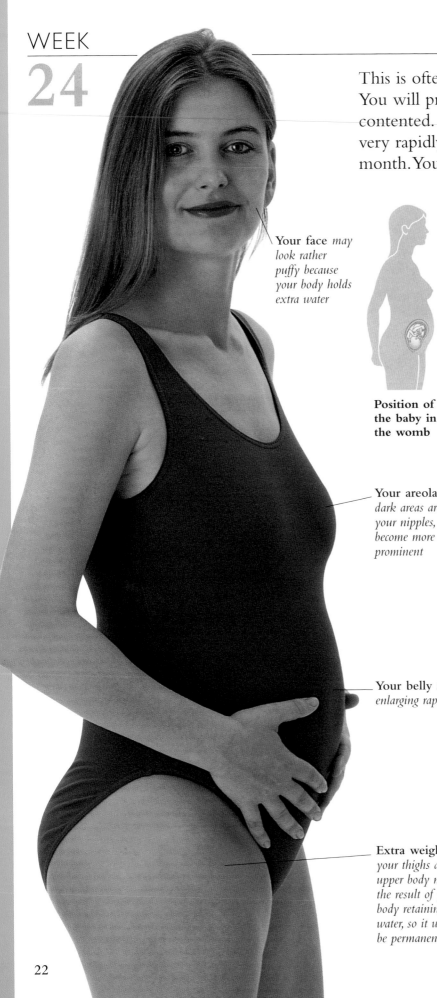

This is often the best month of pregnancy. You will probably look well, and feel happy and contented. If you have not been gaining weight very rapidly so far, you may put on a lot this month. You will start to appear visibly pregnant.

Your face *may look rather puffy because your body holds extra water*

Position of the baby in the womb

Your areolas, *the dark areas around your nipples, may become more prominent*

Your belly *is enlarging rapidly*

Extra weight *on your thighs and upper body may be the result of your body retaining water, so it won't be permanent*

CHANGES IN YOU

★ It's quite common to put on a spurt of weight around this month or the following one.

★ You may find that loose-fitting, unrestricting clothes are more comfortable from now until the end of your pregnancy.

★ Sweating may be a problem because you tend to feel the heat more. Make sure that you drink plenty of water, and try to avoid wearing synthetic materials.

Baby at week 24

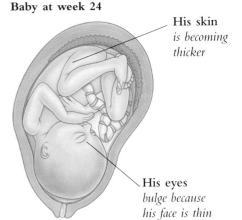

His skin *is becoming thicker*

His eyes *bulge because his face is thin*

YOUR WEIGHT GAIN
at around week 24 of pregnancy
You will probably continue to gain weight at the rate of about 0.5kg (1lb) a week, although if you were underweight when your pregnancy began you might gain at a faster rate than this. Model's weight gain to date: 4.5kg (10lb)

YOUR BABY
Length   33cm (13in)
Weight   570g (1¼lb)

WHAT TO DO

★ If you have flat or inverted nipples, and you want to breast-feed when the baby is born, you should be able to do so; ask your doctor for advice.
★ Put your feet up as much as possible in the day.
★ Continue to exercise gently, but regularly. Stop if you feel any discomfort. Practice relaxation and breathing exercises.
★ If you are working full-time, find a quiet spot in which to take 15-minute breaks.

Q & A
"What is the best kind of bra?"

To give your breasts the support they need in pregnancy, choose a bra (preferably cotton) with a deep band under the cups, broad shoulder straps, and an adjustable back. Check your size regularly, as your breasts will continue to swell throughout pregnancy. By the end, you might fit a cup size two sizes larger than usual. If your breasts become very heavy, wear a lightweight bra at night.

YOUR GROWING BABY

★ No fat has been laid down yet, so the baby is still lean.
★ Sweat glands are forming in the skin.
★ Arm and leg muscles are well developed, and the baby tries them out regularly. He has periods of frenzied activity, when you feel him moving around, alternating with periods of calm.
★ The baby can cough and hiccup; you may feel the hiccups as a knocking movement.

see also:
Prenatal exercises *pages 45–47*
Pregnancy clothes *page 25*
Relaxation and breathing *pages 48–49*

THE BABY IN THE WOMB

While the baby is developing physically, he is also becoming an aware, responsive person with feelings. He lies tightly curled up in the womb, cushioned by the bag of waters that surrounds him, entirely reliant on your placenta for food and oxygen, and for the disposal of his waste products. However, he looks and behaves much the same as a baby at birth.

SIGHT
His eyelids are still sealed, but by week 28, they become unsealed, and he may see, and open and close his eyes.

HEARING
He can hear your voice, and if he's asleep can be woken by loud music. He may prefer some types of music, and show this by his movements. He jumps at sudden noises.

FACIAL EXPRESSIONS
He frowns, squints, purses his lips, and opens and closes his mouth.

LIFE-SUPPORT SYSTEM
The baby is nourished by the placenta and protected by warm amniotic fluid, which can change every four hours. It regulates the baby's temperature, and protects against infection and sudden bumps.

MOVEMENTS
He kicks and punches, and sometimes turns somersaults. He can make a fist.

SLEEPING PATTERNS
He sleeps and wakes randomly, and will probably be most active when you are trying to sleep.

PERSONALITY
The part of the brain concerned with personality and intelligence becomes far more complex over the seventh month, so his personality may soon be developing.

SUCKING, SWALLOWING, AND BREATHING
He sucks his thumb, and swallows the warm water (the amniotic fluid) that surrounds him, passing it out of his body as urine. Sometimes he drinks too much of the fluid and hiccups. He makes breathing movements with his chest, practicing for life outside the womb.

TASTE
His taste buds are forming, and by week 28 he can respond to sweet, sour, and bitter tastes.

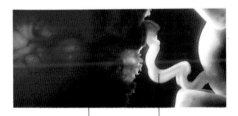

The placenta supplies all the nutrients the baby needs; almost anything entering your body, good or bad, is filtered through to him.

The umbilical cord, a rope of three blood vessels, links the placenta to the baby

WEEK
28

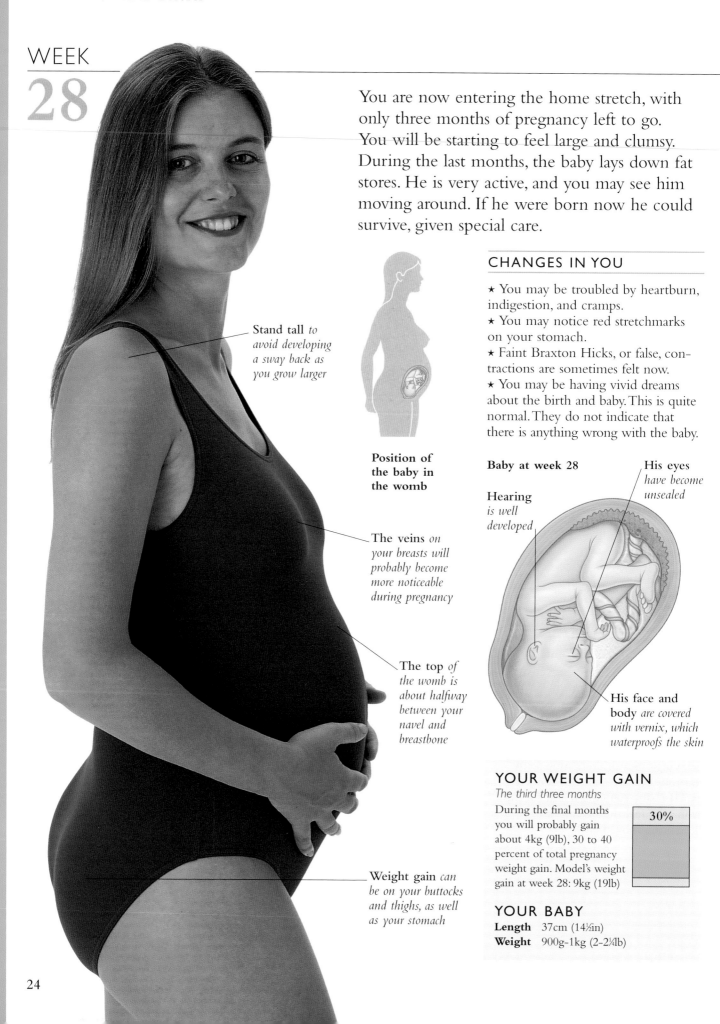

You are now entering the home stretch, with only three months of pregnancy left to go. You will be starting to feel large and clumsy. During the last months, the baby lays down fat stores. He is very active, and you may see him moving around. If he were born now he could survive, given special care.

Stand tall *to avoid developing a sway back as you grow larger*

Position of the baby in the womb

The veins *on your breasts will probably become more noticeable during pregnancy*

The top *of the womb is about halfway between your navel and breastbone*

Weight gain *can be on your buttocks and thighs, as well as your stomach*

CHANGES IN YOU

★ You may be troubled by heartburn, indigestion, and cramps.
★ You may notice red stretchmarks on your stomach.
★ Faint Braxton Hicks, or false, contractions are sometimes felt now.
★ You may be having vivid dreams about the birth and baby. This is quite normal. They do not indicate that there is anything wrong with the baby.

Baby at week 28

His eyes *have become unsealed*

Hearing *is well developed*

His face and body *are covered with vernix, which waterproofs the skin*

YOUR WEIGHT GAIN
The third three months
During the final months you will probably gain about 4kg (9lb), 30 to 40 percent of total pregnancy weight gain. Model's weight gain at week 28: 9kg (19lb)

30%

YOUR BABY
Length 37cm (14½in)
Weight 900g-1kg (2-2¼lb)

WHAT TO DO

★ Make sure you get enough rest in the day, and have as many early nights as possible. If you are still at work, put your feet up during the lunch hour and rest when you come home.

★ If you are still working full-time and in a job that doesn't exhaust you physically, schedule an appointment with the human resources department to discuss your plans. Some women continue on the job until their due date while others need a few weeks to prepare and rest at home before the birth. No matter what you and your employer decide, it's always best to clear the air.

★ Prenatal visits are every two weeks from now until week 36. The baby's heartbeat can be heard from now on, using either a fetal stethoscope or a Doppler ultrasound device.

YOUR GROWING BABY

★ His skin is red and wrinkled, but fat is starting to accumulate beneath it.

★ There have been dramatic develop-ments in the thinking part of the brain, which becomes bigger and more complex. A seven-month-old baby can feel pain, and responds in much the same way as a full-term baby.

★ The baby has far more taste buds than he will have at birth, so his sense of taste is acute.

★ His lungs are still not fully mature, and need to develop a substance called surfactant, which stops them collapsing between each breath.

★ Your partner can feel the baby move if he puts his hand on your stomach, and he may even see the shape of a foot or bottom as the baby kicks and turns.

see also:
Common complaints **pages 40–42**
Protecting your back **page 44**
Stretchmarks **page 42**

YOUR PREGNANCY WARDROBE

Up to five or even six months of your pregnancy, many of your normal clothes may be wearable if they fit loosely or you use a little creativity. However, a few new outfits may greatly improve your morale and you don't have to buy special maternity wear. Look for clothes that are attractive, comfortable, and easy to care for from the standard selection in the shops.

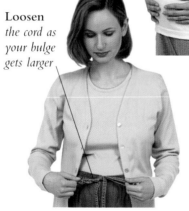

Comfortable tops
Go for stretchy fabrics in soft natural fibers. Some days you may feel happier wearing a baggy sweatshirt.

Loosen *the cord as your bulge gets larger*

Loose-fitting bottoms
Trousers with a drawstring are comfortable and unrestricting; they are convenient as they can be adjusted to fit your expanding waistline.

Dressing up
A simple dress can look casual, but is also easy to dress up. Check that there's enough length in the hem so the dress hangs evenly as you grow larger. Maternity dresses are usually 2.5cm (1in) longer at the front to allow for this.

WHAT TO CHOOSE

You tend to feel the heat more during pregnancy, so look for lightweight, loose-fitting clothes, made of cotton or other natural fibers. If it's cold, put on layers. Avoid anything that is tight around the waist or that restricts blood flow in your legs, such as tight knee-high socks.

Comfortable, low-heeled shoes are essential, although completely flat heels are best avoided. You probably won't be able to wear lace-up shoes soon, because you will have difficulty tying them.

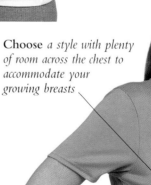

Choose *a style with plenty of room across the chest to accommodate your growing breasts*

A versatile fabric *will stretch to fit your changing shape*

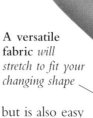

WEEK
32

You need all the rest you can get, so try to lie down in the middle of the day. You will be feeling very bulky, and probably weary of your pregnant state. Now is the time to start going to childbirth classes, which will run until the end of your pregnancy.

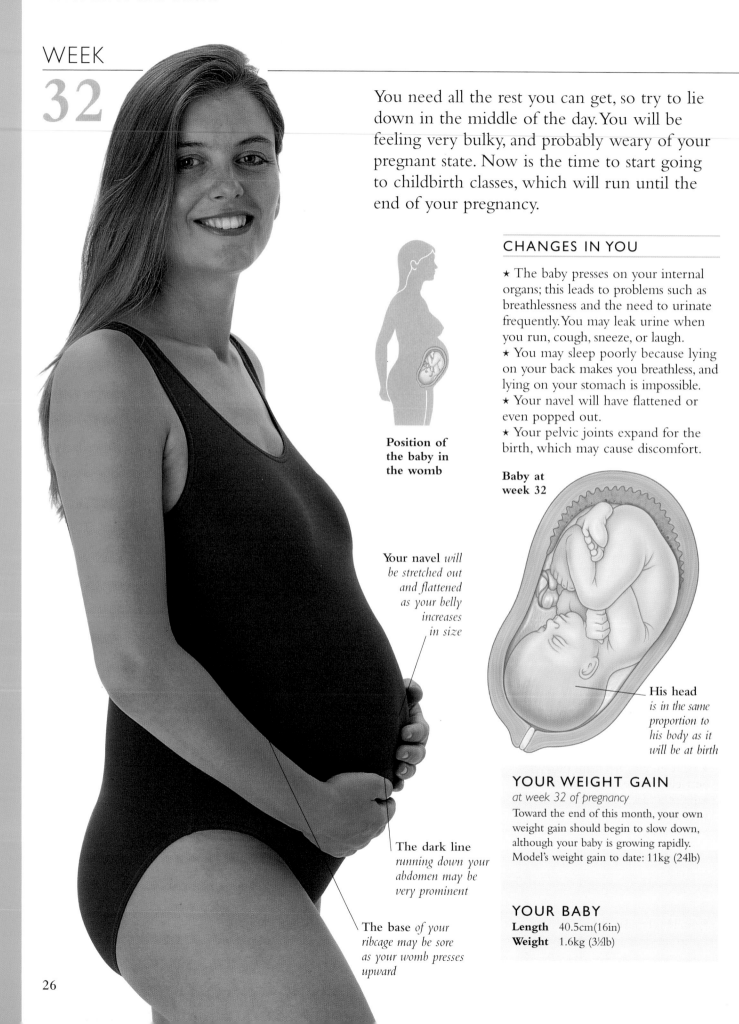

Position of the baby in the womb

CHANGES IN YOU

★ The baby presses on your internal organs; this leads to problems such as breathlessness and the need to urinate frequently. You may leak urine when you run, cough, sneeze, or laugh.
★ You may sleep poorly because lying on your back makes you breathless, and lying on your stomach is impossible.
★ Your navel will have flattened or even popped out.
★ Your pelvic joints expand for the birth, which may cause discomfort.

Baby at week 32

Your navel will be stretched out and flattened as your belly increases in size

His head *is in the same proportion to his body as it will be at birth*

The dark line *running down your abdomen may be very prominent*

The base *of your ribcage may be sore as your womb presses upward*

YOUR WEIGHT GAIN
at week 32 of pregnancy
Toward the end of this month, your own weight gain should begin to slow down, although your baby is growing rapidly.
Model's weight gain to date: 11kg (24lb)

YOUR BABY
Length 40.5cm(16in)
Weight 1.6kg (3½lb)

WHAT TO DO

★ Break up the day by putting your feet up for an hour or two if possible.
★ If you have difficulty sleeping, practice relaxation techniques before going to bed, and sleep on your side, with one leg bent and your stomach supported on a pillow. Try not to worry if you can't sleep; some insomnia is normal at this stage. All the adverse symptoms can conspire against you at night. Don't toss and turn—get up and do something.
★ Keep up with your pelvic floor exercises; this is especially important if you leak urine.
★ Start attending prenatal classes if you haven't already.

Q&A

"I'm worried about harming the baby during intercourse. Is there any danger of this?"

This is a common worry, but an unnecessary one if your pregnancy is normal. The baby is protected and cushioned by the bag of fluid surrounding him, so he can't be harmed when you make love. The doctor will warn you if there are any dangers, such as a low placenta.

YOUR GROWING BABY

★ The baby looks much the same as at birth, but his body still needs to fill out more.
★ He can now tell the difference between light and dark.
★ Because there is less room in the womb, he may have turned into a head-down position by now, ready for birth.

see also:
Prenatal classes *page 17*
Breathlessness *page 40*
Frequent urination *page 41*
Pelvic floor *page 45*
Relaxation techniques *pages 48–49*

ESSENTIALS FOR YOUR BABY

Buy the following basic items for your new baby. You can always add items after the birth.

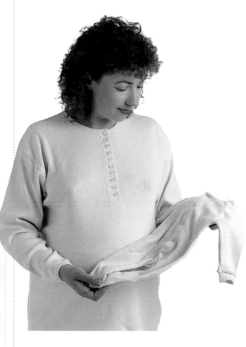

EQUIPMENT
You will need:
★ a crib or bassinet for your baby
★ appropriate bedding
★ a soft blanket
★ bottle-feeding equipment if you are going to bottle-feed
★ baby bathtub
★ two soft towels
★ changing mat or table
★ diaper-changing equipment and diapers
★ an infant car seat, if you have a car; some can double as infant seats.

CLOTHES
Buy a minimum number of "newborn" clothes—your baby will grow fast. You will need:
★ undershirts
★ stretchsuits
★ sweaters
★ infant sleeping or drawstring gowns
★ soft socks or bootees
★ sun hat or warm hat.

ENJOYING SEX

Making love is often particularly enjoyable during pregnancy. Some women become aroused more easily as a result of the increase in hormone levels. And there are no worries about contraception.

OTHER WAYS OF LOVING
There may be times when you lose interest in sex, especially in the first and last weeks. This doesn't mean that you have to stop loving each other physically. Even if you feel too tired or heavy to make love, find other ways to show your affection, such as kissing, cuddling, stroking, and touching.

A CHANGE OF POSITION
In the last weeks of pregnancy, you may find the traditional man-on-top position difficult. Experiment with other positions; perhaps try sitting on your partner's lap, kneeling with him behind, or both lying side by side.

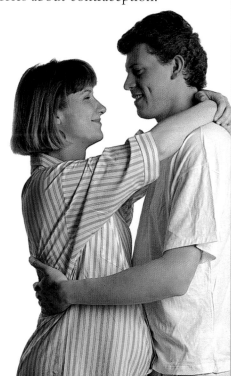

WEEK
36

By now you should have started to wind your life down in preparation for the birth. The baby takes up all the space in the womb, so he kicks and punches rather than shifts his whole body. If he were born now, he would have an excellent chance of survival.

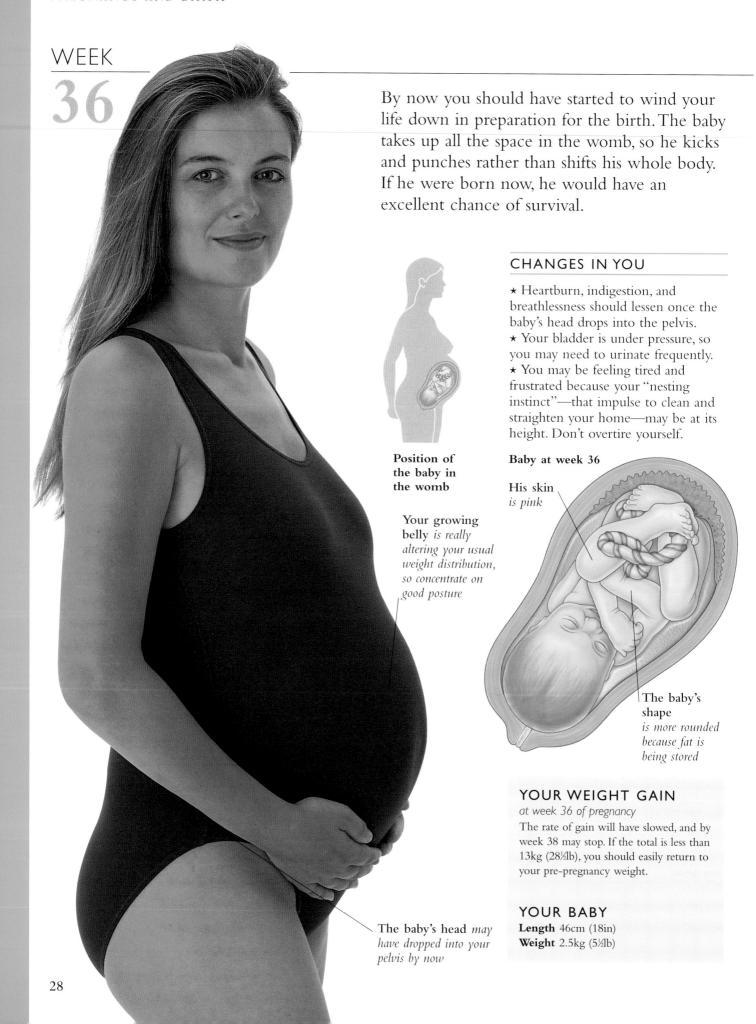

CHANGES IN YOU

★ Heartburn, indigestion, and breathlessness should lessen once the baby's head drops into the pelvis.
★ Your bladder is under pressure, so you may need to urinate frequently.
★ You may be feeling tired and frustrated because your "nesting instinct"—that impulse to clean and straighten your home—may be at its height. Don't overtire yourself.

Position of the baby in the womb

Your growing belly *is really altering your usual weight distribution, so concentrate on good posture*

Baby at week 36

His skin *is pink*

The baby's shape *is more rounded because fat is being stored*

YOUR WEIGHT GAIN
at week 36 of pregnancy
The rate of gain will have slowed, and by week 38 may stop. If the total is less than 13kg (28½lb), you should easily return to your pre-pregnancy weight.

YOUR BABY
Length 46cm (18in)
Weight 2.5kg (5½lb)

The baby's head *may have dropped into your pelvis by now*

WHAT TO DO

★ Put your feet up whenever you can to guard against swollen ankles and varicose veins.
★ Doctor visits may be once a week now.
★ Make sure you take a tour of the delivery room and maternity area.
★ Buy your nursing bras.
★ Go food shopping and stock up on all the basics so they'll be there for your return. If you have a freezer, fill it with easy meals.
★ Pack your suitcase.
★ Don't lie flat on your back. It can decrease the circulation to your uterus.

"Should I have my partner with me during labor?"

Most hospitals and childbirth experts actively encourage this. Labor can be a long process, and a lonely one unless you have someone close to share it with. The natural choice is your baby's father. But if he really doesn't want to be there, it's unfair to put too much pressure on him. It's quite acceptable to have a relative or a good friend there instead.

YOUR GROWING BABY

★ If this is your first baby, his head will probably have descended into the pelvis, ready for birth.
★ Soft nails have grown to the tips of his fingers and toes.
★ In a boy, the testicles should have descended.
★ The baby will gain about 28g (1oz) every day for the remaining four weeks in the womb.

see also:
Essentials for the baby *page 27*
Frequent urination *page 41*
Preparing for the birth *pages 54–55*
Protecting your back *page 42*
Relaxation techniques *pages 48–49*
Swollen ankles *page 42*
Varicose veins *page 42*

RESTING IN LATER PREGNANCY

During the last weeks, you will probably become tired very easily. You may not be sleeping as well as usual, and you will also feel exhausted by the extra weight you have been carrying around. It's important not to fight this tiredness, but to rest and relax as much as possible.

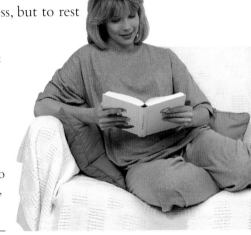

TO AVOID TIRING YOURSELF

Put your feet up whenever you need to during the day. Think of quiet things to do when you rest: practice gentle relaxation exercises, listen to soothing music, read a book or magazine, or perhaps knit something for the baby. It also helps if you try to do things at a slower pace than usual, so that you don't become overtired.

YOUR NURSING BRA

If at all possible, you should breast-feed your baby. You will need at least two front-opening nursing bras. To make sure these are the right size, it's best to buy them no earlier than week 36.

WHAT TO LOOK FOR

There are two main types: one has flaps, which expose the nipple and surrounding breast; the other fastens in front, so you can expose the whole breast. The front-opening kind allows the baby to feel and touch as much of your breast as possible. This helps your milk let-down reflex (see pages 93 and 96). Look for cotton and wide straps.

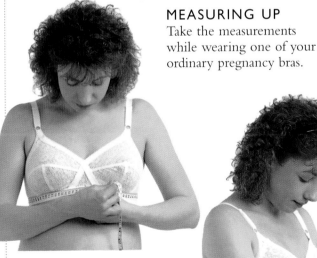

MEASURING UP

Take the measurements while wearing one of your ordinary pregnancy bras.

1 Measure around your body below your breasts. Add 12cm (5in) to get your final chest measurement.

2 Measure around the fullest part of your breasts. If this equals your chest measurement, you need an A cup. If it is 2.5cm (1in) more, you need a B cup. If it is 5cm (2in) more, you need a C cup.

WEEK

40

By this stage, you will feel very ungainly, and will be bumping into objects because of your size. You will be most impatient to give birth, but also excited and relieved that you are nearly there. Rest as much as possible, and enjoy these last baby-free days.

CHANGES IN YOU

★ You will have a feeling of heaviness in your lower adbomen.
★ Your cervix will be softening in preparation for labor.
★ Braxton Hicks contractions may be so noticeable that you think you are in labor, but they won't be regular.

YOUR WEIGHT GAIN
at week 40 of pregnancy
In the final two weeks you may actually lose a little weight. This is a sign that your baby is fully mature, and you can expect labor to start within 10 days. Model's weight gain as at week 36.

YOUR BABY
Length 51cm (20in)
Weight 3.4kg (7½lb)

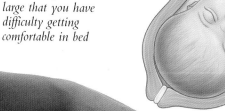

Position of the baby in the womb

Baby at week 40

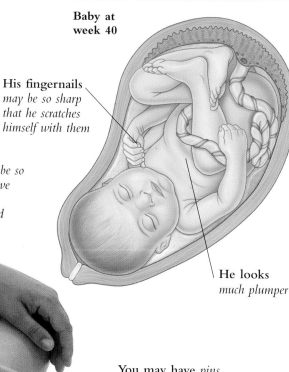

Your skin *will feel stretched and taut across your abdomen, and may be itchy*

His fingernails *may be so sharp that he scratches himself with them*

Your belly *will be so large that you have difficulty getting comfortable in bed*

He looks *much plumper*

You may have *pins and needles in your legs*

WHAT TO DO

★ If you don't feel at least ten movements from your baby in the day, call your doctor.
★ If the Braxton Hicks contractions are noticeable, practice your breathing.
★ Don't worry if your baby doesn't arrive on time; it's perfectly normal for a baby to be born up to two weeks on either side of the expected delivery date.

TOTAL WEIGHT GAIN

The average amount of weight gain during pregnancy varies between 10 and 12kg (22–27lb), but you may put on more or less weight. The total weight gain is made up as follows:

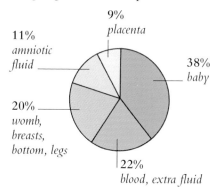

9%
placenta

11%
amniotic fluid

38%
baby

20%
womb, breasts, bottom, legs

22%
blood, extra fluid

YOUR GROWING BABY

★ Most of the lanugo hair has disappeared, though there may still be a little over his shoulders, arms, and legs.
★ He may be covered in vernix, or just have traces in skin folds.
★ A dark substance called meconium gathers in the baby's intestines; this will be passed in his first bowel movement after birth.
★ If this is your second or later baby, his head may engage now.

see also:
Braxton Hicks contractions **page 56**
Breathing techniques **page 49**

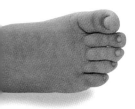

BECOMING A MOTHER

After all the weeks of preparation and planning, you can now hold your baby in your arms. You will probably feel overwhelmingly protective toward this tiny person, who is dependent on you for everything.

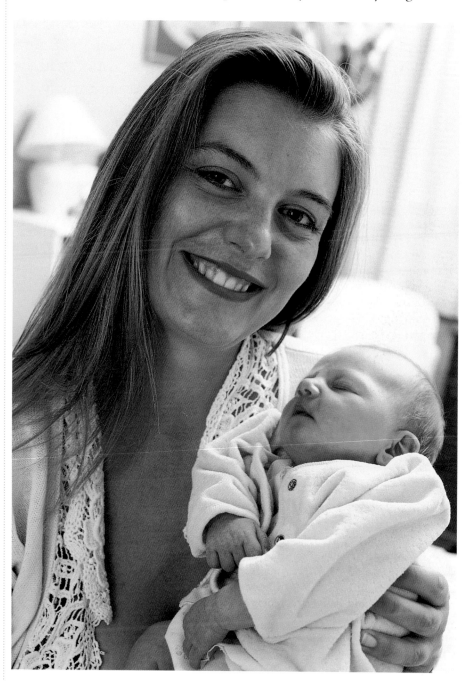

THE FIRST WEEKS

Life in the early weeks following the arrival of your baby revolves around her and her needs, whether she needs feeding, diaper changing, or comforting. But once you get to know each other, and you become more adept at handling your baby and understanding what she requires, she will become more settled, and life will fall into some sort of routine once again.

31

PRENATAL CARE

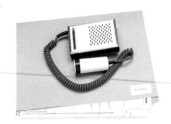

Taking good care of yourself and your growing baby during pregnancy is critical. Soon after you miss your first period or a home-testing kit indicates that you are pregnant, your prenatal care should begin. This modern system of regular visits to the physician who will deliver your baby offers reassuring checks, tests, and a source of answers to any troubling questions. Start your prenatal care early in pregnancy, because the first set of checks and tests provides a baseline for assessing any changes later on. This way, your caregivers can spot any potential problems early on and work with you to achieve the best possible pregnancy and birth for you and your baby.

WHERE TO HAVE YOUR BABY

One of the first decisions you will need to make is where to have your baby. Most babies are born in a hospital. Some hospitals now feature home-like birthing rooms. All hospitals recognize a woman's right to choose the type of birth she would like, provided her wishes are compatible with safety.

HOSPITAL BIRTH
A hospital offers all the equipment and expertise available for giving pain medication, monitoring your baby's progress, intervening in the birth to help you and the baby if necessary, and providing emergency care to both of you. After the birth, a few days in the hospital may give you the rest you need to cope at home later; the average stay is roughly 48 hours. If you are a first-time mother, you may also find the support of staff and other mothers reassuring.

TAKE A HOSPITAL TOUR
Because hospital policies regarding labor and delivery vary tremendously across the country, some women choose to tour nearby medical centers prior to making arrangements for their first prenatal visit. Not all physicians are on staff at, or affiliated to, all the hospitals in a local area. Call ahead and ask if you and your partner can see the obstetrical unit to find out about family-centered births, special labor and delivery rooms, and visiting hours for family members. Seek recommendations from women who have recently become mothers; word-of-mouth tips are often the best. After you settle on a hospital, you can gather the names of physicians whose patients deliver there.

BIRTHING ROOMS
In a traditional hospital birth, a woman labors in one room, and immediately before her baby is ready to be born, she is moved to a special delivery or operating room. However, in recent years, some hospitals have realized that it is not always appropriate to move patients at that critical moment in giving birth. As family-centered births have become more popular, birthing rooms have appeared in many medical centers. Designed for women who are in a low-risk category and expect to deliver their babies normally, these rooms can be more home-like than typical operating rooms, and expectant couples can remain together in an informal setting. A birthing bed, one with a split frame that separates the bottom half from the head of the bed at the time of delivery, is often available, too. Ask about these options; sometimes if you don't enquire you won't be put on a birthing room reservation list.

WHO WILL DELIVER THE BABY?
You can choose a family doctor, or an obstetrician, or in some provinces, a midwife, to deliver the baby. Choose a caregiver with whom you feel comfortable and who really understands your needs. Go to an initial appointment with a written list of questions and be prepared to participate in your prenatal care. Ignorance is never bliss when it comes to having a baby.

GROUP PRACTICES
Some physicians prefer to work in a group. Thus they can relieve each other in giving care that can demand full concentration 24 hours a day. This may mean that you will see various doctors during your pregnancy. There are group practices as small as two and as large as six or even eight physicians.

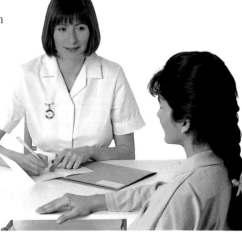

QUESTIONS TO ASK

Hospital facilities vary, so discuss any issues that are important to you with your physician. It's natural to have preconceived ideas about labor and birth, but the reality is often quite different. Even though you may be against pain medication, for example, keep an open mind. In an emergency or under severe strain, you may need it.

ABOUT LABOR

Can my partner or a friend stay with me throughout labor? Will he or she be asked to leave the delivery room at any time?
Will I be able to move around during labor?
What is the hospital policy on pain medication, routine fetal monitoring, and labor induction (see pages 64–66)?
What kind of pain relief will I be offered during labor; are epidural anesthesia or tranquilizers (see pages 64–65) available?

ABOUT THE BIRTH

Will I stay in my labor room or be moved to a delivery area?
Can I give birth in any position I choose to? Are chairs or special birthing beds available?
What is the hospital policy on episiotomies and Cesareans (see pages 66–67)?

AFTER THE BIRTH

How long will I stay in the hospital after the delivery?
Is "rooming-in" available?
What are the visiting hours?
Is there a special care baby unit? If not, where will my baby be taken if special treatment is needed?

UNDERSTANDING THE TERMINOLOGY

Test results and any other details about your pregnancy are kept in your medical files. Do not hesitate to ask for an explanation of any test for which you are scheduled. Test names and other medical facts are generally abbreviated. The following is a sampling of some of the terminology.

Agglu	Blood test.
Alb	Albumin (a protein) found in urine.
BP	Blood pressure.
Br	The baby is bottom down.
C/Ceph or Vx	The baby is in the normal (head down) position.
CS	Cesarean section.
EDD/EDC	Estimated date of delivery/confinement.
ELISA	AIDS test.
Engagement	Relation of the part of the baby to be born first to the brim of the pelvis.

Fe	Iron supplements prescribed.
FH	Fetal heart.
FHH/H or ✓	Fetal heart heard.
FHNH	Fetal heart not heard.
FMF	Fetal movements felt.
Fundus	Top of the womb.
G	Gravida (pregnant).
G2	Second pregnancy.
HBsAg	Hepatitis test.
HgB	Hemoglobin levels in the blood (to check for anemia).
HIV	AIDS test.
LMP	Last menstrual period.
MSS	Maternal serum screen.
MSU	Mid-stream urine sample.
NAD or nil or ✓	Nothing abnormal discovered in urine.
P or Parity or Para	Number of previous births. Thus Gravida 1; Para 0 is a woman in her first pregnancy.
Presentation	Which way up and around the baby is.

Primigravida	First pregnancy.
SGA	Small for dates.
+	A trace found.
U/S	Ultrasound.
VDRL	Test for syphilis.

Abbreviations are used to describe the way the baby is lying in the womb. These are some of the positions:

ROA   LOA

ROP   LOP

A TYPICAL PRENATAL VISIT

Your first visit to your physician should take place soon after you miss your period. You will probably be going once a month until 28 weeks. Visits become more frequent after this; usually every two weeks until you are 36 weeks pregnant, and every week in the last month. A number of routine tests are carried out by the doctor at every visit, to make sure that the pregnancy is progressing normally.

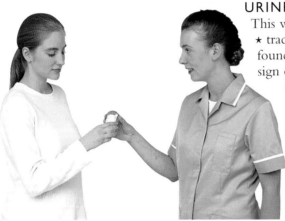

URINE SAMPLE *every visit*
This will be tested for:
* traces of sugar, which, if found repeatedly, could be a sign of diabetes (see page 38)
* traces of protein, which could indicate that your kidneys are not working properly. If protein is found in your urine later in pregnancy, this could be a sign of preeclampsia (see page 38).

HEIGHT
first visit
Your height will be measured, because this is a guide to the size of your pelvis; a small pelvis can sometimes mean a difficult delivery. If you are over 152cm (5ft) tall, you are unlikely to have difficulties giving birth, unless you are carrying an unusually large baby.

WEIGHT *every visit*
You will be weighed at each visit to check that you are gaining weight properly (see Calendar, pages 16–31). Don't worry if you lose some weight during the first three months because of morning sickness. Pregnancy weight gain isn't always predictable or as easily controlled as expectant mothers and their doctors would like.

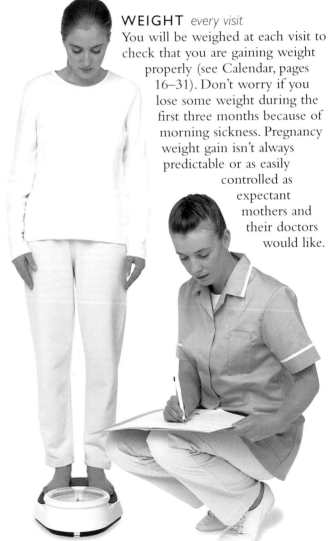

INITIAL APPOINTMENT
At the first visit, the doctor will ask some questions about you and your partner, to find out whether there is anything that could affect the pregnancy or your baby. Routines and procedures vary from place to place, but you can usually expect to be asked about:
* personal details, such as your date of birth, and the work you and your partner do
* your country of origin: some forms of anemia, such as sickle-cell trait or thalassemia, are inherited and affect only certain ethnic groups
* your health: serious illnesses or operations you may have had, whether you are being treated for any disease, and whether you have any allergies, or are taking any drugs
* your family's medical history: whether there are twins or any inherited illnesses in your family or your partner's family
* the type of contraceptives you and your partner used before you became pregnant, and when you stopped using them
* your periods: when they began, whether they are regular, when the first day of your last period was, and the length of your cycle
* any previous pregnancies, including miscarriages and abortions.
A physical examination may include a vaginal examination to check that your reproductive organs and pelvis are normal and to confirm the estimated delivery date.

BLOOD TESTS *first visit*

Some blood will be taken from your arm to check:

★ your blood type and your rhesus, or Rh, factor (see page 38)

★ that you are not anemic (see page 38)

★ that you are immune to German measles (see page 10)

★ that you do not have a sexually transmitted disease, such as syphilis, which must be treated before week 20 if it is not to harm the baby

★ for viruses connected to hepatitis and AIDS (after counseling).

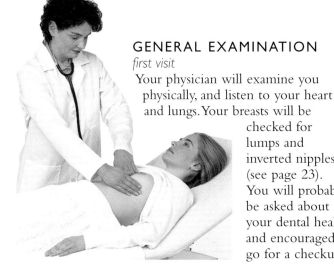

GENERAL EXAMINATION
first visit

Your physician will examine you physically, and listen to your heart and lungs. Your breasts will be checked for lumps and inverted nipples (see page 23). You will probably be asked about your dental health, and encouraged to go for a checkup.

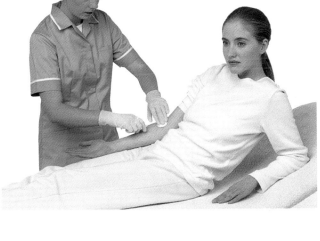

ASKING QUESTIONS

There are bound to be things that puzzle or worry you, or even just interest you, during your pregnancy. Your prenatal visits are your chance to ask about them. It is a good idea to write down any questions before seeing the doctor. Under pressure, it is easy to forget them. Not all doctors are good at explaining medical matters in nonmedical terms. If you don't understand the answer you have been given, ask again, and again if necessary, to clear up any anxieties you may have.

BLOOD PRESSURE *every visit*

Your blood pressure is slightly lower in pregnancy, and it is measured regularly to detect any sudden rises and keep them under control. Normal blood pressure is about 120/70, and there will be cause for concern if your blood pressure rises above 140/90.

Raised blood pressure can be a sign of a number of problems, including preeclampsia (see page 38). However, the stress of a prenatal examination, and waiting for test results, can cause a higher than normal reading, so your blood pressure may be taken again later on during the visit. Ask the doctor or nurse to tell you your blood pressure if she does not automatically do so. It should be written on your chart.

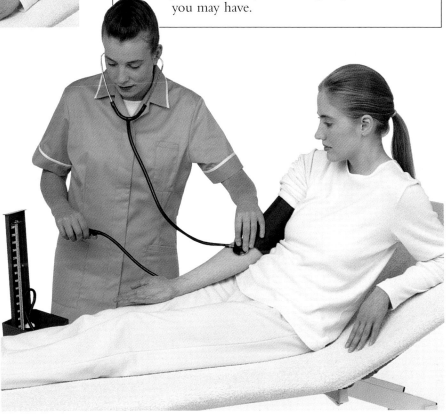

LEGS, ANKLES, AND HANDS *every visit*
The doctor will ask about swelling of your hands, ankles, and lower legs. She may examine them to make sure there is no swelling or puffiness (edema). A little swelling in the last weeks of pregnancy is normal, especially at the end of the day, but if it's excessive it may be a sign of preeclampsia (see page 38).

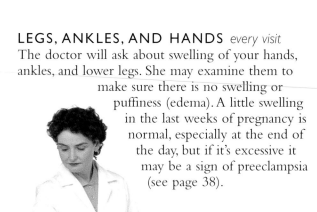

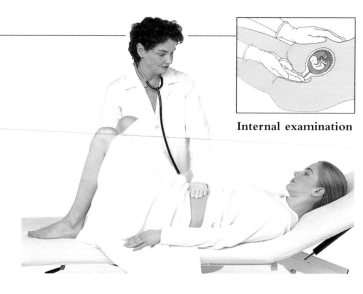

Internal examination

INTERNAL EXAMINATION *first visit*
If your first visit is early in the pregnancy, the doctor may give you an internal examination, to confirm the stage of the pregnancy to check your pelvis for abnormalities. You may also have a Pap smear at the same time to check for abnormal cells; ask for the result at your next visit.

The examination will not hurt you or the baby, and needn't be uncomfortable if you relax. You will be asked to lie on your back with your legs bent and your knees comfortably apart. The doctor will put two fingers of one hand into the vagina, and press your abdomen with the other hand.

LISTENING TO THE BABY'S HEARTBEAT
every visit (after week 14)
From early in pregnancy, this may be done with an electronic instrument (see below), which amplifies the baby's heartbeat so you can hear it, too. After week 28, the doctor may listen with a standard stethoscope.

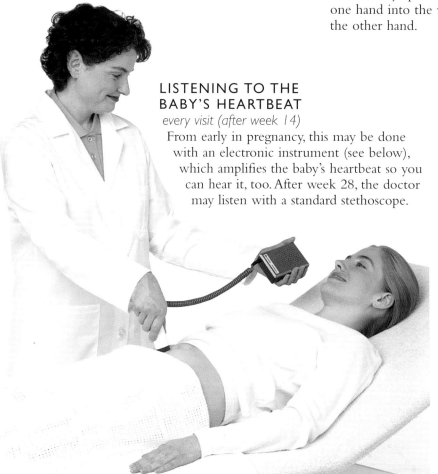

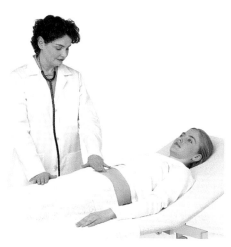

FEELING THE ABDOMEN
every visit
Your abdomen will be felt gently to check the position of the top of the womb, which provides a good clue to the rate of the baby's growth. Later in pregnancy, these physical examinations can indicate the position of the fetus. In the final weeks, the doctor will want to see if the head is dropping into the pelvis (engaging).

EXTRA TESTS

You may be scheduled for an MSS blood test or an ultrasound scan as part of prenatal care. Some tests are offered only in certain circumstances. If you are over 35 years old, amniocentesis might be recommended, for instance. When problems are detected early enough, intervention may be a possible option.

ULTRASOUND SCAN
week 16 (and sometimes later)
This is an exciting test to have, as it enables you to "see" your baby, often moving around, for the first time. If you are scheduled for an ultrasound scan, ask the staff if you can bring your partner with you. The baby becomes a fascinating reality when you both see him on the screen. You may be offered a photograph of the scan, too.

Ultrasound does not always show the baby's gender, but it can be used to:
★ make sure the fetus is growing and developing normally
★ determine the fetus's age and expected delivery date
★ check the position of the baby and placenta, for example, before amniocentesis, or later in pregnancy to make sure the placenta is not blocking the neck of the womb
★ detect some abnormalities, such as problems with the brain and spine
★ find out whether you are carrying more than one baby.

If you are having the test early in your pregnancy, you will be asked to drink plenty of water and arrive with a full bladder, so that the womb is clearly visible on the screen. The procedure takes about 10 minutes, and is safe and painless.

A thin layer of jelly or oil is rubbed over your stomach, and a hand-held instrument, a transducer, is passed over it. This beams and receives sound waves, which are built into an image on the screen.

MATERNAL SERUM SCREEN/TRIPLE (MSS) TEST
week 16
This blood test measures the amount of three hormones in the blood. A high blood level may indicate problems with the baby, such as a malformed spine or Down syndrome. However, it is important to remember that the test is not diagnostic, but rather, it is looking for possible problems. Most women with high test levels go on to have normal babies.

If you have raised MSS levels, you will have an ultrasound scan, and possibly another blood test and an amniocentesis.

AMNIOCENTESIS
weeks 14–18 (and sometimes later)
Amniocentesis can be used to detect some abnormalities in the baby, such as Down syndrome and spina bifida. It is not offered routinely, because there is a risk of miscarriage in about one woman in 100.

Your doctor may suggest the test if:
★ you are over 35, because your risk of delivering a Down syndrome baby rises with your age

★ you have a family history of inherited disease, such as spina bifida
★ you had a raised MSS level.
An ultrasound scan is done to check the position of the baby and the placenta. A hollow needle is inserted through the wall of the abdomen into the womb, and a sample of the fluid that surrounds the baby, and contains some of his cells, is taken. The cells are then tested for abnormality. The test results for amniocentesis can take three to four weeks.

CHORIONIC VILLUS SAMPLING (CVS)
weeks 10–12
Some inherited disorders can be detected very early in pregnancy, by examining a small piece of the tissue that later develops into the placenta. The sample is usually removed through the entrance to the womb.

The advantage of CVS is that it can be done early in pregnancy. The miscarriage rate for the test is slightly higher than for amniocentesis.

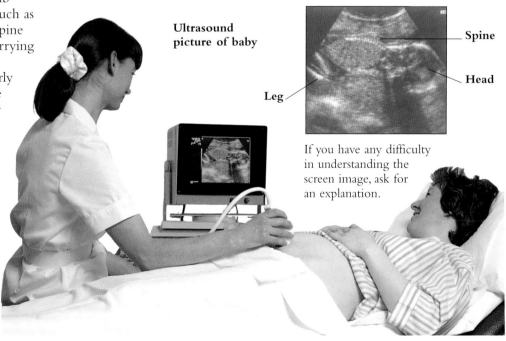

Ultrasound picture of baby

Spine

Head

Leg

If you have any difficulty in understanding the screen image, ask for an explanation.

HIGH-RISK PREGNANCIES

Nearly all pregnancies are straightforward, but occasionally there are circumstances that alert your doctor to possible complications. You might have a general medical condition that puts you into a high-risk category. Or sometimes symptoms develop that warn the doctor that special care is needed.

ANEMIA

Anemia means that you do not have enough red blood cells. Many women are slightly anemic before they become pregnant because they lack iron. It is important to correct this imbalance, so that you can cope with the demands of pregnancy. Being anemic can make you feel tired.

Treatment Try to prevent the problem in the first place by eating a varied diet, with plenty of iron-rich foods (see page 52). If blood tests show you are anemic, your physician can prescribe iron supplements. Some doctors do this as a matter of course. Take iron tablets directly after meals, with plenty of fluid, because they can irritate the stomach and cause constipation, diarrhea, or nausea.

Anemia Eating foods that are a good source of iron, such as tuna fish, legumes, and red meat, will help guard against the problem.

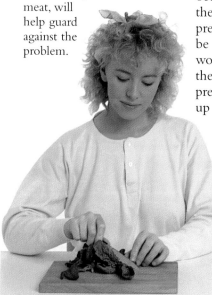

DIABETES

Diabetes must be carefully controlled during pregnancy and your blood sugar level constantly monitored. If this is done, there's no reason the pregnancy shouldn't be normal and straightforward. Some women develop a mild form of the disease for the first time during pregnancy. This nearly always disappears soon after the birth of the baby.

Treatment It's imperative that your blood sugar level remain stable, so the doctor may adjust your insulin intake for the pregnancy. Pay special attention to diet. You may need to visit the doctor more often.

INCOMPETENT CERVIX

In a normal pregnancy, the cervix (neck of the womb) stays closed until labor begins. If miscarriages occur frequently after the third month of pregnancy, the reason could be that the neck of the womb is weak. Under the pressure of a growing pregnancy, the cervix opens up and expels the baby.

Treatment Your doctor may suggest minor surgery to stitch the cervix closed at the beginning of your pregnancy. The stitch is removed toward the end of pregnancy, or as you go into labor.

PREECLAMPSIA

A common but serious problem in late pregnancy, this is a combination of the following symptoms: raised blood pressure above 140/90; excessive weight gain; swollen ankles, feet, or hands; and traces of protein in the urine. If you develop any of these, the doctor will monitor you very carefully.

If blood pressure rises untreated, it could progress to the extremely dangerous condition of eclampsia, where convulsions may occur, putting you and your baby at risk.

Treatment Your doctor may advise bed rest. You may be given a drug to lower your blood pressure, or advised to cut down on salt. If the signs are severe, you will be admitted to the hospital, even though you might be feeling healthy. Labor may be induced (see page 66).

RHESUS NEGATIVE MOTHER

Your blood is tested at the first prenatal visit to see if it is rhesus positive or rhesus negative. About 15 percent of people are rhesus, or Rh, negative, and if you are one of these, you will only have a problem in pregnancy if you give birth to a rhesus, or Rh, positive baby. When blood types are incompatible like this, it won't harm a first baby, but could cause complications in later pregnancies.

Treatment If you are an Rh negative mother, you will be given an injection of anti-Rh immunoglobulin (a protective protein) at 28 weeks, and then again after birth if your baby is Rh positive. You must have these injections with each pregnancy because they stop your immune system from creating antibodies that could hurt your baby.

EMERGENCY SIGNS

Call for emergency help immediately if you have:
★ a severe headache that won't go away
★ misty or blurred vision
★ severe, prolonged stomach pains
★ vaginal bleeding
★ a leakage of fluid, which suggests that your water has broken early
★ frequent, painful urination (drink plenty of water in the meantime).

Consult your doctor within 24 hours if you have:
★ swollen hands, face, and ankles
★ severe, frequent vomiting
★ a temperature of 38.3°C (101°F)
★ no movement, or fewer than 10 kicks, from your baby for 12 hours after week 28.

MISCARRIAGE

A miscarriage is the ending of a pregnancy before 20 weeks, and may happen to one in five pregnancies. Most miscarriages occur in the first 12 weeks, often before the woman has even discovered she is pregnant, and usually because the fetus is not developing normally. Bleeding from the vagina is usually the first sign. Call your doctor immediately and lie down.

Threatened abortion

If bleeding is mild and painless, the pregnancy may continue. Your doctor will probably recommend bed rest, the bleeding may stop, and if you take things easy for a few days, the pregnancy may proceed, without any increased risk of abnormality in the baby. You may be given another pregnancy test or an ultrasound scan (see page 37) to confirm that all is well.

True miscarriage

If the bleeding is heavy and you are in pain, it probably means that the baby has died. You may have to go into the hospital for a D and C, dilatation and curettage, during which your womb is cleaned out.

Your feelings

Even if you miscarry early in pregnancy, you will feel an intense sense of loss. Other people don't always understand that you feel a need to mourn your baby. Worrying about whether you can ever have a normal, healthy baby is common. You may feel guilty too, though you should never blame yourself; it really isn't your fault. It's quite safe to try to get pregnant again as soon as you like, although some doctors suggest waiting until at least three menstrual cycles have passed. Unless you have had a string of miscarriages, there is no reason at all why you shouldn't have a successful pregnancy next time.

"SMALL FOR DATES" BABIES

A baby who doesn't grow properly in the womb and is small at birth is called a "small for dates" baby. This is not a premature baby and it may happen because the expectant mother smokes or eats a poor diet, or because the placenta isn't working properly. (A general medical condition, such as maternal diabetes, may be the cause.)
Treatment If tests during pregnancy show your baby is small, you will be monitored very closely to check his health, and watch the flow of blood to the placenta. If the baby stops growing or appears to be distressed in any way, he will be delivered early, either by inducing labor or Cesarean section (see pages 66 and 67).

TWINS

Your pregnancy and labor will progress normally, although you will have two second stages in labor, and you may go into labor prematurely. There is a greater likelihood of such complications as anemia, preeclampsia, and of the babies lying abnormally in the womb. You may also find that all the common disorders of pregnancy are exaggerated, especially in the last few months.
Treatment Regular prenatal visits are essential if you are expecting twins, so that any complications can be spotted immediately. A multiple pregnancy puts great strain on your body so watch your posture and rest as much as possible, especially in the last few weeks. To avoid problems with your digestion, eat small amounts of fresh, unprocessed food at frequent intervals.

VAGINAL BLEEDING

If you notice bleeding from your vagina at any time in pregnancy, call your doctor without delay and go to bed. Before 20 weeks, it can be a sign of an impending miscarriage. After this time, it may mean that the placenta is bleeding. This can happen if the placenta has started to separate from the wall of the womb (placental abruption) or if the placenta is too low in the womb and covering, or partially covering, the cervix (placenta previa).
Treatment The placenta is the baby's lifeline, so if the doctor thinks there is any risk to it, you will probably be admitted to the hospital immediately, where the position of the placenta can be checked. You may then stay in the hospital until after the birth. If you have lost a lot of blood, you may be given a blood transfusion, and the baby will probably be delivered as soon as possible, by inducing labor or by Cesarean section (see pages 67 and 66). If bleeding is slight and occurs several weeks before the baby is due, the doctor may wait for labor to start naturally, while observing you closely.

Twins You may find this position comfortable to rest in.

COMMON COMPLAINTS

You may suffer from a wide variety of discomforts that exasperate you, but your aches and pains are probably perfectly normal. Many are caused by hormonal changes, or because your body is under extra pressure. A few symptoms, however, should be taken more seriously. Call the doctor if you have any of the signs listed in the box on page 38.

COMPLAINT	SYMPTOMS	WHAT TO DO
Bleeding gums 1 2 3• The gums become softer and more easily injured in pregnancy. They may be inflamed, allowing plaque to collect at the base of the teeth. This can lead to gum disease and tooth decay.	Bleeding from the gums, especially after brushing your teeth.	★ Brush and floss your teeth thoroughly after eating. ★ See your dentist—but you shouldn't have X-rays or general anesthesia.
Breathlessness 3 The growing baby puts pressure on the diaphragm, and prevents you from breathing freely. The problem is often relieved about a month before the birth, when the baby's head descends into the pelvis. Breathlessness can also be caused by anemia.	Feeling breathless when you exert yourself, or even when you talk.	★ Rest as much as possible. ★ Try crouching if there's no chair around and you feel breathless. ★ At night, use an extra pillow. ★ If the problem is severe, consult your doctor.
Constipation 1 2 3 The pregnancy hormone progesterone relaxes the muscles of the intestine, which slows down bowel movements, making you more likely to become constipated.	Passing hard, dry stools at less frequent intervals than usual.	★ Eat plenty of high-fiber foods and drink lots of water. Go to the bathroom often. ★ Exercise regularly. ★ Take any iron supplements you have been prescribed on a full stomach, with plenty of fluid. ★ See your doctor if the problem persists. Avoid laxatives.
Muscle cramps 3 May be caused by a calcium deficiency.	Painful contractions of muscles, usually in the calves and the feet, and often at night. Commonly started by a leg stretch with the toes pointed down.	★ Massage the affected calf or foot. ★ Walk around for a moment or two once the pain has eased to improve your circulation. ★ Discuss the problem with your doctor.
Feeling faint 1 3 Your blood pressure is lower in pregnancy, so you are more likely to feel faint.	Feeling dizzy and unstable. Needing to sit or lie down.	★ Try not to stand still for too long. ★ If you feel faint, sit down and put your head between your knees. ★ Get up slowly from a hot bath, or when sitting or lying down. Turn to one side first when you are getting up after lying on your back.

• The numbers after each complaint relate to the trimester in which you are most likely to suffer from the problem.

Backache see page 44
Skin pigmentation see page 21

Breathlessness
Crouching helps if you suddenly feel out of breath halfway up the stairs. Hold on to the banister.

Cramps
Pull your foot up toward you with your hand, and massage the calf vigorously, to help relieve painful cramps.

COMPLAINT	SYMPTOMS	WHAT TO DO
Frequent urination 1 3 Caused by the womb pressing on the bladder. The problem is often relieved in the middle months of pregnancy.	You need to urinate often.	★ If you find yourself getting up in the night to go to the bathroom, try drinking less in the evenings. ★ See your doctor if you feel any pain because you could have an infection.
Heartburn 3 The valve at the entrance to your stomach relaxes in pregnancy because of hormonal changes, so stomach acid passes back into the esophagus (the tube leading to your stomach).	A strong burning pain in the center of the chest.	★ Avoid large meals, highly spiced or fried foods. ★ At night, try a warm milk drink, and use extra pillows to raise your head. ★ See your doctor, who may advise medication to treat stomach acidity.
Leaking urine 3 Caused by weak pelvic floor muscles (see page 45), and the growing baby pressing on your bladder.	Leakage of urine whenever you run, cough, sneeze, or laugh.	★ Urinate often. ★ Practice pelvic floor exercises regularly. ★ Avoid heavy lifting, and try to avoid becoming constipated.
Morning sickness 1 One of the first signs of pregnancy, nausea is usually worse in the morning, but it can occur at any time of the day. It usually disappears after week 12, but sometimes returns later.	Feeling sick, often at the smell of certain foods or cigarette smoke. Most women find there is a particular time of day when this happens.	★ Try eating small, frequent meals throughout the day. ★ Avoid foods and smells that make you feel sick. ★ Get extra rest.
Hemorrhoids 2 3 Pressure from the baby's head causes swollen veins around the anus. Straining to empty the bowels will make the problem worse. Mild hemorrhoids usually disappear, without treatment, after the baby is born.	Itching, soreness, and possibly pain or bleeding when you empty your bowels.	★ Avoid becoming constipated. ★ Try not to stand for long periods. ★ An ice pack held against the hemorrhoids may ease itching. ★ If hemorrhoids persist, tell the doctor. He or she may prescribe an ointment.
Rash 3 Usually occurs in women who are overweight and who perspire freely. Can be caused by hormonal changes.	Red rash, which usually develops in sweaty skin folds under the breasts or in the groin.	★ Wash and dry these areas often. Use unperfumed soap. ★ Soothe the skin with calamine lotion. ★ Wear loose cotton clothes.
Sleeping difficulty 1 2 3 You may have a problem because the baby is kicking, you have to go to the bathroom frequently, or the sheer size of your baby makes it difficult to get comfortable in bed.	Having trouble going to sleep in the first place, and finding it hard to get to sleep after waking. Some women find they have very frightening dreams about the birth or the baby. Don't worry about dreams; they do not reflect what will happen.	★ Reading, gentle relaxation exercises, or a warm bath before bedtime may help. ★ Experiment with extra pillows. If you sleep on your side, put a pillow under your top thigh.

Heartburn and sleeplessness
This piled-up arrangement of pillows is comfortable if you suffer from heartburn, or are unable to sleep.

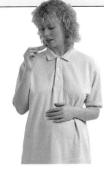

Morning sickness
To counteract nausea, try eating dry crackers, toast, or fruit. Eliminate fried or highly seasoned foods and drink lots of water.

COMPLAINT	SYMPTOMS	WHAT TO DO
Stretchmarks 2 3 These form if your skin stretches beyond its normal elasticity. Excess weight gain can also cause them. The marks may disappear, but are more likely to fade to thin silvery streaks.	Red marks that sometimes appear on the skin of the thighs, stomach, or breasts during pregnancy.	★ Try not to put on weight too rapidly. ★ Rubbing moisturizer into the skin may feel cool and soothing, although creams and ointments won't prevent or heal stretch marks.
Sweating 2 3 This is caused by hormonal changes, and because blood flow to the skin increases in pregnancy.	Perspiring after very little exertion, or waking up in the night feeling hot and sweaty.	★ Wear loose cotton clothes. Avoid man-made materials. ★ Drink plenty of water. ★ Open a window at night.
Swollen ankles and fingers 3 Some swelling (edema) is normal in pregnancy, because the body holds extra water. This is usually no cause for concern.	Slight swelling in the ankles, especially in hot weather and at the end of the day. This shouldn't cause pain or discomfort. You may also notice stiff, swollen fingers in the morning, and your rings may feel tight.	★ Rest often with your feet up. ★ Try gentle foot exercises. Hold your hands above your head; flex and stretch each finger. ★ See your doctor or midwife. Marked swelling could be a warning sign of preeclampsia (see page 38).
Yeast infections 1 2 3 Hormonal changes during pregnancy increase the chances of developing yeast infections. Washing with some soaps can worsen the problem.	A thick white vaginal discharge and severe itching. There may also be soreness and pain when you urinate.	★ Keep the genital area as dry as possible. ★ Wear only cotton or cotton-crotch underpants. ★ Avoid panty hose, tight jeans, and vaginal deodorants. ★ See your doctor, who may be able to advise treatment.
Tiredness 1 3 This is caused by the extra demands that pregnancy makes on your body, and may also be the result of worry.	Feeling weary, and wanting to sleep in the day. Needing to sleep longer at night.	★ Rest as much as possible and practice relaxation exercises. ★ Go to bed earlier. ★ Don't overexert yourself.
Vaginal discharge 1 2 3 You may notice some increase in the amount of mucus produced by the vagina because of the hormonal changes during pregnancy.	Slight increase in clear or white discharge, without soreness or pain.	★ Avoid vaginal deodorants and perfumed soap products. ★ Wear a light sanitary pad. ★ See your doctor if you have any itching, soreness, colored or foul-smelling discharge.
Varicose veins 1 2 3 You are more likely to develop these in a second or third pregnancy, if you are overweight, or they run in your family. Standing for too long, or sitting cross-legged, can worsen them.	Aching legs; the veins in the calves and the thighs become painful and swollen.	★ Rest often with your feet up. Try raising the foot of your bed with pillows under the mattress. ★ Support stockings may help. Put them on before getting up in the morning. ★ Exercise your feet.

Swollen ankles and varicose veins Gently circle your ankles and feet to improve circulation.

Varicose veins Rest with your feet well elevated on at least two cushions if you suffer from this problem. Tuck another cushion into the small of your back.

KEEPING FIT AND RELAXED

Pregnancy, labor, and birth place great demands on your body, so the more you can prepare yourself physically, the better you will feel. You will also find it easier to get back into shape when the baby is born. Relaxation exercises are important too; they will help you calm down and cope more effectively in labor, and they are invaluable for relieving stress and increasing blood flow to the placenta. The exercises on the following pages are designed to make your joints and muscles more supple, in preparation for labor and birth. You can begin prenatal exercises as soon as the pregnancy is confirmed, or earlier if you wish. Practice at home or sign up for an exercise class for expectant mothers. Don't worry if you are well into pregnancy before you begin. Build up gradually until you are exercising for about 20 minutes every day.

EXERCISING SENSIBLY

If you're athletic and have always been so, pregnancy shouldn't slow you down. But there are cautions:
★ Pregnancy is not a time to launch into a fitness blitz; just continue with what your body is used to. If you want to keep on going to your dance or exercise class, make sure the teacher knows you are pregnant.
★ Don't exercise to the point where you feel very tired or out of breath.
★ Avoid any sports where there is a danger of hurting your abdomen, such as riding, skiing, and waterskiing.

★ Be extra careful in the first and last weeks of pregnancy, because you may overstretch ligaments.

Swimming
This is excellent and perfectly safe, since the water supports your body.

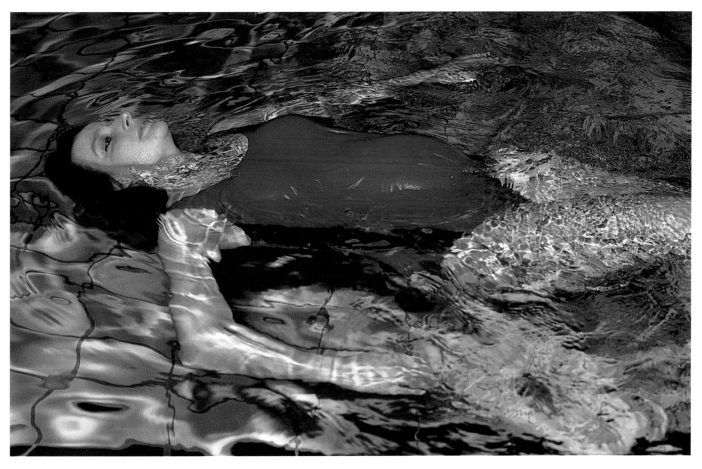

LOOKING AFTER YOUR BODY

During pregnancy, it's important to hold yourself well and avoid strain on your back. You're far more likely to suffer from backache; the weight of the baby pulls you forward, and so there is a tendency to lean slightly backward to compensate. This strains the muscles of the lower back and pelvis, especially toward the end of pregnancy.

Be aware of your body, whatever you are doing. Avoid heavy lifting, and try to keep your back as long as possible. Wear low heels, since high heels tend to throw your weight even further forward.

PROTECTING YOUR BACK

To avoid back trouble, it's equally important to be aware of how you use your body when going about everyday activities such as gardening, lifting a child, or carrying heavy bags. The hormones of pregnancy stretch and soften the muscles of the lower back, and so they are more easily strained if you bend over, get up too suddenly, or lift something the wrong way.

STANDING WELL

You can check that you are standing the right way in front of a full-length mirror. Lengthen and straighten your back, so that the weight of the baby is centered and supported by your thighs, buttocks, and stomach muscles. This will help prevent backache, and tone up your abdominal muscles, making it easier for you to regain your figure after the birth.

Drop *your shoulders and keep them back*

Hold *your back straight*

Lift *your chest and ribs*

Tighten *your stomach muscles*

Tuck in *your bottom*

Bend *your knees slightly*

Stand *with your feet a little way apart*

Bad posture
This is common during pregnancy. As the baby grows, its weight throws you off-balance, so you may over-arch your back and thrust your abdomen forward.

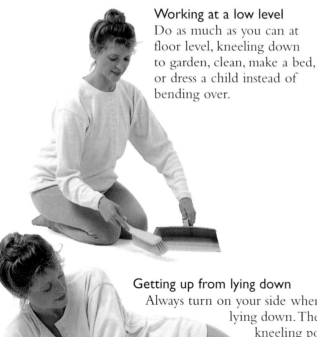

Working at a low level
Do as much as you can at floor level, kneeling down to garden, clean, make a bed, or dress a child instead of bending over.

Getting up from lying down
Always turn on your side when you have been lying down. Then move into a kneeling position. Use the strength of your thighs to push yourself up; keep your back straight.

Lifting and carrying

When lifting an object, bend your knees and keep your back as straight as possible, bringing the object close in to your body. Try not to lift something heavy from up high, as you may lose your balance. If you're carrying heavy bags, divide the weight equally on each side.

Keep *your back straight*

Position *your weight round the object, and face it squarely*

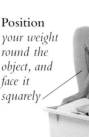

THE PELVIC FLOOR

This is a hammock of muscles that supports the bowel, bladder, and womb. During pregnancy, the muscles go soft and stretchy, and this, together with the weight of the baby pushing down, weakens them, making you feel heavy and uncomfortable. You may also leak a little urine whenever you run sneeze, cough, or laugh. To avoid these problems it's essential to strengthen the pelvic floor.

Hip bone

Tail bone

Pubic bone

Pelvic floor

The pelvic floor
This forms part of the pelvis, cradling and protecting the baby in the womb. The baby passes though it at birth.

Practice
the exercise standing

STRENGTHENING THE PELVIC FLOOR

Practice this exercise often—at least three or four times a day. Once you've learned it, you can do it anytime, anywhere, lying down, sitting, or standing. You will also find it useful in the second stage of labor, when knowing how to relax the muscles can reduce the risk of a tear, by easing the passage of the baby through the pelvis. Lie on your back, with your knees bent and your feet flat on the floor. Now tighten the muscles, squeezing as if stopping a stream of urine. Imagine you are trying to pull something into your vagina, drawing it in slightly, then pausing, then pulling, until you can go no further. Hold for a moment, then let go gradually. Repeat ten times.

Practice
the exercise sitting

DO THIS WHEN:
★ waiting for a bus or train
★ ironing or cooking
★ watching TV
★ having intercourse
★ you have *emptied* your bladder.

PELVIC TILT

This exercise helps you move the pelvis with ease, which is good preparation for labor. It also strengthens the stomach muscles and makes the back more flexible. The pelvic tilt is especially helpful if you suffer from backache. You can do the tilt in any position; remember to keep your shoulders still.

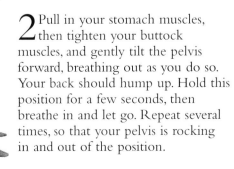

1 Kneel on the floor on your hands and knees. Make sure that your back is flat (at first it helps to use a mirror to check this).

DO THIS WHEN:
★ lying on your back
★ standing
★ sitting
★ kneeling
★ dancing to music.

2 Pull in your stomach muscles, then tighten your buttock muscles, and gently tilt the pelvis forward, breathing out as you do so. Your back should hump up. Hold this position for a few seconds, then breathe in and let go. Repeat several times, so that your pelvis is rocking in and out of the position.

TAILOR SITTING

Tailor sitting strengthens the back and makes your thighs and pelvis more flexible. It will also improve the blood flow in the lower part of the body, and will encourage your legs to fall apart during labour. The main position below is far easier than it appears. This is because your body becomes more supple during pregnancy.

Straighten *your back*

SITTING WITH CUSHIONS
If you find tailor sitting difficult, put a cushion under each thigh, or sit against a wall for support. Remember to keep your back straight.

Stretch *your inner thighs by pressing outward with your elbows*

SITTING WITH CROSSED LEGS
You may find it more comfortable to sit like this. Make sure you change the front leg occasionally.

THIGH STRETCH
Sit with your back straight, the soles of your feet together, and your heels close to your body. Grasp your ankles, and press your thighs down with your elbows. Hold them there for 20 seconds. Do this several times.

Keep *your feet close to your body*

WARNING
When you are doing any exercises, remember these guidelines.
* ★ Don't push yourself beyond your own limits or exhaust yourself.
* ★ If you feel any pain, stop.
* ★ Try not to lie flat on your back in late pregnancy.

SQUATTING

Squatting makes your pelvic joints more flexible, and strengthens the back and thigh muscles. It can also protect your back, if you squat down instead of bending over, and is comfortable if you experience backache. Squatting is also a good position to take up during labor.

You may find it difficult to do a full squat at first, so try holding on to a firm support, such as a chair or window ledge, and place a rolled-up rug or blanket under your heels. Get up slowly, or you may feel slightly dizzy.

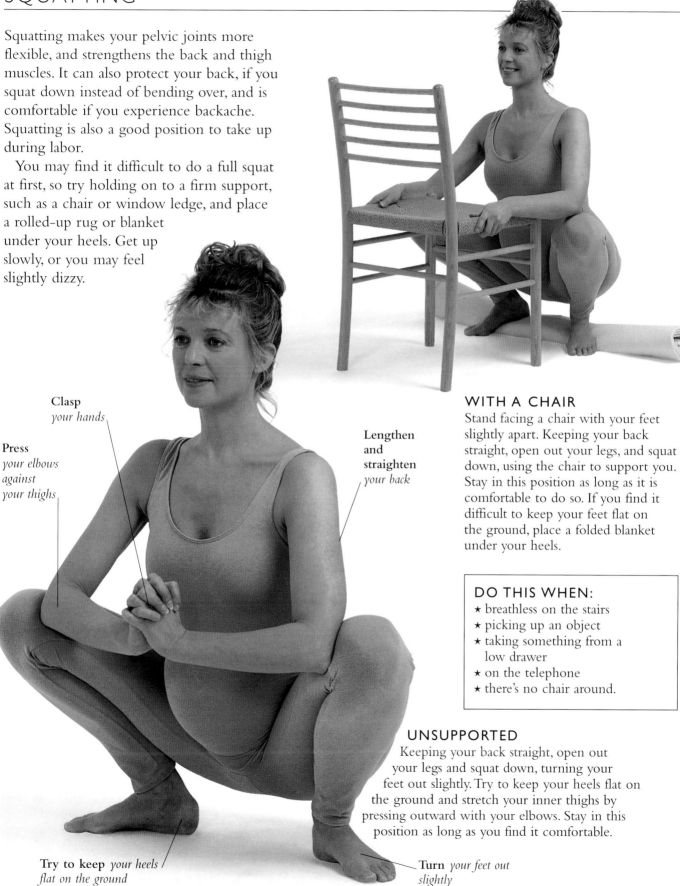

Clasp *your hands*

Press *your elbows against your thighs*

Lengthen and straighten *your back*

Try to keep *your heels flat on the ground*

Turn *your feet out slightly*

WITH A CHAIR
Stand facing a chair with your feet slightly apart. Keeping your back straight, open out your legs, and squat down, using the chair to support you. Stay in this position as long as it is comfortable to do so. If you find it difficult to keep your feet flat on the ground, place a folded blanket under your heels.

DO THIS WHEN:
★ breathless on the stairs
★ picking up an object
★ taking something from a low drawer
★ on the telephone
★ there's no chair around.

UNSUPPORTED
Keeping your back straight, open out your legs and squat down, turning your feet out slightly. Try to keep your heels flat on the ground and stretch your inner thighs by pressing outward with your elbows. Stay in this position as long as you find it comfortable.

RELAXATION AND BREATHING

These relaxation and breathing exercises are among the most beneficial that you can learn. They are invaluable during labor, when knowing how to breathe properly and relax the muscles of your body will help you cope with painful contractions and conserve vital energy. Practice these exercises regularly so that they become a natural response during labor. Relaxation will also help you unwind any time you feel tense or anxious.

HOW TO RELAX
At first it's best to practice this exercise in a warm room where you won't be disturbed. Later you should find it easy to relax anywhere.

Relax your body
Make yourself comfortable, lying on your back, well propped up by pillows, or on your side, with one leg bent and supported on cushions. Now, tense and relax the muscles of each part of your body in turn, starting with the toes and working upward. After doing this for eight to ten minutes, let your body go limp. Try to feel heavy, as though you are sinking into the floor.

Lying on your side
You may be more comfortable, especially during later pregnancy, lying on your side with one leg bent and supported on cushions. Don't place too many pillows under your head, because this is bad for your spine.

WARNING
Try not to lie flat on your back in the late stages of pregnancy, as you can restrict the flow of oxygen to the baby in this position, and may feel faint.

Tilt *your head from side to side, then hold still*

Screw up *your eyes, open, then close*

Pull in *your stomach muscles, then relax*

Arch *the small of your back, then let go*

Clench *your hands, then open*

Squeeze *your buttock muscles, then let go*

BREATHING FOR LABOR

Practice the different levels of breathing with a partner or friend on a regular basis in the weeks leading up to labor. Controlled breathing will help you remain relaxed and calm during labor, and can even control your body during contractions.

Light breathing

This level of breathing will help you at the height of a contraction. Breathe in and out of your mouth, taking air into the upper part of your lungs only. A partner or friend should put her hands on your shoulder blades and feel them move. Practice making the breaths lighter and lighter, but take an occasional deeper breath when you need one.

Deep breathing

This has a calming effect, helpful at the beginning and end of contractions. Sit comfortably and as relaxed as possible. Breathe in deeply through the nose, right to the bottom of your lungs. Your partner or friend should place her hands just above your waistline and feel your ribcage move. Now, concentrate on breathing slowly and gently out. Let the next in-breath follow naturally.

Panting

After the first stage of labor, you will want to push, even though the cervix may not be fully opened. You can resist this by taking two short breaths, and then blowing a longer breath out: say "huff, huff, blow" to yourself.

Tighten *your thigh muscles, then let the tension go*

Bend *your feet at the ankles, then let go*

Relax your mind

While relaxing your body, try to calm and empty your mind. Breathe slowly and evenly, sighing each breath out gently. Do not breathe too hard. Alternatively, repeat a word or sound silently to yourself, or concentrate on some pleasant or peaceful image. Try not to follow any thoughts that arise.

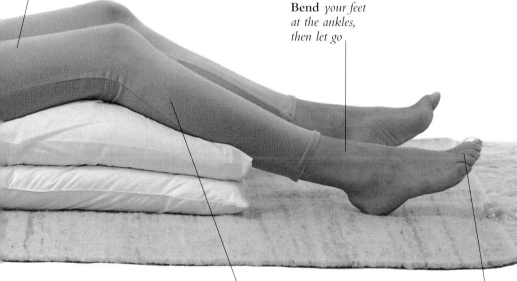

Tense *your calf muscles, then relax*

Curl *your toes, then relax*

EATING FOR A HEALTHY BABY

A baby has only one source of food—you. During pregnancy, more than at any other time, it is essential that you have a varied and balanced diet. You do not need to plan this specially, nor do you have to eat for two. All you have to do is eat a range of fresh, unprocessed foods from the selection below, to ensure that you get all the nutrients you need. Once you are, or know you want to become, pregnant, think about the foods you eat regularly. Do you eat or drink anything that may harm the baby? Increase your intake of raw vegetables and fresh fruit, and cut down on sugary, salty, and processed foods.

ESSENTIAL NUTRIENTS

CALCIUM

This is important to ensure the healthy development of your baby's bones and teeth. You will need roughly twice as much calcium as normal. Good sources include milk, cheese, yogurt, and leafy, green vegetables. However, dairy products are high in fat, so choose low-fat varieties, such as skim milk. Almonds and brazil nuts are a good source of calcium, but are also high in fat.

Get the extra calcium you need in a day from: 3oz (85g) hard cheese or 1 glass of milk plus a 6oz (170g) yogurt cup.

PROTEIN

During pregnancy, your need for protein increases, so try to eat a good variety of protein-rich foods. Fish, meat, nuts, beans, and dairy foods are all good sources of protein. Animal sources can also be high in fat, so choose lean cuts of meat and lower-fat milk products whenever possible.

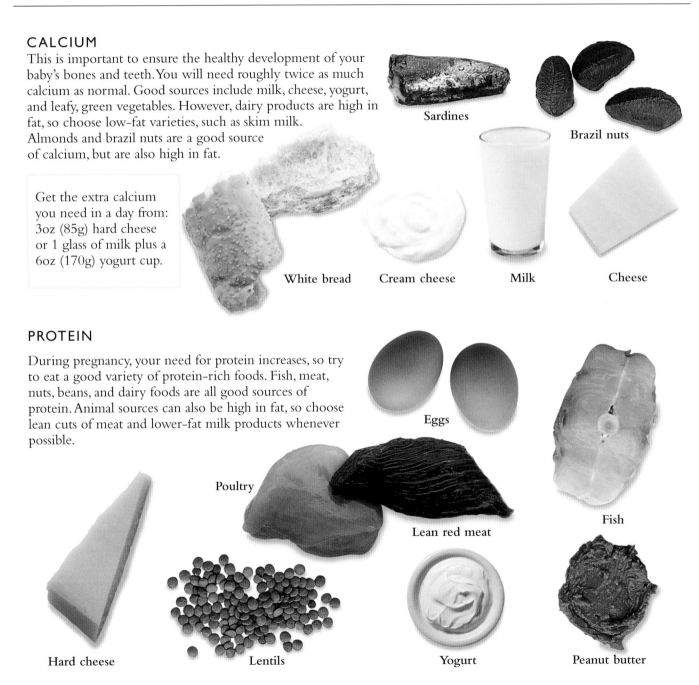

Sardines

Brazil nuts

White bread   Cream cheese   Milk   Cheese

Eggs

Poultry

Lean red meat

Fish

Hard cheese   Lentils   Yogurt   Peanut butter

VITAMIN C

This will help build a strong placenta, enable your body to resist infection, and aid in the absorption of iron. It is found in fresh fruit, vegetables, and juices, and supplies of the vitamin are needed daily, because it cannot be stored in the body. A lot of vitamin C is lost by prolonged storage and cooking, so it's best to eat fresh produce, and steam green vegetables or eat them raw.

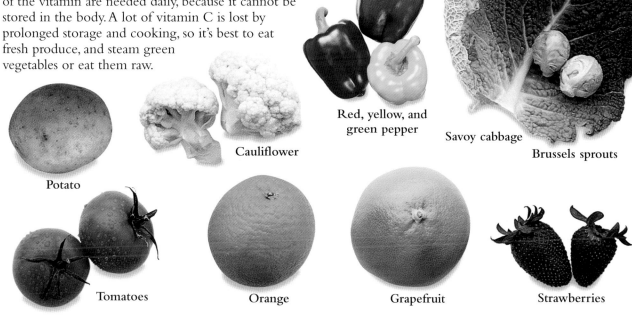

Red, yellow, and green pepper

Savoy cabbage

Brussels sprouts

Cauliflower

Potato

Tomatoes

Orange

Grapefruit

Strawberries

FIBER

This should form a large part of your daily diet, since constipation (see page 40) is common in pregnancy and fiber will help prevent it. Fruit and vegetables are key sources, and should be used plentifully. Bran, in moderation, is useful.

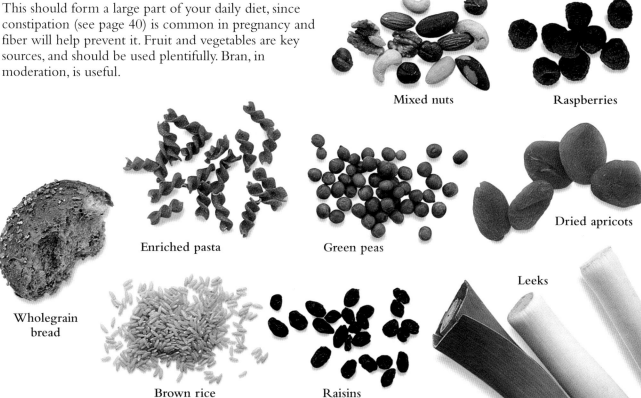

Mixed nuts

Raspberries

Enriched pasta

Green peas

Dried apricots

Leeks

Wholegrain bread

Brown rice

Raisins

FOLIC ACID

Folic acid is needed for the development of the baby's nervous system. Supplements should be taken before and during the first three months of pregnancy. Ask your doctor for recommendations. The body cannot store folic acid, so it's essential to have a daily supply. Fresh dark green, leafy vegetables are a good source, but steam them, or eat them raw, because a lot of the nutrient is destroyed by cooking. Other sources are cooked beans (fava, kidney, pinto, roman, soy, white or navy), chickpeas, lentils, orange juice, canned pineapple juice and sunflower seeds.

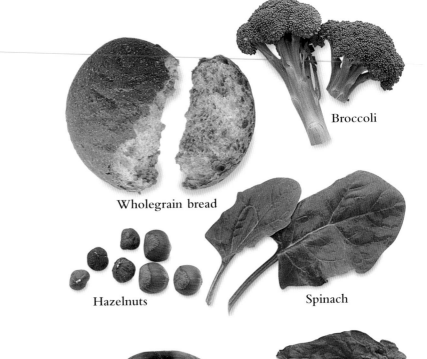

Broccoli

Wholegrain bread

Hazelnuts

Spinach

IRON

Iron is needed in increased amounts. The baby will need to build up stores of iron after the birth, and the extra blood your body produces needs iron to carry oxygen. Iron from animal sources is absorbed more easily than it is from foods such as beans and dried fruit, so if you do not eat meat, combine iron-rich foods with those rich in vitamin C to allow maximum absorption.

Tuna fish

Spinach

Lean red meat

Dried apricots

VEGETARIAN DIET

If you eat a variety of protein-rich foods and fresh fruit and vegetables every day, you should provide the baby with all that he needs. The only nutrient you may lack is iron; the body has great difficulty absorbing iron from plant sources, so you may be given supplements of the mineral to compensate. If you have also eliminated dairy foods from your regular diet, you may be prescribed calcium, and vitamins B12 and D.

SALT

Most people consume too much salt. Health Canada recommends that all Canadians reduce their salt intake. In pregnancy, excess salt can aggravate preeclampsia and swelling (see pages 38 and 42).

FLUID

It is essential to consume lots of fluids during pregnancy in order to keep your kidneys healthy and avoid constipation. Water is best; drink as much as you like.

TOP FOODS

These foods are all sources of at least one nutrient. Try to eat some of them each day:
★ Cheese, milk, yogurt for calcium and protein
★ Dark green, leafy vegetables for vitamin C, fiber and folic acid
★ Lean red meat for protein and iron
★ Oranges for vitamin C, folic acid and fiber
★ Poultry for protein and iron
★ Fish such as flounder, tuna, salmon, or bluefish for protein
★ Wholegrain bread for protein, fiber, and folic acid
★ Enriched pasta for iron and folic acid, and brown rice for fiber.

VITAMIN AND MINERAL SUPPLEMENTS

Pregnancy has particular nutritional needs. Eat a well-balanced diet with plenty of fresh, unprocessed foods. Your doctor may prescribe vitamin supplements. If you are found to be anemic it will be essential that you take these (see page 38).

PROTECTING YOUR BABY

Almost everything you consume during pregnancy—both good and bad—can make its way to your baby via the placenta.

PROCESSED FOODS
Avoid convenience foods that have been highly processed. Some processed foods have excess sugar and salt added, and may contain a lot of fat, as well as unnecessary preservatives, artificial flavors and colors. Read labels carefully, and also check the product's date of expiry.

FOUR FOOD GROUPS
Plan your meals around the basic food groups: meat and alternatives; fruits and vegetables; grain products; milk products. Use oils that are high in polyunsaturated fats, such as corn oil and sunflower oil.
Avoid processed luncheon meats, potato chips, salted nuts, soy sauce, excess mustard and ketchup. Fruit drinks may contain little fruit, so buy pure, 100 percent juice brands.

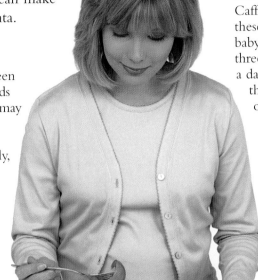

COFFEE, TEA, AND HOT CHOCOLATE
Caffeine, a stimulant that is found in all these drinks, is rapidly absorbed by the baby. Limit your intake to no more than three cups of caffeinated drinks a day, and if possible, gradually cut them out altogether. Drink plenty of water instead.

HERBAL TEAS
If you want to drink herbal teas during your pregnancy, it is sensible to check first with your doctor. Most prepackaged teas will not harm the baby—raspberry leaf tea, for example, is a traditional remedy to ease labor—but some may have unwanted effects.

SUGAR
Sugary foods, such as cakes, cookies, candies, sodas, and colas are low in essential nutrients. Get your energy from starchy carbohydrates, such as wholegrain bread, and cut down on the sugar.

CRAVINGS
It's common in pregnancy to find that you suddenly develop a taste for certain foods, such as pickled onions or ice cream. If you long for a particular food, go ahead and indulge yourself within reason, provided it isn't fattening and doesn't cause indigestion.

ALTERNATIVES TO ALCOHOL
Any alcohol that you drink during pregnancy is passed through the placenta into your baby's bloodstream, and can cause physical defects and developmental delay. The extent of these risks has only been recognized in recent years. Bear in mind that even small amounts of alcohol may disrupt normal development, resulting in such conditions as low birth weight. So it's best to cut out alcohol altogether and make your own fresh fruit cocktails, milkshakes, and fruit juice drinks.

ESSENTIAL FATTY ACIDS
Essential fatty acids (EFAs) are vital for the development of your baby's brain, nervous system, and retina. The fetus can't manufacture these for itself, and relies on an efficient supply from the mother across the placenta and, after birth, from breast milk. Oily fish such as salmon and mackerel are by far the richest source of EFAs. Nuts, seeds, vegetable oils and eggs are other sources.

GENETICALLY MODIFIED FOODS
Genetically modified foods (also called genetically engineered foods or biotechnology-derived foods) are foods that have been modified by genetic manipulation. All GM foods are studied by Health Canada, which is responsible for ensuring that all foods are safe prior to being introduced to Canada.

PRACTICAL PREPARATIONS

About a month before your due date, make sure that everything is ready. Go food shopping and start planning for meals and other essentials that will make your life easier after the birth. Start assembling the things you'll want to take for the birth. Some doctors or hospitals offer a list of what to bring. Buy or borrow equipment for your baby.

HELPFUL THINGS FOR LABOR

All the items below may be useful in labor and immediately after birth. Pack them separately, because you will want them during labor.

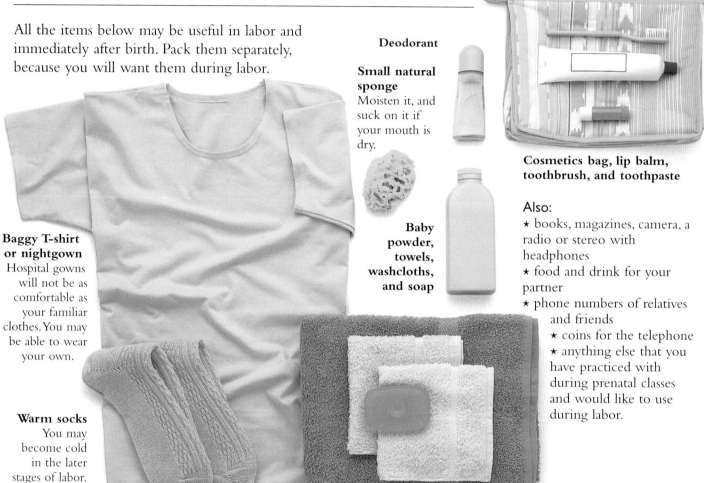

Deodorant

Small natural sponge
Moisten it, and suck on it if your mouth is dry.

Baby powder, towels, washcloths, and soap

Cosmetics bag, lip balm, toothbrush, and toothpaste

Baggy T-shirt or nightgown
Hospital gowns will not be as comfortable as your familiar clothes. You may be able to wear your own.

Warm socks
You may become cold in the later stages of labor.

Also:
★ books, magazines, camera, a radio or stereo with headphones
★ food and drink for your partner
★ phone numbers of relatives and friends
★ coins for the telephone
★ anything else that you have practiced with during prenatal classes and would like to use during labor.

GOING TO THE HOSPITAL WHEN YOU ARE IN LABOR

It's always a good idea to make trial runs to the hospital or birthing center long before you feel those first pains of labor. When you and your partner are under the stress of imminent childbirth or you are counting contractions, you don't want to get lost or stuck in unfamiliar territory. Knowing which door to enter when you arrive and where you'll be headed inside can be a relief. Ask about the preliminary papers you'll need to fill out. And, if you'll be using a big city hospital, have a good idea of what rush hour traffic conditions might be like.

In the last few weeks, make sure your car always has enough gas to get you there. Put money or tokens for road tolls or emergency calls in your car ahead of time.

If you aren't going to be driving in your own car, keep the name and phone number of a 24-hour taxi service posted by the telephone. If someone has volunteered to drive you to the hospital, make sure that they will be able to respond instantly at any hour of the day or night. Post their phone number in a handy location by your telephone where you can find it quickly and easily.

FOR AFTER THE BIRTH

This checklist will help you as you pack;
if you go into labor unexpectedly and haven't
packed your suitcase, these are the items your
partner should assemble. The hospital will
probably provide all the essentials for the
baby during your stay.

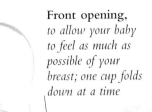

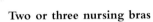

Front opening, *to allow your baby to feel as much as possible of your breast; one cup folds down at a time*

Wide *support straps*

Two or three nursing bras

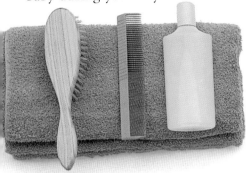

Brush, comb, shampoo, towel

Also:
* tissues
* hairdryer
* hand mirror for
freshening up at bedside.

Nursing pads
Slip these inside your bra to
absorb leaking milk. Shaped
ones are best.

Body lotion
This relieves
dry skin

One box
*should be super-
absorbent for
the first few days*

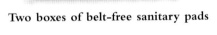

Two boxes of belt-free sanitary pads

**Six pairs of
underpants**
Buy cotton
pants. You may
go through
several pairs a
day so pack
a pile.

**Two to three machine-
washable nightdresses
and a dressing gown**
These should be made of
cotton because it is the
most comfortable
fiber.

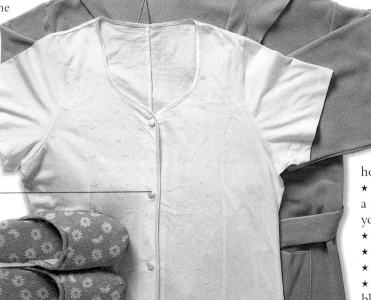

Front opening,
*with buttons that
undo well below
the breasts, if
breast-feeding*

**Low-heeled
slippers**

COMING HOME
Choose an outfit for your
partner to bring when it's
time for you to be
discharged. Don't pick
anything too tight fitting; you
may not be back to your pre-
pregnancy size. The baby
needs clothes for coming
home, too, so set aside:
* two diapers (don't forget
a pin and plastic pants if
you're not using disposables)
* undershirt
* stretchsuit or nightgown
* sweater and hat
* receiving blanket or a warm
blanket for cold weather.

LABOR AND BIRTH

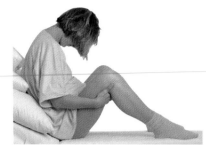

Labor and delivery are the culmination of your pregnancy, and the moment when you first see your baby is now only hours away. You may be excited, yet apprehensive. If you have prepared yourself and understand what is happening to your body and your baby at each stage, it won't be so frightening. Stay calm and save energy. The pain of labor can be intense or mild but you should never be made to feel like a failure. There are no perfect standards for having a baby, so as you practice your breathing and relaxation techniques, don't be too hard on yourself. You are bringing a little human being into the world.

KNOWING YOU ARE IN LABOR

Every woman's experience is different, but first-time mothers often worry that they won't recognize true labor. In late pregnancy, you may be plagued by short, irregular pains, called Braxton Hicks contractions, and there's always the possibility of confusing these with the real thing.

SIGNS OF LABOR
A show
The plug of thick, blood-stained mucus that blocks the neck of the womb in pregnancy usually passes out of the vagina, either before or during the early stages of labor.
What to do The show may happen a few days before you go into labor, so wait until you start to feel regular pains in your stomach or back, or your waters break, before calling the doctor.

Your waters break
The bag of fluid that surrounds the baby can break at any time during labor. It may be a sudden flood, but it's far more common to notice a trickle of fluid. If the baby's head descends into the pelvis, it may stem the tide.
What to do Call the doctor immediately. Go to the hospital even if you don't have contractions, because there is a risk of infection. Meanwhile, wear a sanitary napkin.

Contractions
These may start off as a dull backache, or you may have shooting pains down your thighs. As time goes by you will have contractions in your stomach, rather like bad menstrual cramps.
What to do When the contractions seem to be regular, time them. If you think you are in labor, call the doctor. Unless contractions are coming very frequently (every five minutes), or are very painful, there is no need to go to the hospital immediately. A first labor usually lasts about 12 to 14 hours, and it is often better to spend several hours of this time at home. Move around gently, resting whenever you need to. Perhaps relax in a warm bath, if your waters haven't broken, or eat a light snack. The hospital will probably suggest that you wait until the contractions are quite strong and occurring every five minutes or so before you leave home.

FALSE STARTS
Throughout pregnancy, the womb contracts. In the last weeks, these Braxton Hicks contractions become stronger, so you may think you are in labor. However, true labor contractions occur very regularly, and grow stronger and more frequent, so you should be able to tell when the real thing begins.
Occasionally contractions start and then die away. If you stay active, they may begin again.

TIMING CONTRACTIONS
10 minutes — Contraction
20 minutes
15 minutes — Interval between contractions
15 minutes

Time contractions for an hour, noting when each one starts and ends. They should become stronger and more frequent, and last for at least 40 seconds. The diagram shows intervals between contractions in early labor.

THE FIRST STAGE

During this stage, the muscles of your womb contract to open up the cervix (neck of the womb) to allow the baby to pass through at birth. It takes an average of 10 to 12 hours for a first baby.

Don't be surprised if at some time in the first stage you suddenly feel panic-stricken. However well prepared you are, the feeling that your body has been taken over by a process that you can't control can be frightening. Stay calm and try to go with your body. It is now that you will most appreciate having your partner or a good friend by your side, especially if they understand labor, and have gone to prenatal classes.

After admission
When initial checks are over, some hospitals allow a shower.

ADMISSION TO THE HOSPITAL

It's useful to have a partner alongside you all the way. He or she can act as a kind of intermediary between you and the medical staff, which will help when you don't feel like talking. Once you reach the hospital, a nurse or technician will carry out several routine admission procedures.

Checking you

After you have changed into the hospital gown or the clothes you brought with you for the birth, the nurse may take your blood pressure, temperature, and pulse, and give you an internal examination to check how far the neck of the womb has opened. You will also give a urine sample, to be tested for traces of protein and sugar.

Checking the baby

The nurse checks the baby's position by feeling your abdomen, and listens to his heartbeat with an obstetric stethoscope or a special instrument (see page 65).

The nurse or doctor may attach an external or internal fetal monitor to record the baby's heartbeat. It will indicate that your baby is receiving enough oxygen during contractions.

Optional hospital routines

Some hospitals routinely offer enemas to women in labor in preparation for delivery. This "prep" can be a personally demeaning way to begin your childbirth experience, and studies say it has little effect on the progress of labor.

Another "prep" that is administered occasionally is shaving the pubic area of the expectant mother. It is performed to make the perineum area clear during birth, but if you don't want to be shaved, tell your physician. When pubic hair is growing back after childbirth it can make you feel itchy and uncomfortable.

INTERNAL EXAMINATIONS

The doctor may give you regular internal examinations to check the position of the baby, and to check how much the cervix is dilating (opening up). Ask for progress reports. It is encouraging to find that your cervix is widening, but this may not happen at a steady rate.

The examination is usually done between contractions, so tell the nurse if you feel one coming. You may be asked to lie on your back, propped up with pillows, but if this is uncomfortable, try your side. Relax as much as possible. Don't pressure yourself to be perfect. Getting through labor can be tough.

THE CERVIX IN LABOR

This is normally kept closed by a ring of muscles. Other muscles run from the cervix up and over the womb. These contract during labor, drawing the cervix into the womb, and then stretching it so it is wide enough for the baby's head to pass through.

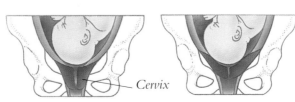

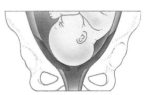

Cervix

1 The tough cervix is gradually softened by hormonal changes.

2 Gentle contractions then efface (thin) the cervix.

3 Once it is fully effaced, stronger contractions dilate it.

POSITIONS FOR THE FIRST STAGE

Try a variety of positions during the first stage of labor, since different positions will probably be comfortable at different times. Practice these positions beforehand, so that you can follow your body's natural cues with ease.

Staying upright

During early contractions, support yourself on a nearby surface, such as a wall, chair seat, or the hospital bed. Kneel down if necessary.

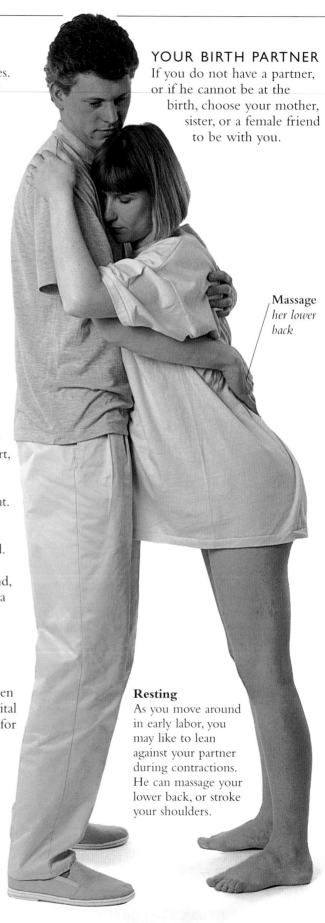

YOUR BIRTH PARTNER

If you do not have a partner, or if he cannot be at the birth, choose your mother, sister, or a female friend to be with you.

Massage
her lower back

Sitting forward

Sit facing the back of a chair, and lean over it on to a cushion or pillow. Rest your head on your folded arms.

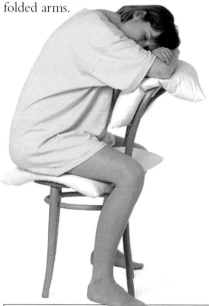

WHAT YOUR PARTNER CAN DO

★ During contractions give her plenty of praise, comfort, and support. Don't worry if she becomes annoyed with you; you are important.
★ Remind her of the relaxation and breathing techniques she has learned.
★ Mop her brow, give her sips of water, hold her hand, massage her back, suggest a change of position, or do anything else that helps. Learn what sort of touch and massage she likes beforehand.
★ Act as a mediator between your partner and the hospital staff. Stand by her wishes, for example on pain relief.

Resting
As you move around in early labor, you may like to lean against your partner during contractions. He can massage your lower back, or stroke your shoulders.

WHIRLPOOLS

Immersion in water at body temperature can help you to relax and may help ease pain during labor. Some hospitals provide whirlpool baths for this purpose. If you want to use a whirlpool in labor, check early in your pregnancy if the birthing unit you plan to attend has one.

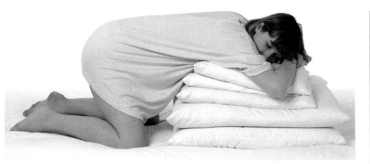

Kneeling forward
Kneel down with your legs apart, and relax forward on to a pile of cushions or pillows, or a bean bag. Try to be as upright as possible. Sit to one side between contractions.

BREATHING FOR THE FIRST STAGE

Deep even breaths   Light breaths   Deep even breaths

IN

OUT

Peak

Length of contraction

At the beginning and end of a contraction, breathe deeply and evenly, in through the nose and out of the mouth. When the contraction peaks, try a lighter, shallower kind of breathing. Both in and out breaths should be through your mouth. Don't do this for too long, because you will feel dizzy.

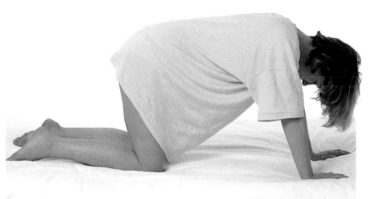

On all fours
Kneel down on your hands and knees on the floor (you may find a mattress more comfortable), and tilt you pelvis up and down. Do not arch your back. Between contractions, relax forward and rest your head in your arms.

BACK LABOR
When the baby is facing toward your abdomen, instead of away from it, his head tends to press against your spine, causing backache. To relieve pain:
★ during contractions, lean forward with your weight supported, such as on all fours, to take the baby's weight off your back, and rock your pelvis up and down, move around between contractions
★ ask your partner to massage your back, or hold a hot-water bottle to the base of your spine between contractions.

WAYS TO HELP YOURSELF
★ Keep moving between contractions; this helps you cope physically with the pain. During contractions, take up a comfortable position.
★ Try to stay as upright as possible, so the baby's head sits firmly on the cervix, making your contractions stronger and more effective.
★ Concentrate on your breathing, to calm you and take your mind off a contraction.
★ Relax between contractions (see pages 48 to 49) to save energy for when you need it.
★ Sing, or even moan and groan, to release pain.
★ Look at a fixed spot or object to help take your mind off a contraction.
★ Take one contraction at a time, and don't think about the contractions to follow. Perhaps see each contraction as a wave, which you have to ride over to reach the baby.
★ Urinate often, so your bladder doesn't get in the way of the baby.

Lower back massage
This will relieve backache, and calm and reassure you. Your partner should massage you at the base of the spine, using the heel of his hand to make firm, circular movements. Baby powder will help prevent friction.

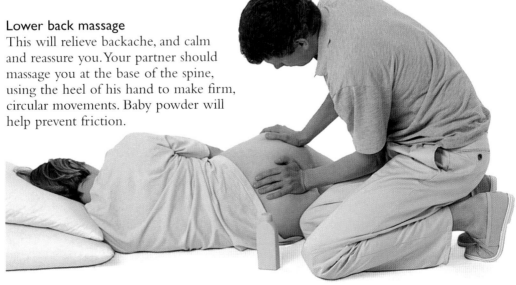

TRANSITION

The most difficult time in labor is often at the end of the first stage, when contractions are strongest. They last about a minute, and may be only a minute apart, so there is little time to rest after one before the next is upon you. This phase, which often lasts about half an hour, is known as transition. You will be tired, and may feel disheartened, tearful, excitable, or just bad-tempered. You will probably lose all sense of time and doze off between contractions. Nausea, vomiting, and shivering are common, too.

Eventually, you may have a strong urge to push. If you do this too early, the cervix can become swollen. Tell the doctor or nurse you are ready to push. He or she may examine you to determine whether your cervix is fully dilated.

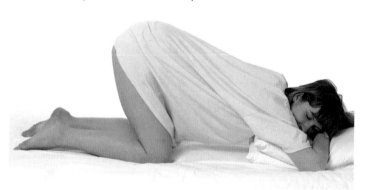

To stop yourself pushing
If the doctor or nurse says you are not fully dilated, say "huff, huff, blow" (see above, right) in this position. You may also find gas and air useful (see page 64).

Kneel down, and lean forward, resting your head in your arms; stick your bottom in the air. This reduces the urge to push, and also makes pushing more difficult.

BREATHING FOR TRANSITION

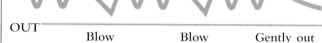

Short breaths   Short breaths   Short breaths
IN

OUT
        Blow   Blow   Gently out

If you want to push too early, say "huff, huff, blow" to yourself, taking two short in- and out-breaths, and blowing a longer breath out. When the need to push fades, give a slow, even breath out.

WHAT YOUR PARTNER CAN DO
★ Try to relax her, encourage her, and wipe away any perspiration; if she doesn't want to be touched, stay back.
★ Breathe with her through contractions.
★ Put thick socks on her legs if they start to shake, and hold them still.
★ If she feels an urge to push, call the doctor immediately.

THE CERVIX IN LABOR

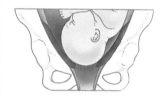
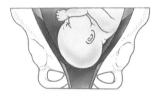

At 7cm (2¾in), the doctor feels the cervix quite well stretched out round the baby's head.

When the doctor can't feel the cervix (at about 10cm/4in), you are fully dilated.

THE SECOND STAGE

Once the cervix has dilated and you can push, the second stage of labor has begun. You can now add your own efforts to the powerful contractions of the womb, and help push the baby out. If the baby is lying in a slightly different position, you may not feel this urge to push, but the doctor will guide you so that you push when it is most needed. He or she will also help you find the most comfortable position in which to push. Even though the contractions are stronger, they don't feel as bad as before. Pushing is hard work but satisfying; each effort brings your baby's birth closer. This stage usually lasts about an hour for a first baby.

BREATHING FOR THE SECOND STAGE

Deep breaths   Deep even breaths   Even breaths
IN
        Push   Push

OUT

When you want to push (this may happen several times during a contraction), take a deep breath and hold it for a short time as you bear down, if this helps the push; it's important to do what your body tells you. Between pushes, take a few deep calming breaths. Relax slowly as the contraction fades.

POSITIONS FOR DELIVERY

Try to be as upright as possible when you are pushing during the second stage of labor, so you are working with gravity, rather than against it.

Sitting upright

A common delivery position is to sit on the bed propped up by pillows, some beds can be raised or lowered to suit you. Keep your chin down, and grip under your thighs as you push. Between contractions, try to relax back on the pillows.

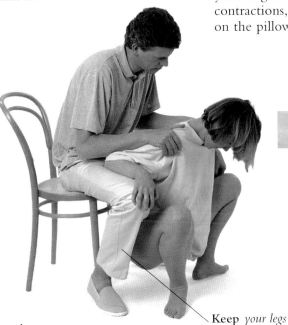

Keep your legs comfortably apart

WAYS TO HELP YOURSELF

★ Push smoothly and steadily during a contraction.
★ Try to relax the muscles of your pelvic floor, so you feel as if you are letting go completely.
★ Keep your face relaxed.
★ Don't worry about trying to control your bowels, or about any leakage of water from the bladder.
★ Rest as much as possible between contractions, so you save all your energy for pushing.

Squatting

This is an excellent position for delivery, because it opens the pelvis wide and uses gravity to help push out the baby. But unless you have practiced it beforehand (see page 47), you may find it tiring after a while. If your partner sits on the edge of a chair, with his legs apart, you can squat between his knees, resting your arms on his thighs for support.

Kneeling

This may be less tiring than squatting, and is also a good position to push from. A helper on each side will make you feel more stable. You may also find kneeling down on all fours comfortable; keep your back straight.

WHAT YOUR PARTNER CAN DO

★ Try to relax her between the contractions, and continue to give encouragement and support.
★ Tell her what you can see as the baby's head emerges, but don't be surprised if she doesn't notice you during the birth.

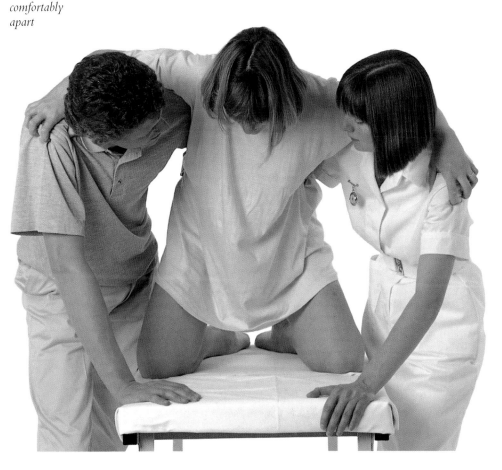

THE BIRTH

The climax of labor has now arrived, and your baby is about to be born. After all your hard work, you can actually touch your baby's head for the first time as it emerges, if you want to.

Your partner's company may calm you and give you confidence during the long hours of labor and delivery. If you have both been to childbirth classes, you have trained together for this moment. Your partner can coach and support you and remind you of breathing and relaxation techniques. The sheer force of the muscular contractions can make you feel that your body has been taken over and rendered powerless. You experience physical sensations that are completely new to you. Your partner can rub your back, sponge your brow, and count you through the contractions so that you can push with them. His involvement will help him to feel that he is a more integral part of the birthing process. If your partner is not able to be there, you will appreciate the help of a close friend or relative.

You will hold your baby very soon and will probably feel a great sense of physical relief, but there may also be wonder, emotional tears of joy, or perhaps a feeling of great tenderness toward your baby. Exhausting, painful and emotionally overwhelming, the birth of your baby will certainly be one of the most memorable and extraordinary experiences of your life.

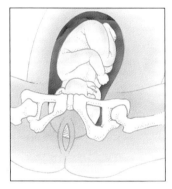 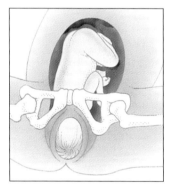 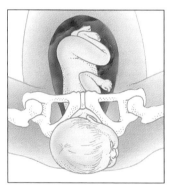 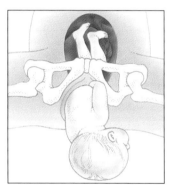

1 The baby's head moves nearer the vaginal opening, until eventually your partner will be able to see the bulge where it is pressing against the pelvic floor. Soon the head itself will be seen, moving forward with each contraction, and perhaps slipping back slightly as the contraction fades. Don't be discouraged if this happens; it is a perfectly normal.

2 When the head "crowns" (the top is visible), the doctor will ask you not to push, because if the head is born too quickly, your skin might tear. So, relax, and pant like a dog for a few seconds. If there is a risk of a serious tear, or the baby is distressed, you will have an episiotomy (see page 66). As the head widens the vaginal opening, there will be a stinging feeling, but this only lasts for a short while, and is soon followed by numbness because the tissues have been stretched so much.

3 The head is born face down. The doctor will probably check the umbilical cord, to make sure it isn't looped around the baby's neck (if it is, the cord can usually be slipped over the head when the body is delivered.) Then, the baby turns her head to one side so that it is in line with her shoulders. The doctor cleans her eyes, nose, and mouth, and, if necessary, sucks out any fluid from her upper air passages through a tube.

4 The body comes sliding out within the next two contractions. The doctor will usually lift the baby up under her armpits and deliver her onto your stomach, while the cord is still attached. Your baby will probably look rather blue at first. She may be covered in vernix, a sticky, grayish-white substance, and streaks of blood. She may be crying. The umbilical cord is usually clamped and cut at this point. The doctor may clear the baby's airways again to make sure she can breathe easily.

"What is Group B Strep? How can I protect my baby?"

Q&A

Group B Streptococcus (GBS) is a bacterium that is present in the vagina in one-fifth of pregnant women and can be contracted by the baby during the birth. Antibiotics are given in labor in high-risk situations, such as a fever in the mother.

"Should I breast-feed my baby immediately after the birth?"

Q&A

Try offering your baby the breast but leave it up to her. There will not be any actual milk at this stage, but a newborn baby's urge to suck is often quite strong right after birth, as sucking is comforting. It can also be a wonderful way for you to get to know your baby.

THE APGAR SCORE

Immediately after birth, the doctor will assess the baby's breathing, heart rate, skin color, movements, and response to stimulation, and give her an Apgar score of between 0 and 10.

Most babies score between 7 and 10. The test is done again about five minutes later, so even if the score was initially low, it may improve the second time around.

THE THIRD STAGE

Your birth experience is not complete until the placenta is also delivered. It may take only a few seconds for it to separate spontaneously from the wall of your uterus and contractions will reduce it in size dramatically. Or it might take up to half an hour. You may lose a little blood as this happens. You may also have to push a bit to rid your body of it, but the pushes will be nothing in comparison to what you have just gone through. Your physician may push down gently on your abdomen and tug on the umbilical cord still attached at one end to the placenta. Occasionally, oxytocin is administered to speed up this third stage. Your physician will make sure the placenta is complete because if pieces of it remain in your uterus, they can cause excessive bleeding later.

AFTER THE BIRTH

You will be cleaned up, and the physician will stitch any tears or surgical cuts you've sustained (see page 66). Your baby will be weighed and measured, and checked for any abnormalities. Sometimes, the baby is given vitamin K at this time to prevent a rare bleeding disorder.

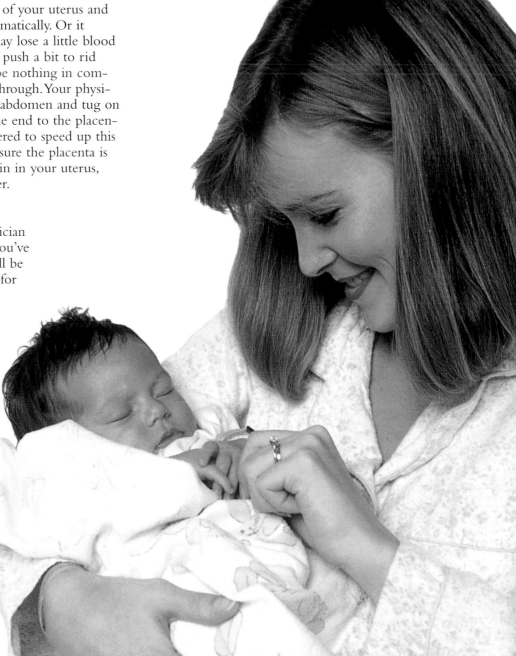

Becoming a family
After the birth, you can relax and spend a few quiet moments alone gently cuddling your new baby.

PAIN RELIEF

Although labor is not usually pain-free, the pain does have a purpose; every contraction brings you one step nearer to the birth of your baby. At the start you may be determined to have a completely natural birth with no pain medication, but keep an open mind. Whether you need it or not depends very much on your labor and your ability to deal with pain—and pain is always worse if you try to fight it. You may be able to cope using the self-help methods on pages 59 and 61. But if the pain is more than you can bear, ask for pain medication and don't feel like a failure.

Gas and air
You regulate the gas that you breathe, and can move around freely.

Hold *the mask firmly against your face*

EPIDURAL

An epidural is a kind of anesthesia that relieves pain by temporarily numbing the nerves in the lower body. Not all hospitals offer epidurals, and they are administered by a specially trained anesthetist.

Epidural, or caudal, anesthesia numbs you from your waist to your toes. It can interfere with your ability to push your baby out and can make it more likely that your physician will use forceps at delivery. It can slow the baby's heartbeat and lower your blood pressure, and take hours to wear off afterward. However, it may also be exactly what you need to get you through a physically demanding experience. Talk to your physician and weigh the pros and cons.

An epidural takes about 20 minutes to start working. You will be asked to curl up in a ball, with your knees tucked under your chin, so your back is as rounded as possible. The anesthesia is injected through a catheter inserted in your lower back. A tube may be taped in place, so that you can be given additional medication at a later stage. You will be hooked up to an intravenous (IV) line in your arm, and you will be monitored continually. You should have no pain and remain aware throughout. Some women may feel faint, and have a headache.

Giving the anesthetic
A hollow needle is inserted between the vertebrae of your spine. A fine tube is passed through the needle, and local anesthetic fed directly into this.

Vertebra
Hollow needle
Spinal cord
Epidural space

SADDLE BLOCK

A saddle block, like an epidural, is a type of spinal anesthesia. It is usually used for delivery only, and often for a Cesarean section. The numbness can extend up to your ribcage but you'll be awake for the delivery. The medication is injected into the spinal fluid of your back.

DEMEROL

Also called meperidine, this is a synthetic narcotic that may be used in the hospital during labor. With small dosages, you remain awake and able to participate in all aspects of the birth. With an average dose, it takes about 20 minutes for you to feel the effect, but it will last up to three hours and it gives some women the strength or willpower to stay on top of difficult contractions. In that brief interval between contractions, you can actually nap. However, some women report that they end up feeling nauseated or disoriented by Demerol. Unfortunately, narcotics like Demerol do cross the placenta and end up in the baby's system. At birth this may inhibit the newborn's ability to breathe deeply, but this effect can be minimized by keeping dosages small. Medication is always available in the delivery room for any infant suffering from a drug-induced side effect such as this.

ENTONOX *(gas and air)*

This is a mixture of oxygen and nitrous oxide, which gives considerable, although not complete, pain relief. You inhale the gas through a hand-held mask, attached by tubing to a cylinder. The gas takes about 30 seconds to reach a peak, so you need to take a few deep breaths of the gas at the beginning of a contraction. The gas only takes the edge off the pain, so this may not be enough. You may feel light-headed or sick while inhaling.

LOCAL ANESTHETIC

These pain inhibitors may be used at various stages during labor and delivery. A paracervical block might be injected into the tissue next to your cervix during labor to numb it. Another type, the pudendal block, will work on the nerves that supply the vagina and perineum, or that space between the vagina and rectum. Sometimes, these locals are administered because your doctor has decided on a forceps delivery. A local anesthetic will also be administered if you've had an episiotomy, when the surgical cut is stitched up.

GENERAL ANESTHESIA

Unless your baby is suddenly in distress and you are being rushed in for an emergency Cesarean section, you are unlikely to have general anesthesia.

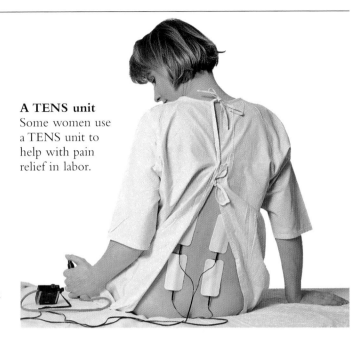

A TENS unit
Some women use a TENS unit to help with pain relief in labor.

MONITORING

Throughout labor your baby's heartbeat will be monitored. This will be done with either a hand-held standard obstetric stethoscope, an electronic monitor attached to your stomach, or an internal fetal monitor inserted into your vagina and clipped to the baby's scalp.

OBSTETRIC STETHOSCOPE

A nurse or doctor may place the instrument on your stomach at regular intervals throughout labor to listen to the baby's heartbeat.

ELECTRONIC FETAL MONITORING (EFM)

This is a way of recording the baby's heartbeat and your contractions using sophisticated electronic equipment. Some hospitals routinely monitor women throughout labor. Others do so at intervals if:
★ your labor was induced
★ you are having an epidural
★ you have a problem or condition that puts you or your baby at risk
★ the baby is distressed.
External or internal EFM is not usually painful, but it does restrict your freedom to move around, which may make your contractions more uncomfortable.

The procedure is safe for you and your baby. If you are unsure as to why it is being used, ask your doctor.

What happens

You will probably be asked to sit or lie on the hospital bed with your trunk supported by pillows, and small pads will be strapped to your abdomen to monitor the baby's heart-beat and to measure your contractions. These appear on a paper printout attached to the monitor. Later in labor, when your water has broken, the baby's heartbeat can be measured directly by clipping an electrode to his head. This internal method is the most accurate way to monitor the progress of labor. Monitors look for abnormalities in the baby's heart rate, check that the fetus is getting enough oxygen, and insure that the umbilical cord isn't twisted or wrapped around his neck.

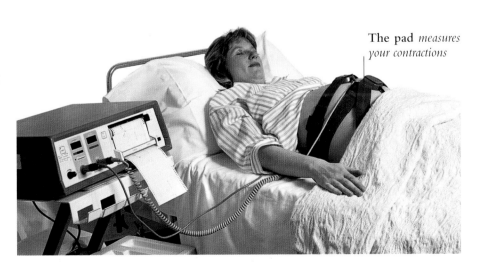

The pad *measures your contractions*

SPECIAL PROCEDURES

EPISIOTOMY	ASSISTED DELIVERY	INDUCTION
This small cut widens the vaginal opening and prevents a tear. Some hospitals perform episiotomies more often than others, so speak to your physician about routine practices in the hospital you have chosen. To avoid an episiotomy or a tear: ★ learn how to relax your pelvic floor muscles (see page 45) ★ stay upright during the delivery.	Sometimes the baby has to be helped out with forceps or by suction. Forceps are used only when the cervix is fully dilated, and the baby's head has engaged (descended into the pelvis), although suction or a vacuum extractor may be used occasionally before full dilation has been reached, if labor is prolonged.	If you are induced, labor is started artificially. Various methods may be used to speed up labor if it is going slowly. Hospital policies on induction vary from place to place, so ask your physician about his policies on induction.
When used An episiotomy may be needed if: ★ the baby is breech, premature, distressed, or has a big head ★ you have an assisted delivery ★ you are having difficulty controlling your pushing ★ the skin around your vaginal opening hasn't stretched enough.	**When used** You may have an assisted delivery if: ★ you cannot push the baby out, perhaps because he has a big head ★ you or the baby shows signs of distress during the labor ★ your baby is breech or premature; the forceps protect his head from pressure in the birth canal.	**When used** Labor may be induced if: ★ you are long past the baby's due date, and he shows signs of being distressed or the placenta starts to fail ★ you have high blood pressure, or another problem or condition that puts you or the baby at risk.
What happens Your pelvic floor area will probably be numbed with an injection of local anesthesia, and a small cut is made from the bottom of the vagina, usually slightly out to one side, at the peak of a contraction. Sometimes there is no time for an injection, but the stretching of the tissues also numbs them, so you shouldn't feel any pain. Stitching up after an episiotomy or a tear may take some time, because the different layers of skin and muscle have to be carefully sewn together. It can be painful, too, so ask for more anesthesia if you need some. The stitches will dissolve so they won't have to be removed.z	**What happens** ★ **Forceps** You will probably be given an injection of local anesthesia into your pelvic floor area, and an episiotomy. The doctor positions the forceps on either side of the baby's head and gently pulls to deliver it. You can help by pushing. The rest of the body is delivered normally. **Forceps** These form a cage around the baby's head, protecting it from pressure and damage. ★ **Vacuum** A small plastic cup, connected to a vacuum pump, is passed into the vagina and attached to the baby's head. The baby is gently pulled through the birth canal as you push.	**What happens** Induction is always planned in advance, and you will be asked to go into the hospital. If the cervix is not dilated, your doctor may insert a gel containing a substance called prostaglandin to soften and help open the cervix before starting induction. Labor may be induced in either of two ways: **1** Breaking your water or performing an amniotomy. The doctor makes a small hole in the bag of fluid surrounding the baby, using a special instrument that passes through the cervix. Most women don't feel any pain. Contractions nearly always start soon afterward. **2** Giving you a hormone such as oxytocin, which makes the womb contract. This is fed through an IV in your arm at a controlled rate. Sometimes, the drug is administered to speed up a labor that has slowed considerably or stopped altogether.
Effects Some discomfort and soreness is normal after an episiotomy, but pain can be severe if an infection develops. The wound should heal within 10 to 14 days, but if you are sore after this time, ask your doctor. There is less pain with a tear.	**Effects** ★ The forceps may leave pressure marks or bruises on either side of the baby's head, but these are harmless and disappear within a few days. ★ The vacuum cup will cause slight swelling, and later a bruise, on the baby's head. This gradually subsides.	**Effects** ★ Amniotomy is usually painless and labor ordinarily begins soon after the membranes have been broken. ★ When artificial hormones like oxytocin are used, labor can come on with full immediate force, so you are much more likely to need pain medication.

CESAREAN SECTION

BREECH BIRTH

A breech baby is born bottom, or occasionally feet, first. About four in 100 births are breech. During a normal vaginal delivery, the baby's head puts tremendous pressure on the birth canal, forcing it to dilate. The head itself decreases in diameter during labor, making it easier to emerge at birth.

In a breech presentation, however, the baby's bottom or feet don't put enough pressure on the birth canal to dilate it sufficiently, and the baby's head doesn't have the chance to change shape during labor so that it will fit through the mother's pelvis without stress. That's why some hospitals automatically suggest performing C-sections when they see a baby in the breech position. Turning the baby (external version) may be attempted to enable a vaginal birth.

TWINS

There is always an increased risk of complications when twins are on the way, so they should be born at a hospital. Sometimes, they arrive prematurely or the stress of carrying them brings on preeclampsia (see page 38). One of the babies may be in a breech or some other awkward position.

A woman carrying twins will go through one first stage, but have two second stages as she pushes first one baby out, and then the other. The second twin is usually born 10 to 30 minutes after the first.

With a Cesarean birth, the baby is delivered abdominally. You may know you are going to have a Cesarean in advance, or it may be an emergency operation because of problems in labor. If a Cesarean is planned, you can have it under an epidural (see page 64), so you are awake throughout and can hold your baby right away. This may also be possible if you are told in labor that a C-section is imminent. In a real emergency, however, general anesthesia is often necessary so the doctor can deliver the baby quickly.

It's only natural to feel disappointed, and perhaps cheated, if you need a Cesarean. But these feelings can be minimized if you understand the reasons for the decision. Ask if your physician if your partner can be with you throughout.

WHAT HAPPENS

Your pubic hair will be shaved and you will be hooked up to an IV. A catheter will also be inserted into your bladder. If the C-section was planned, you may have an epidural. If it's an emergency, you might need general anesthesia. There are two types of incisions: a vertical cut from your navel to your pubic hairline or a horizontal cut near your pubic hairline. The head is delivered and mucus may be suctioned from his mouth before his feet are visible. The operation should take approximately 45 minutes.

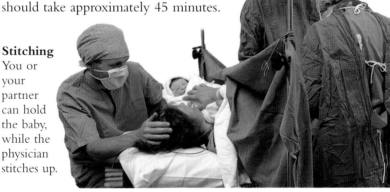

Stitching
You or your partner can hold the baby, while the physician stitches up.

The incision
The "bikini" cut is usually made horizontally, just above the pubic hairline, and it is almost invisible when it heals.

AFTER THE OPERATION

You will be encouraged to walk soon after the birth. The incision will be painful for a few days, so ask for pain medication. Moving won't open it up. Stand tall, and cup your hands over the wound. It may help to hold your stomach when you laugh, sneeze, or cough. Use a footstool to get in or out of bed. Ask your doctor before exercising (see page 72). The stitches will be removed several days later, unless they're soluble, and you'll feel much better after a week. Don't strain yourself for at least six weeks. The scar usually fades within six months.

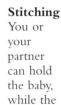

How to breast-feed
Support your baby on one or two pillows beside you, so he is not resting on the wound.

YOUR NEW BABY

Your baby will probably look very different from what you expected. He will probably seem smaller than you imagined, and very vulnerable. The shape of his head may seem rather strange, and you are bound to notice spots, blotches, and changes of color, all of which are perfectly normal. Ask your doctor or midwife if anything worries you. They should soon put your mind at ease. You may love your baby immediately. But if you don't feel this strongly at first, allow yourself time. Once you get to know your baby, to care for him and cuddle him, when you find that he responds to you and is soothed by the sound of your voice, love will grow naturally.

FIRST IMPRESSIONS

Don't be dismayed if your baby doesn't look perfect—few babies do at birth. You may notice some red marks and other blemishes, but most of these will disappear by the time the baby is about two weeks old.

HEAD
A strange shape is usually caused by the pressure of birth. The head should look normal in two weeks.
On the top of the head is a soft spot (fontanelle), where the bones of the skull have not yet joined together. They should fuse by the time the child is 18 months.

EYES
These are usually blue at birth. True eye color may not develop until the baby is about six months old.
Puffy eyelids are usually caused by the pressure of birth, but ask the doctor or nurse to check your baby's eyes, since there is sometimes an infection.
Cross-eye is common. The baby may look cross-eyed at times in the first months.

TONGUE
This may seem anchored to the floor of the mouth, so that the tip looks slightly forked when the baby sticks it out. The tip will grow forward in the first year.

HANDS AND FEET
These may be bluish (see page 217) because the baby's circulation is not working properly yet. If you move your baby into another position, they should turn pink.
The fingernails are often long at birth.

Red marks are caused by pressure from the birth, or because the baby's skin is still immature

BREASTS
Your baby's breasts may be swollen and even leak a little milk. This is perfectly normal in both sexes. The swelling should go down within two days; do not squeeze the milk out.

GENITALS
These look large on both male and female babies.
A baby girl may have discharge from her vagina. This is caused by the mother's hormones and will soon disappear.
The testicles of a baby boy are often pulled up into his groin. If worried, see your doctor.

The fontanelle *cannot be damaged through everyday handling*

Your baby *may have a good head of hair, or he may be bald*

His hands *will be clenched*

The umbilical cord *stump drops off in about ten days*

The baby can see *you at birth if you hold him about 20cm (8in) away from your face*

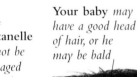

CHECKS ON THE BABY

SKIN

Spots and rashes are very common, and should vanish of their own accord.

Peeling skin, especially on the hands and feet, should vanish in a couple of days.

Downy body hair (lanugo) may be noticeable, especially if the baby was born early. This rubs off within two weeks.

Greasy white vernix is the substance that protects the baby's skin in the womb, and may cover him completely. It can be easily wiped off.

Birthmarks usually vanish. These include:

★ red marks, often found on the eyelids, forehead, and at the back of the neck; they take about a year to disappear

★ strawberry birthmarks, which can be worrying since they gradually increase in size; they usually disappear by the time the child is five

★ blue patches, often found on the lower backs of babies with dark skin

★ port wine stain, a bright-red or purple mark, which is permanent.

STOOL

At birth, the baby's bowel contains a dark, sticky substance called meconium. Once he starts to feed, the stool changes color.

The baby's legs
often look bowed because he has been curled up in the womb

Your baby will be examined several times in the first week. Your doctor will do a quick check right after delivery, and a more thorough check later in the nursery. The hospital nursery staff will weigh him regularly, and check him daily for any problems or signs of infection. This is a good time to discuss any worries that you may have.

GENERAL EXAMINATION

The doctor will check the baby from head to toe to ensure there is nothing abnormal.

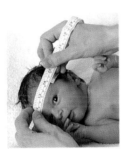

1 The doctor may measure the head, and looks for any abnormalities. He checks the fontanelle, and feels the roof of the mouth to make sure it is complete.

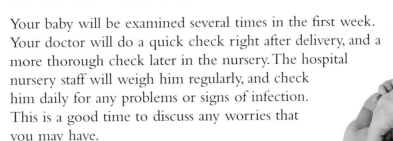

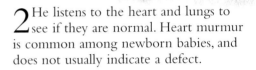

2 He listens to the heart and lungs to see if they are normal. Heart murmur is common among newborn babies, and does not usually indicate a defect.

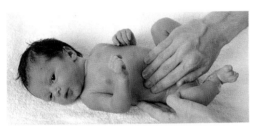

3 By putting his hand on the baby's tummy, the doctor checks that the abdominal organs are the right size. He also feels the pulses in the baby's groin.

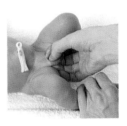
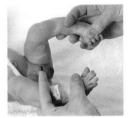

4 The genitals are checked for abnormality. If you have a boy, the doctor will be looking to see if both testicles have descended.

5 He gently moves the baby's limbs to and fro, and checks that the lower legs and feet are in alignment, that the legs are the right length, and that the baby doesn't have a club foot.

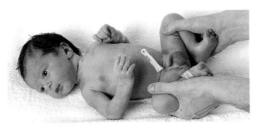

6 The doctor checks the hips for any dislocation, by bending the baby's legs up and gently circling them.

SPECIAL TESTS

A blood sample taken via a small prick on the baby's heel is tested for PKU (a rare cause of mental disability), and thyroid deficiency. Both these disorders are treatable if diagnosed early.

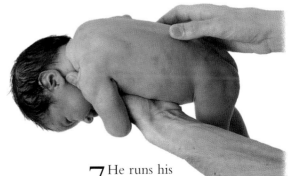

7 He runs his thumb down the baby's back, making sure that all the vertebrae are in place along the spine.

BABIES NEEDING SPECIAL CARE

Some babies need special care after birth. This is usually because they are premature (babies born before 37 weeks), or small for dates (see page 39). These babies are more likely to have problems with breathing, feeding, and maintaining their temperature, and so need special treatment and monitoring. The time that your baby has to spend in special care is bound to be difficult for you. Not only will you be separated from her before you have got to know her, but you will have to become used to seeing her surrounded by the intimidating array of equipment that is keeping her safe. This can seem quite frightening at first, but it helps if you ask the staff to explain what the equipment is for.

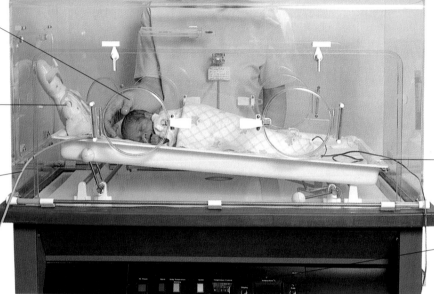

Portholes, *so you can touch your baby and talk to her*

You may like *to bring along a soft toy for your baby*

Feeding tube, *which passes into the baby's stomach; you can express your own milk to be fed to the baby*

The baby in the incubator
Your baby needs just as much love and attention as any normal healthy baby.

Tilting tray, *to help with respiration and feeding*

Control, *to regulate the temperature inside the incubator*

GETTING TO KNOW YOUR BABY
It's important to spend as much time with your baby as possible; many hospitals have special rooms you can stay in, so you are near to your baby and can take part in her daily care. At first, she may look so small and vulnerable that you worry about touching her. But, all babies respond to loving handling, and even if she can't be taken out of the incubator and cuddled, which some babies can, you can still talk to her and stroke her through the portholes in the side. You may even be able to help with changing her diaper and dressing her.

ASKING QUESTIONS
Ask the doctor or nursing staff about anything that worries you. Often parents don't ask questions, because their baby looks so frail that they are afraid of the reply. But with modern intensive care, even babies born before 28 weeks can survive.

FEEDING
If the baby can suck, you may be able to feed her normally. Otherwise, she will be fed through a tube, which is passed through her nose or mouth and down into her stomach.

JAUNDICE
Many newborn babies develop very mild jaundice about three days after birth, which turns their skin and the whites of the eyes slightly yellow. This happens because a baby's liver is still immature, and a pigment called bilirubin accumulates in the blood faster than the liver can dispose of it.

Jaundice usually clears up in a few days of its own accord, although the baby may be more sleepy than usual, so wake her up often, and encourage her to feed. It also helps if her crib is near a window so she is exposed to sunlight. Sometimes jaundice has to be treated with a special light (phototherapy). This can usually be done in the newborn nursery, and only in a few severe cases is the baby taken into special care.

STILLBIRTH
Very rarely, a baby is born dead. What makes this so hard to bear is that you never knew your child. It's probably a good idea to see him after birth; by holding him, and giving him a name, you can grieve for him as a person, and you need to do this. You will probably feel angry, and want to know what went wrong, and find something or someone to blame. Shame and guilt are also quite common. Ask your doctor to put you in touch with a therapist or a self-help group.

GETTING BACK TO NORMAL

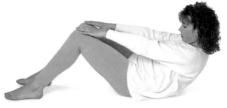

For the first week after delivery, try to get some rest whenever you can. Don't be tempted to use your spare time to catch up on all the things you haven't had time to do. Do not hesitate to call your doctor if you have any problems before your postpartum checkup. You may be rather dismayed when you see your body after birth. Your belly will be gone, but your stomach won't be flat yet. Your breasts will still be large, and the tops of your legs will feel heavy. But if you practice your postnatal exercises from the first day after birth (unless you have had a Cesarean section), you should soon look and feel better.

HOW YOU WILL FEEL

You will probably have some discomfort, and even pain, in the first days after birth. Ask the doctor if anything worries you.

AFTER PAINS
You may feel cramping pains in your stomach, especially when breast-feeding, as the womb contracts back to its pre-pregnant size. This is a good sign that your body is returning to normal. The pains may last several days.
What to do If contractions are severe, a mild pain-killer such as acetaminophen may ease them.

BLADDER
It's normal to urinate more in the first days, as the body loses the extra fluid gained in pregnancy.

What to do Urinating may be difficult at first, because of soreness, but try to do so as soon as possible after birth.
★ Get up and about to encourage the flow.
★ Take a long shower as soon as you feel you are steady on your feet. The warm water will relax your muscles.
★ If you have stitches, try pouring warm water over them as you pass urine to stop your skin stinging.

BLEEDING
You may have vaginal bleeding for anything from two to six weeks. This usually stops more quickly if you are breast-feeding. The bright-red discharge is heavy at first, but over the next few days it gets less and gradually becomes brownish. Often the

discharge continues until the first menstrual period.
What to do Wear sanitary pads to catch the flow; don't use internal tampons, they can cause infection.

BOWELS
You may not need to empty your bowels for a day or more after the birth.
What to do Get mobile as soon as possible: this will start your bowels working.
★ Drink plenty of water and eat high-fiber foods to stimulate your bowels.
★ When you want to open your bowels, do so at once, but don't strain or push.
★ It is most unlikely that any stitches will tear when you move your bowels, but holding a clean sanitary pad against the area while you do so may feel good and give you confidence.

STITCHES
These may be very sore for a day or two. Most dissolve in about a week.
What to do The following suggestions will help.
★ Practice pelvic floor exercises as soon as possible after birth to speed up healing.
★ Keep stitches clean by relaxing in a warm bath. Dry the area thoroughly afterward.
★ Soothe soreness by applying an ice-pack to the area.
★ Lie down to take pressure off the stitches, or sit on a rubber ring.

COPING WITH THE BLUES
Many women feel low a few days after delivery, usually when the milk comes in. One cause is the sudden change in hormone levels, another is the feeling of anti-climax that inevitably occurs after birth. These postnatal blues usually vanish. If you feel depressed for more than four weeks, or your depression is very severe, see your doctor right away.

Thinking positively
The sheer pleasure and delight of having your newborn baby will probably more than compensate for the after-effects of birth.

SHAPING UP AFTER BIRTH

With some gentle exercising every day, your figure can return to normal again in as little as three months after the birth, although your stomach muscles may not be as firm as before. Build up your exercise program slowly at first, since your ligaments are still soft and stretchy, and always stop straight away if you feel pain or tiredness. It's best to exercise a little but on a regular basis.

WARNING

If you have had a Cesarean, you won't be ready to start the exercises for your stomach muscles until much later after birth. Check with your doctor first before practicing these exercises, and stop immediately if you feel any pain. Begin with the week one routine, regardless of time since birth.

WEEK ONE

You can begin to strengthen the stretched, and possibly weakened, muscles of your pelvic floor and stomach from the first day after birth. The pelvic floor and foot pedalling excercises are also good if you have had a Cesarean.

PELVIC FLOOR EXERCISE *from day one*
Practice gentle squeezing and lifting exercises (see page 45) as often as possible every day to stop yourself from leaking urine involuntarily. It's important to do this before you go on to the exercises in week two. If you have had stitches, strengthening the pelvic floor will help them heal.

FOOT PEDALLING *from day one*
This will guard against swelling in the legs and improve circulation. Bend your feet up and down at the ankle. Practice hourly.

STOMACH TONER *from day one*
A gentle way to strengthen these muscles is to pull them in as you breathe out, hold them in for a few seconds, then relax. Try to do this as often as possible.

From day five after birth, if you feel all right, practice the following exercise twice a day, too:

1 Lie on your back, with your head and shoulders supported on two pillows, and your legs bent and slightly apart. Cross your arms over your stomach.

2 Lift your head and shoulders, and as you do this, breathe out and press gently on each side of your stomach with the palms of your hands, as if pulling the two sides together. Hold this position for a few seconds, then breathe in, and relax. Repeat three times.

WEEK TWO

After about a week, try the following exercises as a daily routine, and continue for at least three months. Repeat each exercise as many times as is comfortable. Begin with the curl downs, and when you can do these easily, move on to the other exercises. If you find the new exercises strain you, practice the curl downs for a few days longer. Remember to keep practicing the exercise for your pelvic floor.

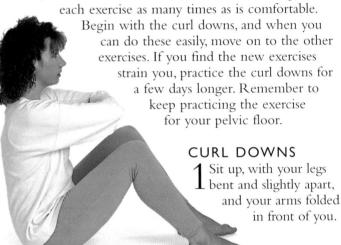

CURL DOWNS

1 Sit up, with your legs bent and slightly apart, and your arms folded in front of you.

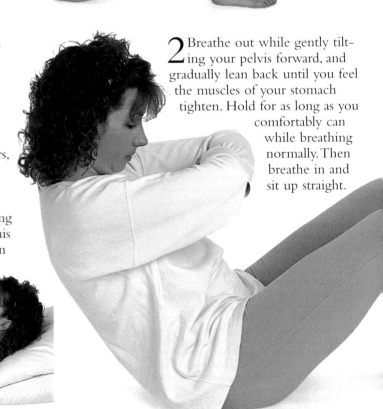

2 Breathe out while gently tilting your pelvis forward, and gradually lean back until you feel the muscles of your stomach tighten. Hold for as long as you comfortably can while breathing normally. Then breathe in and sit up straight.

SIDE BENDS

1 Lie flat on your back with your arms by your side, and the palms of your hands resting on the outsides of your thighs.

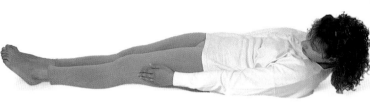

2 Lift your head slightly, and bending to the left, slide your left hand down your leg. Lie back and rest for a moment, then repeat on your right side. As this becomes easy, try bending to each side two or three times before you lie back and rest.

CURL UPS

1 Lie flat on your back on the floor, with your knees bent and your feet slightly apart. Rest your hands on your thighs.

2 Breathe out, and lift your head and shoulders, stretching forward to touch your knees with your hands. Don't worry if you can't reach far enough at first, you will with practice. Breathe in and relax.

WHEN THIS IS EASY, TRY:

★ lifting yourself up more slowly and holding the position for longer
★ placing your hands on your chest as you lift your head and shoulders
★ clasping your hands behind your head as you lift yourself up.

CHECKING YOUR PELVIC FLOOR

By three months after birth, these muscles should be strong again. Test them by skipping. If any urine leaks, practice the pelvic floor exercises for another month and try again. If leaking is still problem after four months, see your doctor.

HOW YOUR BODY RECOVERS

Your body won't be fully recovered for at least six months after the birth of your baby. However, by the time you have your six-week check-up, your body should be getting back to normal. Your womb may have shrunk back to its pre-pregnant size and you may have started your periods again. If you have been practicing your postnatal exercises regularly, your muscles should be in far better shape.

THE SIX-WEEK CHECK-UP

About six weeks after the birth you will have a check-up with your physician. It is a good time to discuss any worries or concerns that you may have.

What happens

★Your blood pressure, weight, and a sample of urine will be checked.
★Your breasts and stomach will be examined. The doctor will check that any stiches have healed.
★You will have an internal examination to check the size and position of the womb, and may be given a Pap smear.
★The doctor will discuss contraception; you can be fitted with a diaphragm or IUD.

YOUR PERIODS

The first period after the birth is often longer and heavier than usual. When it arrives depends on how you are feeding your baby. If you are breast-feeding, your periods may not start until after your baby is weaned. If you are bottle-feeding, the first period usually comes four to six weeks after the birth.

Q&A

"When can we resume our sex life?"

The best time to start making love again is when you are both ready. You may feel too sore and tender to resume sex until after the postnatal check-up, or you may want to try sooner—it's up to you.

When you resume your sex life, take it slowly. Relax as much as you can, and use extra lubrication, because your vagina may be slightly drier than normal.

Q&A

"I'm breast-feeding my baby; do we still have to use contraception?"

Even if you are breast-feeding or haven't started your periods again, you need to use contraception. The doctor will discuss this with you soon after the birth. If you want to go on the pill, make sure the doctor knows you are breast-feeding; if you previously used a diaphragm, you must have a new one fitted because your cervix will have changed shape.

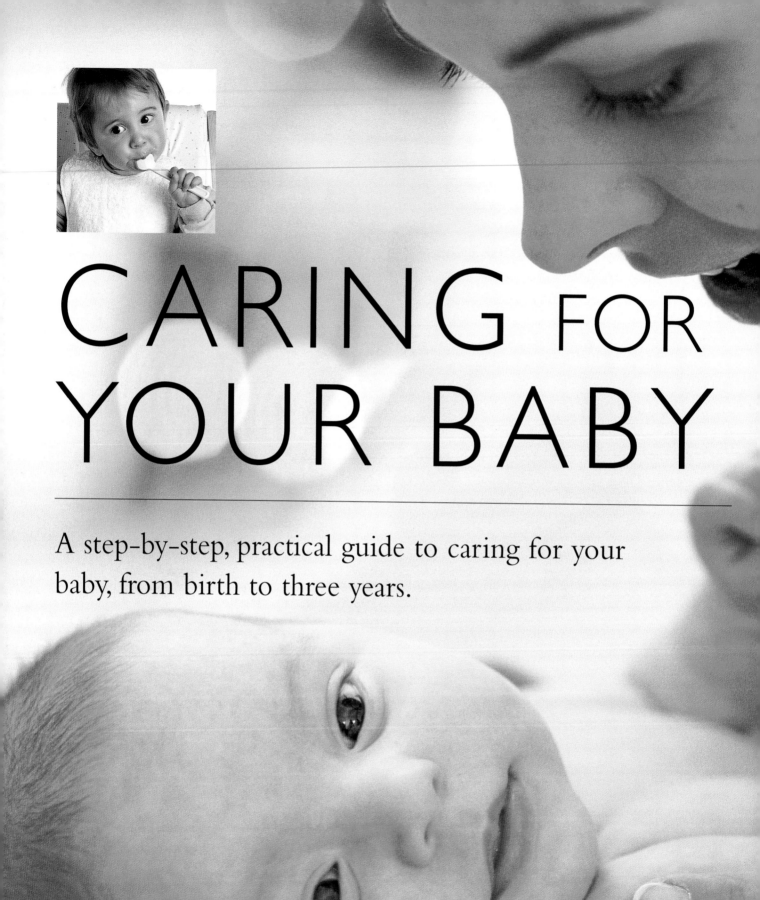

CARING FOR YOUR BABY

A step-by-step, practical guide to caring for your baby, from birth to three years.

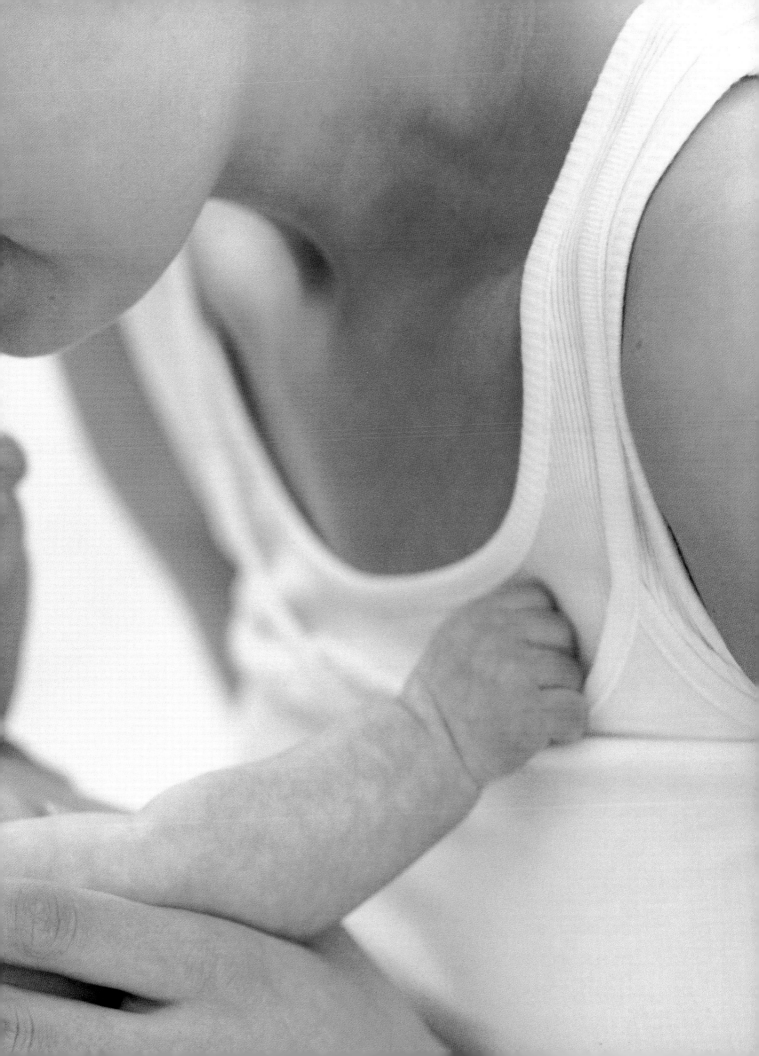

THE FIRST WEEKS OF LIFE

Nothing can really prepare you for the reality of having a child. The first weeks of your baby's life can seem like a chaotic whirlwind of new experiences and sensations as you get to know this new person in your lives and adapt to the feeling of being a parent. You have so much to learn: how to feed and nourish your baby, how to dress her and care for her skin, what she likes and what she doesn't like.

Looking after a new baby involves a combination of warmth, attention, and stamina. Although some of this will be instinctive, at other times you may both feel lost. In fact, you'll learn new skills: before long, eating with one hand while your baby feeds will come naturally. The early phase of adjustment and chaos doesn't have to last long. This chapter tells how one couple and their new baby, Amy, coped in the first few weeks.

"The first weeks weren't easy. You think you're a capable, confident person, then you have a helpless baby to look after and you feel like jelly!"

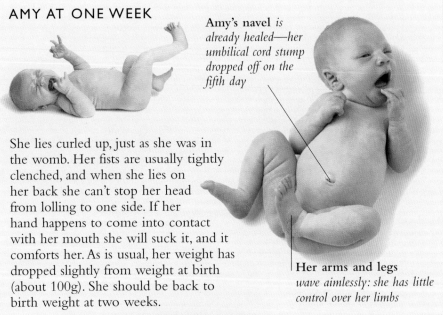

AMY AT ONE WEEK

Amy's navel *is already healed—her umbilical cord stump dropped off on the fifth day*

She lies curled up, just as she was in the womb. Her fists are usually tightly clenched, and when she lies on her back she can't stop her head from lolling to one side. If her hand happens to come into contact with her mouth she will suck it, and it comforts her. As is usual, her weight has dropped slightly from weight at birth (about 100g). She should be back to birth weight at two weeks.

Her arms and legs *wave aimlessly: she has little control over her limbs*

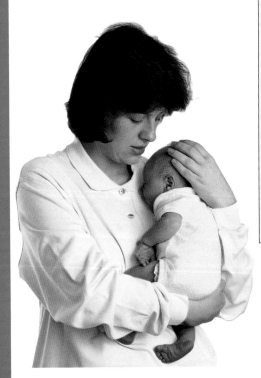

Amy's one-week checkup
Now that moms and their babies often leave the hospital within a day or so of the birth, many doctors like to see the baby one week afterward. This provides an opportunity to check the newborn for problems, such as jaundice, that may not have been apparent at discharge.

Amy asleep
Newborn babies sleep an average of 16 hours a day, but Amy sometimes slept as little as 10 or 11 hours in total, with a long, stormy period from late afternoon to late at night when she only dozed for short periods. During her times of deep sleep she was oblivious to her surroundings. Within five weeks she adopted a more sociable sleep pattern, with a longer sleep at night and an earlier bedtime.

BECOMING A FAMILY

Now there are three of you, and everything changes. Your partner is no longer just your lover, he's your companion and ally in this new adventure of parenthood—and she's as much his baby as yours. Your tried and tested family relationships will subtly change too: you're not just a son or a daughter any more, you're a parent, with a new life depending on you. No matter how topsy-turvy your life seems at this time, try to make time for your partner. Often the new father is shell-shocked in the days immediately following the birth, and he needs your support as much as you need his. Let him share in the care of the baby: he may be more nervous than you when handling her floppy body, but, with practice, he will grow more confident.

"The first days were such a tangle of conflicting feelings—elation and overwhelming pride at being a father, anxiety about Ruth, exhaustion from the round-the-clock demands of our new baby, even a tiny regret that our happy, carefree life together seemed to be at an end."

AMY'S DAY

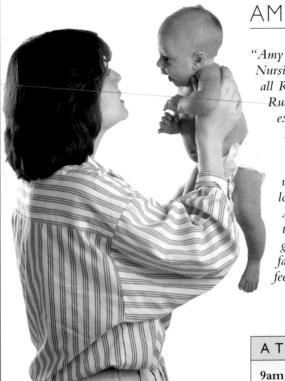

"Amy seemed insatiably hungry. Nursing Amy seemed to take up all Ruth's time and energy. Once Ruth had to miss a feeding, so she expressed milk into a bottle, and I fed Amy in Ruth's absence. I took over the diaper-changing too, to give Ruth a break. I was surprised to find I even loved that—it was one way Amy and I built a closeness together. We would play little games, or I would pull funny faces, or introduce her to her feet and hands."

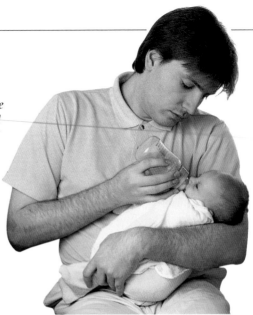

Building a loving relationship

Right from the beginning, your relationship with your new baby is an intense, two-way one that will grow into a real and lasting love. As you bring her up close to talk and coo to her, she will gaze raptly at your face—and eye contact plays a big part when you are falling in love. She will reward your efforts to calm her by quietening at the sound of your voice. And when she's miserable, she wants you to comfort her.

A TYPICAL DAY AT AROUND THREE WEEKS OF AGE

9am	**Ruth is woken** by Amy crying next to her in the bed: she had a feeding there at 5am, and they both fell asleep together. Amy has another feeding now.	1pm	**Amy cries** for a feeding, and afterward they doze off together on the sofa.
10am	**Ruth takes Amy** into the bathroom to change her diaper and clothes, and sponge bathe her. Then she puts Amy in the infant seat and chats to her while she dresses herself.	3:30pm	**A friend** comes to visit and, as she rings the doorbell, Ruth wakes up. She shares some baby stories with Ruth, then they wake Amy to admire her.
11am	**Amy falls asleep.** Ruth puts the washing in the washing machine and cleans up, then she puts her feet up, but doesn't sleep.	4pm	**Her friend** leaves, but Amy is cross from being woken, so Ruth feeds her to soothe her.
12:30pm	**Ruth has** some lunch.	5:30pm	**Ruth puts Amy** in the baby carriage then she walks to the bus stop to meet Tim as he comes home from work. The movement puts Amy to sleep.

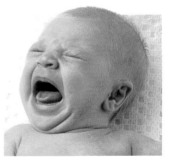

"Rubbing her stomach was a good way to soothe her, provided we rubbed fast and firmly—yet my instincts were to be very gentle. You soon learn how tough babies are."

Amy crying

Crying is your baby's way of expressing her need for love and comfort. Always respond—don't leave her.

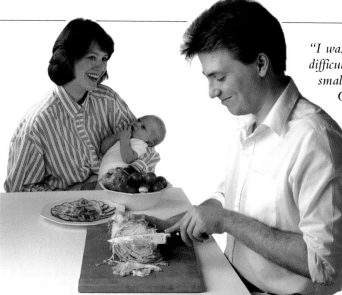

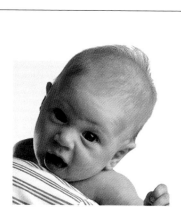

Amy wakeful
Held against your shoulder
your baby has a good view
of the world, and will
enjoy her wakeful times.

*"I was astonished at how
difficult it was to get any
small job finished during the day.
Once Tim got home from
work it was down to him
to get the supper ready—
sometimes I wouldn't
even be dressed! It was
odd for me to be so
disorganized, I wasn't
used to having so little
time for myself."*

6:15pm	**Home again**, and Amy starts to cry. Ruth feeds Amy, changes her, then rocks her in her arms. Feeding is the only thing that really soothes Amy at this time of day, but Ruth is getting tired. Tim snatches some sleep.	**10pm**	**Amy is still crying;** she will be soothed for a while, then cry again. Ruth lets her suck, walks her around, and pushes her to and fro in her carriage.
8:30pm	**Tim wakes up** and he and Ruth take turns to carry Amy around and prepare some food. Amy dozes off for a few minutes at a time, then wakes and cries—so dinner is interrupted by short feedings at the breast and walking Amy around.	**2am**	**Amy falls asleep** at last. Tim and Ruth, exhausted, go to bed.
		4am	**Amy wakes** and cries, so Ruth takes her into bed for a feeding. Tim wakes up too and helps to rock Amy back to sleep again after her feed.
		7am	**The alarm goes off** and Tim gets up to go to work— he's had four hours' sleep plus two in the evening.

Involving other family members
Your parents, sisters, brothers, and
other members of your family will all
be extremely keen to meet the new
baby; but don't feel guilty about
limiting visitors if you want to.

Getting plenty of rest
Every new mother has to
learn how to cope with too
little sleep. Plenty of rest
whenever you can snatch it is
the only answer—and this is
especially important if you're
breast-feeding your baby. Rest
whenever your baby is asleep,
even if you don't go to sleep
yourself. Your body isn't strong
enough yet for strenuous
work, and the housework
can go undone for now.

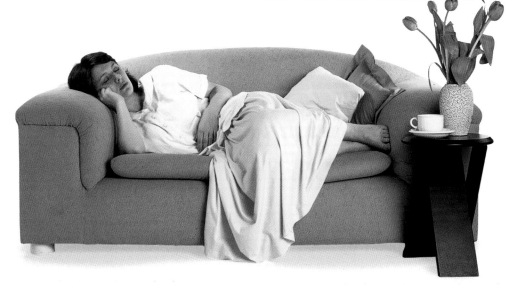

SIX WEEKS OLD

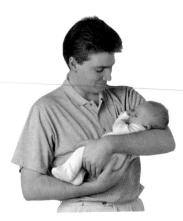

"By six weeks Amy was a real person—nothing like the greedy, screaming bundle of only weeks before. She responded to each of us in her own way: her first, crooked smiles were just for me, usually when I changed her, but at times only Ruth would do. We were lucky, Amy was very responsive and she helped us to love her; and you certainly learn fast when you have a new baby reliant on you for every need."

PREMATURE BABIES

Your baby's first six weeks at home may be especially difficult if she was born prematurely. She may cry incessantly and refuse to be comforted; or be very sleepy and reluctant to feed. In addition to your natural anxiety about your new baby, you may feel rejected by her: she doesn't make you feel that she loves you, so it's that much harder to love her in return. Your preterm baby will need extra care from you: she loses heat quickly, so you need to keep your home warm for her, especially when bathing or changing her, and she will need frequent feeding to help her grow. Even though she may have a small appetite and be a troublesome feeder, offer her a feeding frequently, letting her take as much as she wants at each feed. Concentrate on giving the care she needs: in time your baby will grow more responsive to you, and you will learn to understand your baby better.

AMY AT SIX WEEKS

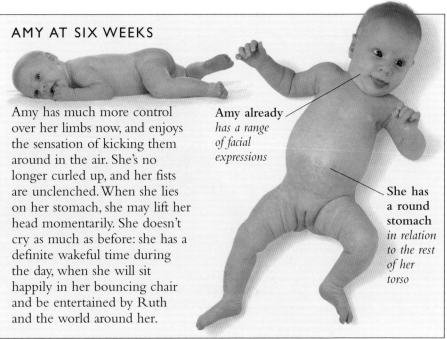

Amy has much more control over her limbs now, and enjoys the sensation of kicking them around in the air. She's no longer curled up, and her fists are unclenched. When she lies on her stomach, she may lift her head momentarily. She doesn't cry as much as before: she has a definite wakeful time during the day, when she will sit happily in her bouncing chair and be entertained by Ruth and the world around her.

Amy already *has a range of facial expressions*

She has a round stomach *in relation to the rest of her torso*

AMY'S SIX-WEEK CHECKUP

The one-month or six-week checkup is the first of the major development checks for a new baby. Your doctor will perform the check in a friendly, informal atmosphere.

1 General assessment The doctor discusses Amy's general well-being and demeanor with Ruth. She wakes Amy and talks to her to assess how she responds to the stimulus of a new face. The doctor is looking for that magical early smile, a sure sign that Amy is developing a normal, sociable personality. She checks Amy's sight by moving a rattle across her field of vision. Amy follows it with both eyes, demonstrating healthy eyesight with no sign of cross-eye.

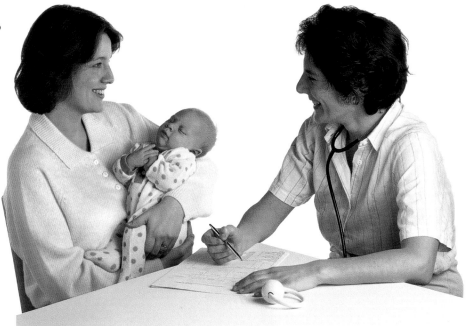

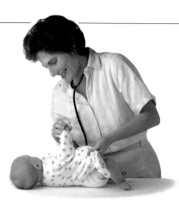

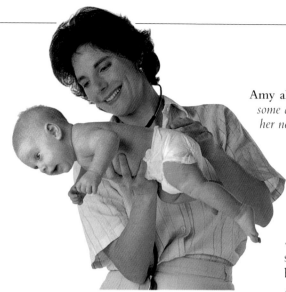

Amy already has some control over her neck muscles

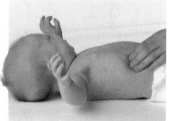

2 Limbs and muscle tone
The doctor undresses Amy herself, so she can observe her muscle tone and how she moves her limbs.

3 Control of head The doctor holds Amy in the air to see that she holds her head in line with her body. Then she watches as she pulls Amy into a sitting position.

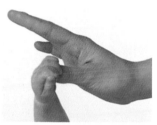

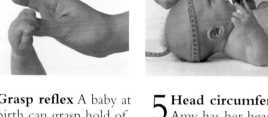

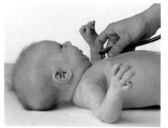

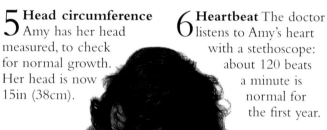

4 Grasp reflex A baby at birth can grasp hold of a finger put into her palm and hold on strongly. By six weeks it's normal for her birth reflexes to begin to disappear, as Amy's have.

5 Head circumference Amy has her head measured, to check for normal growth. Her head is now 15in (38cm).

6 Heartbeat The doctor listens to Amy's heart with a stethoscope: about 120 beats a minute is normal for the first year.

7 Internal organs A good feel around Amy's stomach reassures the doctor that her liver, stomach, and spleen are all growing normally, and none is too big or the wrong shape.

9 Weighing Amy has been weighed in her diaper at regular intervals up to now, and she will be weighed at every visit to the doctor's office, or whenever Ruth requests: normal weight gain usually means a healthy baby. Amy's weight chart will be an important record for years to come.

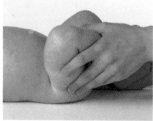

8 Hip check Hip dislocation is a possibility still, so the doctor tests the action of the joints with her middle fingers, as she manipulates Amy's legs.

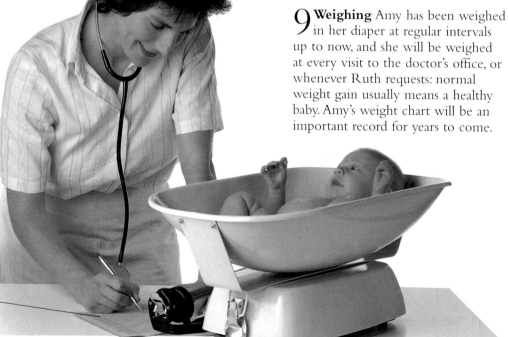

Amy's weight is recorded on her personal chart

HANDLING YOUR BABY

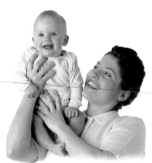

From an early age, your baby needs closeness and comfort as well as food, warmth, and sleep. Talk to your baby as you handle him—your voice is familiar and reassuring. Remember that until he is about eight weeks old, he cannot control his head or muscles. You need to support his body all the time. Your normal, careful handling won't hurt him; even the soft fontanelle on his head has a tough membrane to protect it. But you may startle him if you pick him up suddenly, making him fling his limbs out. It won't be long before you're much more confident of each other. As he gains control over his muscles, your baby may enjoy boisterous games—at five months he may love to be swung above your head or perched high on your shoulders. If he's timid, respond by handling him gently until he is more outgoing.

PICKING UP AND PUTTING DOWN A NEWBORN BABY

Always put your baby on his back to sleep. In this position, he will run a much lower risk of crib death. Babies who sleep on their backs are not at more risk of choking. However, during periods when he is awake, he should spend some time each day lying on his front.

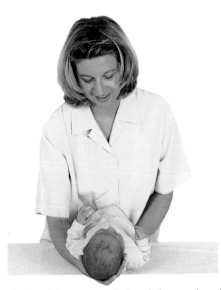

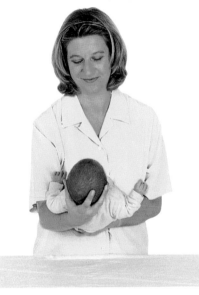

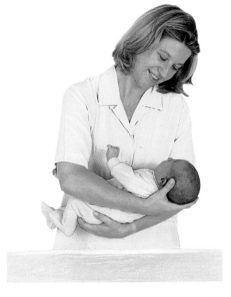

1 To pick up your baby, slide one hand under his lower back and bottom, the other under his head and neck.

2 Lift him gently and slowly, so that his body is supported and his head can't loll back.

3 Carefully transfer his head to the crook of your elbow or your shoulder, so that it is supported.

PUTTING YOUR BABY DOWN

1 Put one hand underneath his head and neck, then hold him under the bottom with the other. Lower him slowly, gently supporting him until the mat or mattress is taking his weight.

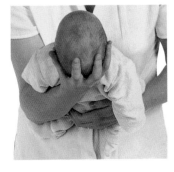

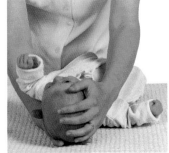

2 Slide your nearest hand out from under his bottom. Use this hand to lift his head a little so you can slide out your other hand, and lower his head down gently. Don't let his head fall back on to the surface, or jerk your arm out quickly.

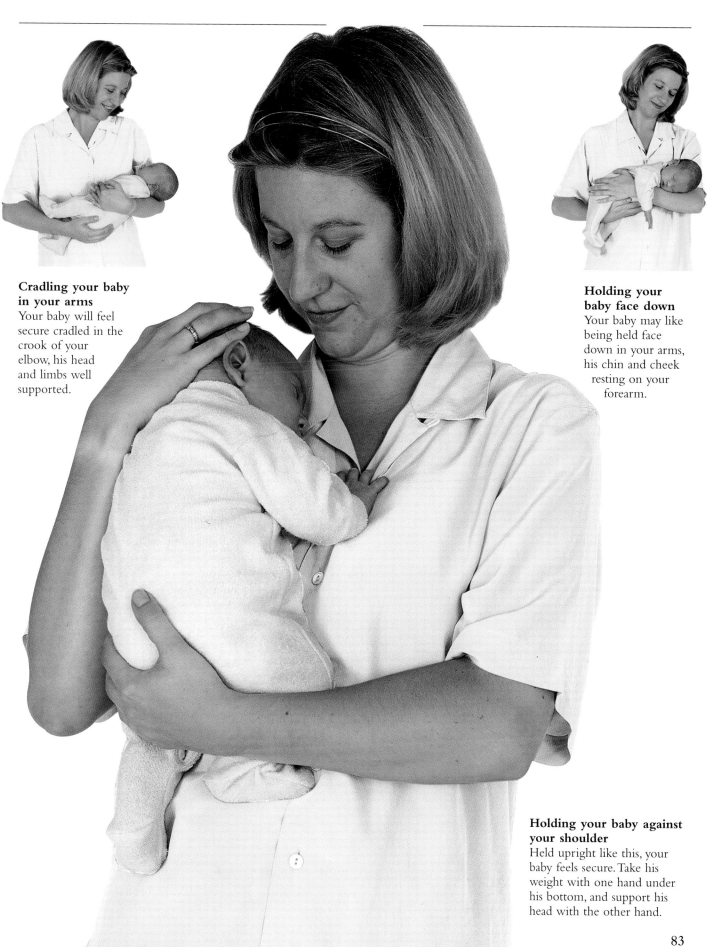

**Cradling your baby
in your arms**
Your baby will feel
secure cradled in the
crook of your
elbow, his head
and limbs well
supported.

**Holding your
baby face down**
Your baby may like
being held face
down in your arms,
his chin and cheek
resting on your
forearm.

**Holding your baby against
your shoulder**
Held upright like this, your
baby feels secure. Take his
weight with one hand under
his bottom, and support his
head with the other hand.

83

PICKING YOUR BABY UP FROM HER SIDE

1 When asleep, your baby is safest lying on her back. But if she is awake and on her side, pick her up by sliding one hand under her neck and head, the other under her bottom.

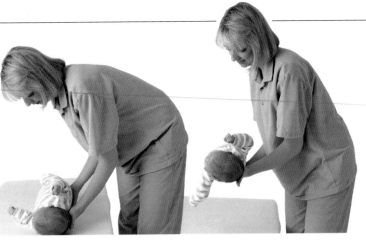

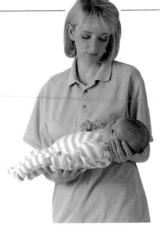

2 Scoop your baby into your arms, making sure her head doesn't flop. Lift her slowly and gently.

3 Hold her against your body, then slide your forearm under her head.

4 Now her head is supported in your elbow, and she feels secure.

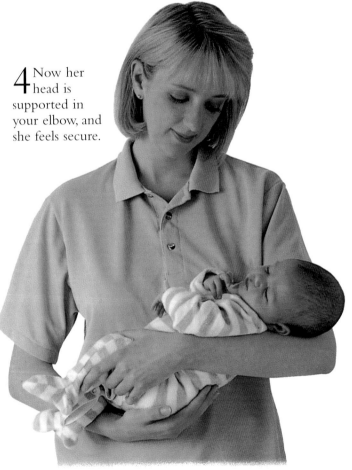

SAFETY FIRST

You will often want to lay your baby down for a few moments, either for her own amusement or because you need to do something. Whether in your own home or visiting family or friends, follow these simple precautions to ensure that your baby keeps safe and sound at all times:

★ Never place your baby's chair, basket, or infant seat on a raised surface—only the floor will be completely safe.
★ Never put your baby next to a radiator, fire, or open window. She may burn herself or overchill.
★ Never leave your baby alone with a dog, cat, or other animal.
★ Never place your baby within reach of unstable furniture or other heavy objects. She may pull them over and hurt herself.
★ Never leave your baby unsupported on a bed, sofa, or chair—always use a pillow to prevent her rolling off.
★ Favorite toys will keep your baby entertained —but take care not to leave anything sharp in her reach. Avoid toys that are small enough to fit into her mouth, or heavy enough to hurt her.

PICKING YOUR BABY UP FROM HER FRONT

1 If your baby is lying awake on her stomach, lift her by sliding one hand under her chest, so your forearm supports her chin, the other under her bottom.

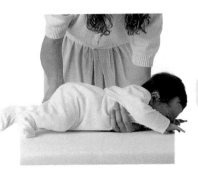

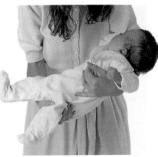

2 Lift her slowly, turning her toward you. Bring her up to your body and slide the arm supporting her head forward, until her head nestles comfortably in the crook of your elbow. Put your other hand under her bottom and legs, so she is cradled and secure.

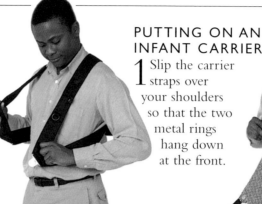

INFANT CARRIERS

An infant carrier is an excellent way of carrying your baby around in the first three months. The contact with your body and the motion as you walk will soothe and comfort her. An added advantage is that it leaves your arms free. It's not difficult to put one on when there's no one to help you; take it off using the same method in reverse.

PUTTING ON AN INFANT CARRIER

1 Slip the carrier straps over your shoulders so that the two metal rings hang down at the front.

2 Attach the padded triangular section by snapping the circular fasteners on the straps into place.

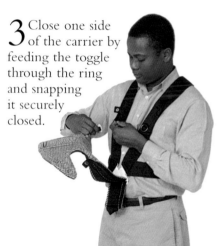

3 Close one side of the carrier by feeding the toggle through the ring and snapping it securely closed.

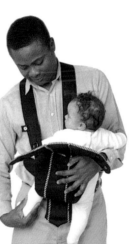

4 Hold your baby so that she faces you. If she is very young, support her head with your hand. Feed her leg through the hole on the fastened side of the carrier. Keep your arm around her on the open side to ensure that she doesn't fall.

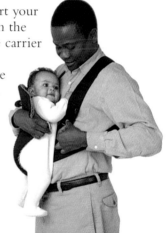

5 Support your baby in the seat of the carrier with one hand while you fasten the toggle and snap under her arm with the other.

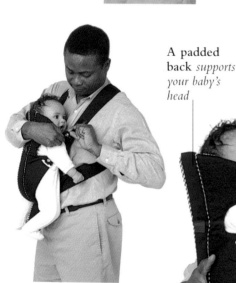

6 Close the top fasteners so that an arm hole is created on each side. The back flap supports a younger baby's head and neck.

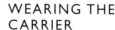

A padded back *supports your baby's head*

WEARING THE CARRIER

After three months, your baby may prefer to face forward. Follow the same sequence, but start with your baby facing forward. With the front flap folded down, she can get a better view of the world around her.

Wide shoulder straps *are the most comfortable*

A machine-washable fabric *is a good idea*

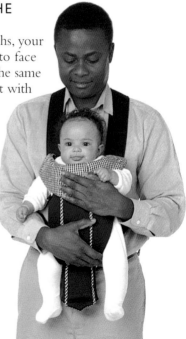

HANDLING AND PHYSICAL PLAY

LET HER FACE FORWARD

Your alert three-month-old has a good view of the world facing forward. Put one hand between her legs, the other round her chest. She doesn't need you to support her head any more.

PLAY BOUNCING GAMES ON YOUR LAP

Your four-month-old baby will love the feeling of being jogged gently up and down by your knees, in time to a favorite rhyme. Hold his arms in case he jerks backward.

LET HER KICK

It's best not to let your baby become too dependent on being held. Let her spend some time kicking on the floor —and get down to her level instead.

SIT HIM ON YOUR SHOULDER

Sit your six-month-old on your shoulder so he's taller than you are: he will be exhilarated by this new perspective.

EYE-TO-EYE CONTACT

Your baby will love you to swing her up high. Your face is always the best entertainment of all.

PLAY ROCKING GAMES

Rock her back and forth, going higher and higher if she likes the game. This type of rocking motion is a good way to soothe her, too.

WINDING DOWN

However boisterously you play with your baby, have a few minutes of gentle, quiet hugs afterward. Always take your cue from your baby, and forget the playtime for today if he's not responding with his usual giggles of pleasure.

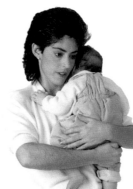

FEEDING YOUR BABY

One of the decisions you and your partner will have to make is whether to breast-feed or bottle-feed your baby. Breast-feeding is recommended for all infants with very few exceptions because breast-fed babies are generally healthier, with fewer ear, chest, gastrointestinal and urine infections. They also suffer fewer allergies, asthma, eczema and diabetes. Breast-fed babies are easier to settle and more convenient to travel with.

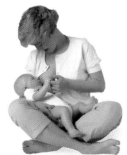

Breast-feeding also has health benefits for you. By nursing your baby as soon as you are able to after delivery, you will reduce the risk of excessive uterine bleeding. Continuing to breast-feed will help you return more quickly to your pre-pregnant weight and reduce your chances of breast, uterine and ovarian cancer and osteoporosis. If you have concerns about breast-feeding, talk to your doctor.

WHAT MOTHERS SAY ABOUT BREAST-FEEDING

Some women know early on in pregnancy that they want to breast-feed. Others are unsure. Either way, it is best to learn about breast-feeding before your delivery. You can talk to other mothers who breast-fed, your doctor, your community health nurse, lactation consultants and your local breast-feeding support group. Breast-feeding clinics are also useful if you have any particular concerns.

"I knew that by breast-feeding I was giving him the best possible milk he could have. I could tell he was digesting it easily, and I knew it had exactly the right blend of nutrients."

Breast milk contains substances that help protect your baby from disease until his own immune system has matured, and protects against allergies —which is important if there is an allergy in your family.

"I loved the convenience of breast-feeding my baby: the milk was always there, always sterile, always at the temperature she liked."

If you are out visiting friends or places, traveling or just enjoying a day in the park, breast milk is the ultimate convenience food.

"The breast was always the best method of soothing my baby whenever he cried."

Breast-fed babies are less fussy than bottle-fed babies. They have less constipation, less gas and suffer less illness.

"I was worried that my breasts would become saggy with breast-feeding but my obstetrician told me that if the breasts are going to go saggy, the changes already happen during pregnancy."

During the first few months, breasts will be fuller as feeding time nears. After that, you'll notice only occasional feelings of fullness, such as after your baby's had a longer sleep.

"I was tired and sore after my Cesarean section and the baby was nursing often. My mother and husband helped a lot and it worked out very well."

All mothers need help in the weeks after delivery. They need the time to focus on the baby and get to know this new little person in their lives.

"I was convinced that I wouldn't be able to breast-feed—my bust was so small. But I had plenty of milk, and my baby certainly didn't mind my small breasts."

Nearly all mothers have enough milk. If there is not enough, your baby will not gain weight adequately. If you are unsure, see your doctor.

"At first, I found it really hard nursing at night but then the lactation consultant showed me how to nurse lying down. Now we sleep together and the baby nurses whenever he needs to."

Nursing lying down is a great way for you to rest and even sleep. Babies can nurse on their side but should be turned onto their backs for sleep. Mothers and babies should not sleep together if the mother's breasts are very large, if either parent is a smoker, using sedating medication, alcohol or street medication. Avoid letting your baby sleep on a soft surface, such as on a waterbed or sofa and having loose covers in the bed. There should be no spaces that could trap your baby, such as between bed and wall.

"My husband was a great help after the baby came, but said he felt left out by the breast-feeding. I told him how good he made me feel by all the things he was doing and how much I loved him. It was a special moment for both of us."

Fathers and mothers are equally important in the lives of their children but their role is different.

ESSENTIALS OF FEEDING

DEMAND FEEDING

Feeding on demand means giving your baby the breast or a bottle when he is hungry, not following timetables. Babies who are hungry will act a little anxious, will turn their heads toward any cheek stimulation and open their mouths like little birds. If they are not fed at that point, they will go on to cry. There is nothing to be gained by keeping your baby waiting once he has acted hungry. You are not spoiling your baby by meeting his needs; you are caring for him and showing you love him by feeding him when he says he is hungry.

How often will he feed?

During the first two days, your baby may tend to feed every two to four hours, 15 to 30 minutes on one or both sides. By the third day, he'll be much more awake and his tummy will be ready for the extra milk you should be making. He'll tend to nurse every 2 to 3 hours, for 15 to 30 minutes on each side.

How do I know he is getting enough?

Babies will not act normally if they are not getting enough milk. They will be excessively sleepy at the breast and feeds will be very short and infrequent or excessively long. When awake, they will be very unhappy.

Your baby should lose no more than 7 percent of his birth weight, should be back at birth weight by day 10 to 14 and gain roughly 1oz (30g) a day during the first months. As he gains, his cheeks, tummy and thighs fill in and he may get a double chin. Every baby is a little different. If you are not sure yours is gaining well, see your health care provider.

Your baby will soon establish his own feeding pattern. Most babies take both breasts at each feed but if the mother has a very large supply, sometimes they only take one. Some babies are snackers and some are eight-square-meals-a-day babies. If your baby looks chubby, is gaining well and happy, relax and let him show you what he needs.

SPECIAL CASES

Premature babies Preterm babies are very varied in their ability to feed. The younger the baby, the more health and feeding problems he can have. Preterm babies tend to be very sleepy and may not wake and demand food even though they need it, so when applicable, wake your baby every three hours and offer a feeding.

If your baby is too sick to feed at the breast, start pumping as soon as you can with a high-quality electric pump and use an attachment that lets you pump both breasts at the same time. You will need to pump regularly and often to maintain your milk supply until the baby can nurse. See your physician, nurse or lactation consultant for help with this.

Twins It's perfectly possible to breast-feed twins. Most mothers have more than enough milk. Feed them one at a time at first. Then when you are more confident, it will make your life easier to nurse them together.

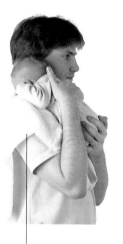

Protect your clothes
with a clean cloth diaper

IF YOUR BABY IS FUSSY

Babies can be fussy at the breast for a number of different reasons. Some have stomach cramps, some might need a little break and others might need a little burp. If your baby is suddenly unsettled at the breast, try giving him a little break by putting him up on your shoulder and gently rubbing upward on his back until he is a little calmer.

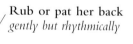

Rub or pat her back
gently but rhythmically

Holding your baby

You can hold a baby of any age across your lap to help him bring up gas. By three months, you can also jiggle him on your lap while rubbing his back.

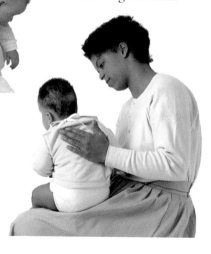

Can I overfeed my baby?

No. Babies take the amount of milk that they need. If they are full, they simply won't latch on to the breast. Babies need a lot of time at the breast during the first months. The breast provides food, as well as warmth, security and an easy way to get to sleep when they are tired. If your baby is unhappy, always offer the breast. Most of the time, that will be what he wants. If he does not settle, try other things like different holding positions such as laying your baby across your lap face down, rocking and gentle massage.

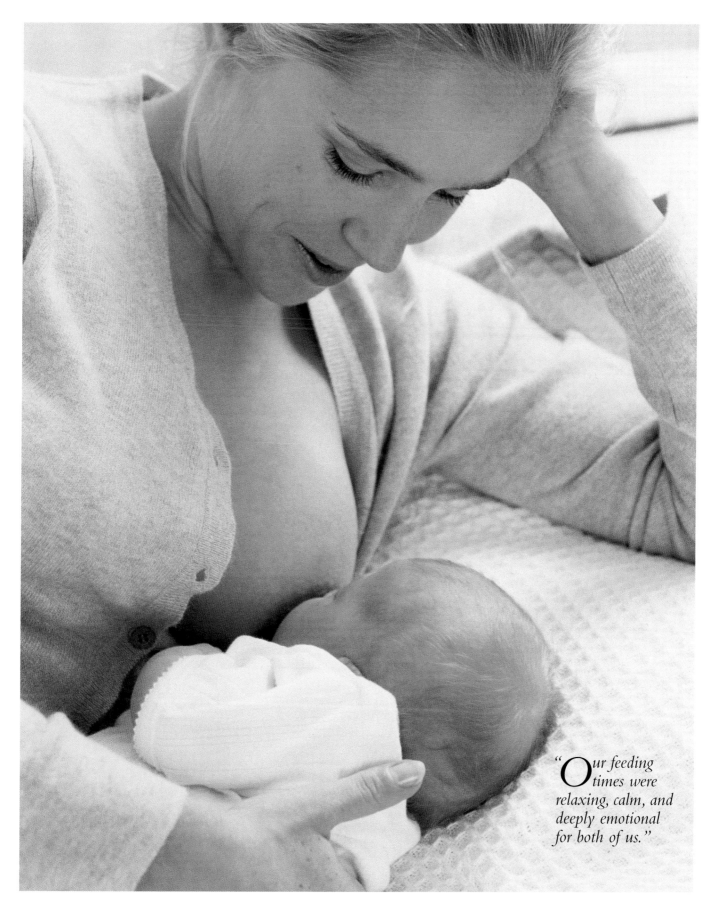

"*Our feeding times were relaxing, calm, and deeply emotional for both of us.*"

BREAST-FEEDING YOUR BABY

Breast-feeding can be a supremely rewarding aspect of caring for your baby, and you'll be giving her the best nourishment nature can provide, so don't be deterred if you have a few problems in the early days. You and your baby have to learn this new skill together, so be patient. Part of the wonderful experience of parenthood is finding out who your baby is and what works for both of you. Try getting together with other nursing moms. Most communities have mom-to-mom support groups like La Leche League. You can also get information from your health center. For help with specific problems, see your physician, nurse, lactation consultant, or breast-feeding clinic. It's worth persevering for successful and satisfying nursing.

FINDING THE NIPPLE

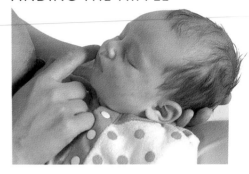

1 Your baby has a reflex that makes her open her mouth when the area is touched. Position her so that her mouth is in front of the nipple. If she turns away from you, bring out the rooting reflex by lightly stroking the cheek closest to the breast. This will make her turn toward your nipple.

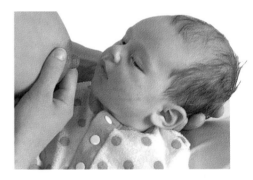

2 If your baby is very young and sleepy, you can put a little milk on her lips, remove her clothing or massage her a little to help her wake up.

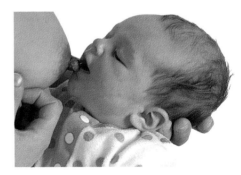

3 Insure that your baby's mouth is right in front of the nipple. Stroke the baby's top lip with your nipple. This will tell the baby that it is time to latch on.

GETTING COMFORTABLE

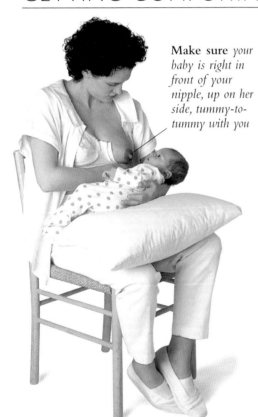

Make sure your baby is right in front of your nipple, up on her side, tummy-to-tummy with you

Nursing your young baby
Sit comfortably in an upright position with your back supported. A padded chair with low arms and firm, low back is ideal. Pillows are useful to bring your baby up to the level of your nipples, and help you avoid back and neck ache. Use a nursing pillow, or adapt a regular pillow by pinning a towel to one side of it, running it behind your back and pinning it to the other side. A footstool may be helpful, too.

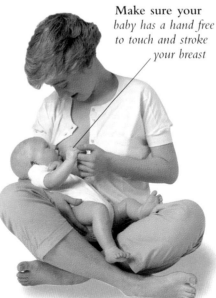

Make sure your baby has a hand free to touch and stroke your breast

Nursing your older baby
Once you are both used to breast-feeding, you will find positions that work best for you. Don't be afraid to experiment until you find the right one for you.

HOW TO BREAST-FEED

LATCHING ON

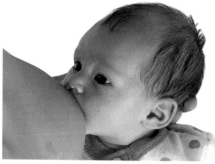

Once your baby's mouth opens widely, quickly bring her head forward onto the areola. The baby's mouth will close and she'll create a vacuum and start to "milk", suck, or squeeze the breast with her jaws by pressing on the reservoirs of milk under the areola. If you feel pain, unlatch your baby and try again.

From your viewpoint, your firmly latched-on baby will open her jaws wide as she nurses and her mouth will be full of your breast. You can tell she is nursing properly when you see her temples and ears moving with each squeeze.

NURSING

Babies tend to squeeze or suck the breast in rhythmic bursts of four to eight sucks, followed by a little pause. As the feeding progresses, your baby will become sleepier until she is no longer sucking. Tickle or rub her gently. If this does not result in further sucking, your breast feels softer, and your baby has nursed an appropriate amount of time for her age, she will fall off the breast or can be taken off.

During the first few weeks each feeding may take up to an hour. Insure you are comfortable before latching her on. Check that your feet, arms, and your baby are all supported. Cradle your baby on her side, and make sure that her mouth is right in front of the nipple.

BONDING

Most babies will explore the mother's body with their hand while they are feeding. This is part of the bonding process for babies. Babies enjoy the act of sucking as much as feeding, and the smell of your skin, the sound of your voice and the sight of your face are all important parts of feeding your baby.

THE LET-DOWN REFLEX

Your baby's sucking action stimulates your breasts to bring milk from the breast to the areola, where the baby can get it. This is called the let-down reflex. The sensation of the reflex varies greatly; it can burn, tingle, feel like a very hard squeeze or not have any feeling associated with it. Some mothers, especially during the first month, will leak from both breasts during a let-down.

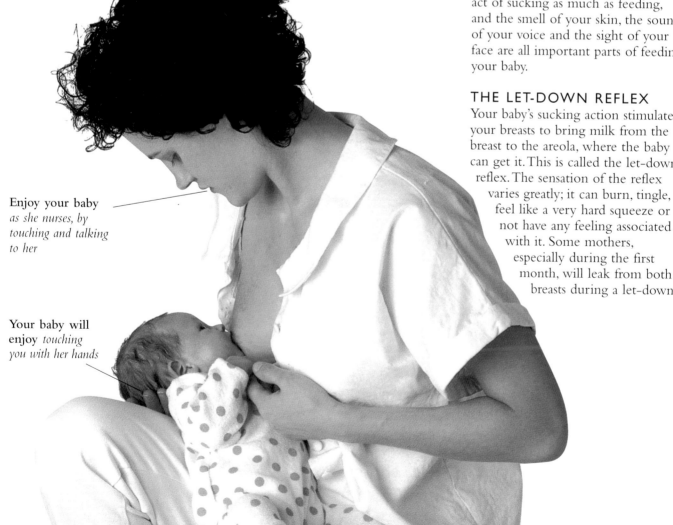

Enjoy your baby *as she nurses, by touching and talking to her*

Your baby will enjoy *touching you with her hands*

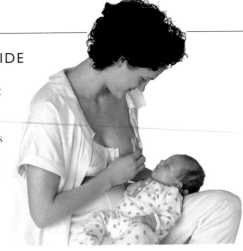

NURSING THE FIRST SIDE

1 Let your baby nurse for as long as she wants at the first breast. Usually this will be less than 30 minutes. As she nurses, she will become progressively sleepy. If she is just doing one suck at a time, instead of a several 5- to 10-second bursts of sucking, or has stopped altogether, stimulate her by rubbing her. She may just fall off the breast at this point. If she doesn't want to let go and she has nursed well, take her from the breast by slipping your little finger between her jaws to break the suction.

Use your clean *little finger to break your baby's suction*

2 Always alternate the starting side for each feeding. If you can't remember which side you last nursed, feel your breasts. The fuller one should be nursed first. You could also try using memory aids, such as attaching a safety pin to your bra strap or slipping a tissue in your bra.

OFFER THE OTHER BREAST

1 After a little shoulder cuddle, your baby may often start to act hungry by becoming a little vocal and by active sucking on anything around her mouth. She is showing that she's ready for the second side.

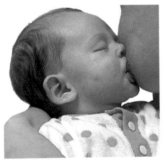

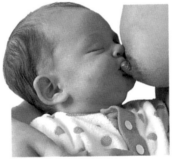

2 Often the second side is not nursed as vigorously or as long. Some babies don't even want the second side and that's fine. Just don't withhold it if she wants it. When your baby's had enough, she will stop sucking just like on the first side.

HOW YOUR BREASTS WORK

Your breasts make food that is just right for your baby. In the first few days after the birth, they produce colostrum. This is a low-volume protein-rich food that's perfect for those first three to four days while your baby's stomach is getting used to eating. After that, the breasts start to produce milk. Breast milk isn't all the same—it becomes more fatty toward the end of each nursing. As your baby grows, the milk will look more like skim milk and is exactly what your baby needs.

Breast milk production works on a supply and demand system: the more often your baby nurses, and the more she takes, the more your breasts will produce. The key to a good milk supply is feeding your baby when she wants to be fed— and in the early days that means nursing at two- or three-hour intervals. As your baby grows, she'll figure out what works best for her. Feedings will take less time and your baby will become more distractible. This shows that she's becoming aware of the world around her.

Supplementary bottles of formula will undermine this system: if your baby's hunger is satisfied by a bottle, she won't be eager to suck and your breasts won't be stimulated.

Will my breast make enough milk?

Nearly all mothers have enough milk for their babies. There are a small number who don't, and this includes some mothers who have had breast reduction surgery, hormone problems such as infertility and thyroid problems, and mothers who are very ill after surgery. If any of these apply to you, see your doctor, nurse, lactation consultant or breast-feeding clinic.

The vast majority of mothers have excess milk, and your milk supply will not decrease without a very good reason.

WHEN YOUR MILK COMES IN

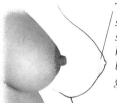

The areola *is swollen and firm, so it may be hard for your baby to grasp*

Normal breast **Engorged breast**

1 Around the third or fourth day after delivery, your breasts start to produce milk, rather than colostrum. You may note your breasts becoming larger, hard and uncomfortable. This is engorgement, and it may last for a few hours to a few days. Your baby will find it hard to latch on because the nipple isn't sticking out, but is held tightly against the hard areola. Continue to nurse your baby as often as she will feed, offering both breasts at each feeding. The following tips should help to lessen the engorgement.

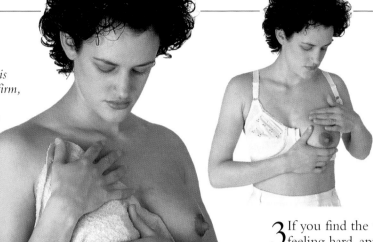

Draw your fingertips down towards the areola

2 If you note a full area developing, massage the breast with your fingers or thumbs in steady strokes from behind the full area, over it, and up to the nipple. A warm cloth over your breast or a shower can help to start the let-down.

3 If you find the whole breast feeling hard, apply the same massaging techniques to the whole breast. You can help your fingers slide more easily by using a little unscented oil or cream on your fingers.

4 When you put your baby to the breast, you can soften the areola by massaging it with your fingers. Make sure your baby opens widely before latching. If nursing and massaging are still not easing the engorgement, try to pump your breasts (see page 95).

"When my baby was one month old, he started being very fussy for several hours every evening. My breasts don't feel very full during that time. Is he not getting enough?"

Many breast-feeding babies follow this pattern. It is called cluster feeding and is normal. It starts at one month, and goes on for two to three months afterward. He is actually drinking lots of extra milk during this time, to get ready for a longer nighttime sleep. That is why your breasts feel empty. They are making milk as he is nursing instead of storing it. Once your baby starts this pattern, your nights will get a whole lot better!

"How will breast-feeding affect my body?"

Breast-feeding will help your body return to its prepregnant start more quickly. This is because the hormones triggered by nursing will help your uterus contract more quickly. The fat reserves that your body stored during pregnancy are used in the production of breast milk and the calories you share with your baby will mean you lose weight more quickly.

"Can I take medication while I am breast-feeding?"

Most medications are fine while nursing because only a little bit of what you take will get into the milk. There are a very few select drugs that are a problem. Consult your doctor, nurse, lactation consultant or breast-feeding clinic. Also remember that scientists are constantly doing new research so try to get the most recent information you can. There are also some phone services for such information. Remember, breast milk is the best food for your baby. Breast milk with a small amount of medication in it is usually still much better than formula.

EXPRESSING MILK

At some point you might need to be separated from your baby and will need to have breast milk available. By experimenting, you will find the best way for you to express milk. Some mothers find manual expression works best, others like pumping and some find both that work equally well. There are also some mothers who find neither works because, unlike the baby, pumping and manual expression do not stimulate the breast as effectively. It takes time and experience to learn how to stimulate the let-down, so *low expressed milk volumes do not mean that you don't have enough milk.* The best test of your milk supply is your baby's weight, appearance and behavior.

HAND EXPRESSING

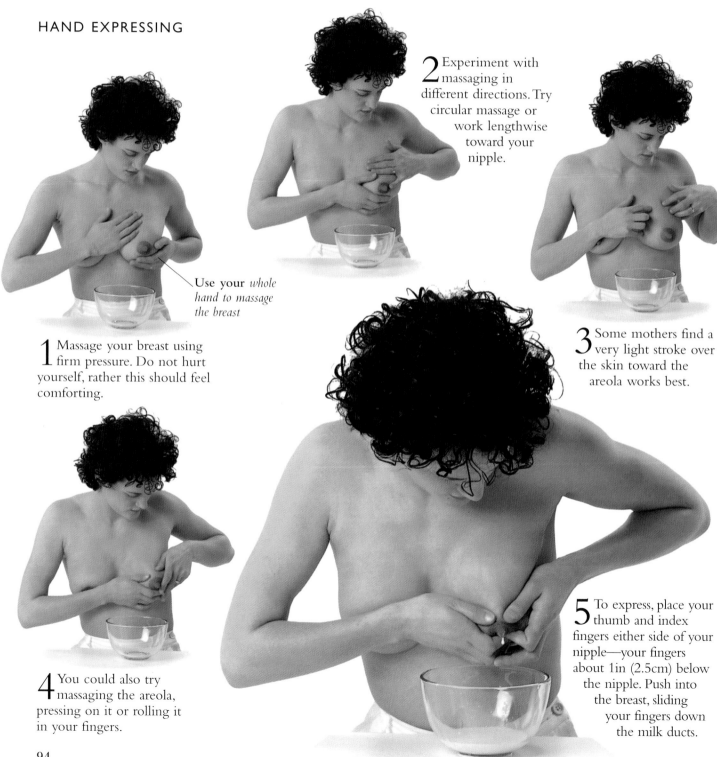

Use your *whole hand to massage the breast*

1 Massage your breast using firm pressure. Do not hurt yourself, rather this should feel comforting.

2 Experiment with massaging in different directions. Try circular massage or work lengthwise toward your nipple.

3 Some mothers find a very light stroke over the skin toward the areola works best.

4 You could also try massaging the areola, pressing on it or rolling it in your fingers.

5 To express, place your thumb and index fingers either side of your nipple—your fingers about 1in (2.5cm) below the nipple. Push into the breast, sliding your fingers down the milk ducts.

EXPRESSING MILK USING A PUMP

Pumps are available in various styles. Consider ease of use, durability, and suction adjustment before you buy one. Speak with your health care provider. If you are frequently separated from your baby, as with a sick infant, you might consider using a double-sided electric pump. These offer more stimulation in half the time. During pumping, make yourself comfortable in a chair with good back support and try to rest your arms on a pillow or armrests.

1 Prepare your pump. Stimulate your breasts before starting to pump, as described in the facing page. Place the funnel of the pump over the areola so that it forms an airtight seal. Ensure your nipple is in the middle of the funnel.

2 Gently apply the vacuum and hold it for five to 10 seconds until the milk stream stops. Release and reapply the vacuum.

3 Store milk in the fridge (five days), upstairs freezer (six months) or chest freezer (one year). To avoid waste, freeze small amounts.

PUMPS

Manual pumps These type of pumps are hand operated and have a device that needs to be worked manually to create suction. They can be quite hard work. Ask your healthcare provider for advice.

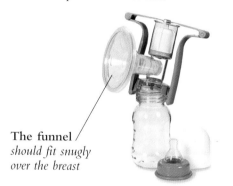

The funnel /
should fit snugly over the breast

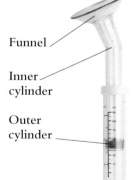

Funnel

Inner cylinder

Outer cylinder

Battery pump
Suction tends not to be as powerful with battery operated pumps as an electric pump, but they are useful if you have a good, well-established milk supply. Some come with an adaptor so that they can be operated by electricity.

Battery

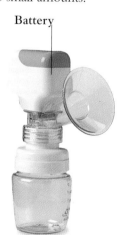

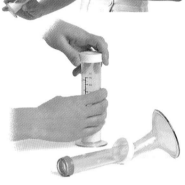

DIOXINS IN BREAST MILK

Recent studies have shown that dioxins—widespread environmental pollutants—are present in breast milk and can pose a variety of risks to humans and animals. Research on animals has shown that they can affect sperm production. While the precise nature of the risk to humans remains controversial, accumulating evidence suggests that exposure to dioxins may affect the developing reproductive organs and immune system.

Babies are particularly susceptible to these toxic effects because of their dependence on breast milk for food, the high degree of absorption of substances found in milk, and the unique sensitivity of certain biological processes in early development. However, the important advantages of breast-feeding must be weighed against a baby's susceptibility to dioxins. In almost all cases, the proven benefits will exceed the risks, and breast milk remains much healthier than any alternative.

BREAST-FEEDING PROBLEMS

If your have any problems with breast-feeding, get help quickly from your healthcare professional. In addition to community nurses and physicians, breast-feeding clinics exist in most major cities. Breast-feeding should not hurt. Some of the problems you may encounter are easy to fix; others need specialized attention. Struggling alone is discouraging and deprives you of the treatment and support you need. Some mothers will resort to expressing instead of nursing when faced with a problem. Remember that expressing and pumping is a lot of work and can lead to sore nipples, engorgement and then a low milk supply. Finally, a baby who is not fed at the breast for a time, might not want to resume nursing.

LEAKING BREASTS

Your breasts may leak copiously between feedings in the early weeks before supply has matched demand. Leaking is normal, and helps to ease engorgement.
Treatment Nursing pads inside your bra will absorb some drips, but change the pads frequently because continually being wet may make your nipples sore.

Disposable breast pad
A breast pad will absorb drips and small leaks.

BLOCKED DUCTS

These feel like a row of marbles going towards the nipple or like a hard lump anywhere on the breast. They are tender and develop quickly, especially if you've been expressing instead of nursing.
Treatment Massage the milk out from the outer side of the lump towards the nipple after each feeding and, if necessary, several times between feedings. It usually clears within two days.

MASTITIS

Experienced by 15 percent of mothers, the most typical sign of mastitis is the sudden extreme tenderness in one area of one breast and overlying redness. You may also develop fever. You are most likely to get it if you have a cracked nipple or a large milk supply.
Treatment Continue nursing, and if you have no nipple cracks and no fever, try expressing milk and massaging out the area. If you have fever, are not better in 24 hours or have a cracked nipple, you require antibiotics.

SORE OR CRACKED NIPPLES

Some mothers have sensitive nipples that will tend to be tender and even break down with each baby. They will note a sharp pain when they latch the baby on and this can sometimes even continue during the feeding. Start by nursing the baby in a different position at each feeding. This will distribute the stress on your nipple. Ask your health care professional to insure your baby is well positioned and latched. Usually, this pain starts to settle by the third day after delivery. If you find the pain is getting worse, you could use a nipple shield to help with the pain. The best shield is one with a large-sized cone. As a last resort, you can express for a minimal number of feedings.
Treatment If your nipples are blistered, scabbed or bloody, apply a bland ointment after each feed. Do not air-dry your nipples. If your nipples are not feeling and looking much better by the third day, it's important to see your doctor for treatment.
Mammary yeast Some mothers develop yeast infections of the areola and nipple. The treatment is either a cream for a mild infection, or a one- to two-week prescription for an antifungal tablet. Babies do not need to be treated unless they have the white lacy patches of thrush on the inside of their cheeks and lips. A small number of babies also get thrush on their tongue.

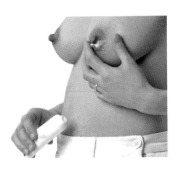

Medicated cream
An antiyeast cream may be prescribed for a mild infection, if needed.

ASK FOR HELP

Other breast-feeding problems include areolar eczema and milk pimples. Remember that you are not alone. Never be shy to ask for advice from your doctor, community health nurse, a lactation consultant or breast-feeding clinic. With a little help, these problems can be settled and you will be able to enjoy this special time with your child.

FEEDING THE OLDER CHILD

Until the age of about six months, babies only need milk. After that, they are ready and able to start complementary foods. Milk will still be the most important food for the first year of life and an important food afterwards. When you start complementary foods, remember that you can make your own healthy foods for your baby, easily and inexpensively. Talk to your health care provider on how to do this. Start by offering your baby solids in small amounts and at the same time you have your own family meals if practical, so that her routine will coincide with the rest of the family. She will continue to nurse whenever she needs to and for as long as she needs to.

How often will she nurse?

As your baby grows, her feedings will become more varied in duration and frequency. She'll nurse for hunger, thirst, when cold, tired and when she just wants a snuggle. Some babies nurse more often and some less. Just let your baby decide. Remember that her varied nursing pattern does not mean that your milk is drying up. That just doesn't happen without a very good reason. Rather, your baby is just starting to grow up, and this is a normal pattern.

Going back to work

If you are returning to work, you can continue to breast-feed, and supply your baby with breast milk. It means a little bit of work each day but may actually save you time as your baby will have less illness.

You will need to get your baby used to receiving milk occasionally from a bottle, if she is less than seven months. Have a different person than yourself do this feeding so that she associates bottle-feeding with that person and breast-feeding with you. If your baby refuses, try again another day. A different nipple may help, or moisten the nipple with some breast milk. She will soon learn.

If you are returning to work during the first year, you will need to express milk one or more times during the day or you will feel too full. Also, it is best if you can pump several times during each day in order to maintain your milk supply. Talk with your employer and co-workers. Some mothers shorten their lunch times and increase their coffee breaks so they can pump three times a day. You will soon find out what works for you, your family and your work place.

Get used to pumping before you go back to work. Pump occasionally if your breasts feel full. Mornings are often the best time as you'll probably be fuller then and your baby often will only nurse a little on the second side—try pumping one side and nursing on the other one for that feed. Pumping after a baby has nursed well will not result in a lot of milk. Store expressed milk in the freezer.

Once you are back at work, you can keep your milk in a fridge at work or in a cooler bag with an ice pack. Find a quiet, private place to pump. The older your baby becomes, the less you will feel you have to pump. However, it is best to continue pumping at work in order to maintain the supply.

How long should I nurse for?

The more breast milk a baby gets, the healthier she will be. No international group or organization has put a limit on the duration of breast-feeding and all encourage extended breast-feeding. The World Health Organization recommends two or more years for as long as mutually desirable. When your baby is ready to stop, she will just nurse less and less.

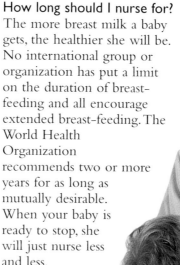

Continuing breast-feeding
You can continue to nurse your baby for as long as you feel comfortable doing so.

How do I wean?

Gradually replace one breast-feeding at a time, with milk by bottle or cup (depending on the age of your child). See page 106 for suggested guidelines when switching to bottle-feeding. If your baby is less than nine months of age, replace breast milk with formula; otherwise, check with your doctor. You may want to stop the night time breast-feeding last, as this is often a special time for you and your baby. Especially if you have gone back to work, continuing to breast-feed your baby in the evening will be a time for you to relax and enjoy a quiet time with your child.

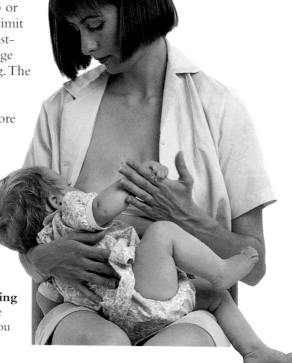

BOTTLE-FEEDING YOUR BABY

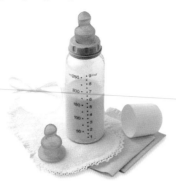

If you decide to bottle-feed your baby, you must be very vigilant about protecting your baby from bacteria that might cause stomach upsets or diarrhea. There are different types of bottles and nipples. Your local public health unit will have information and be able to advise you. You will need to suppress your own milk supply, too. You may be surprised at how full and uncomfortable your breasts feel once you go over to bottle-feeding. Medication to suppress milk production is no longer used, nor is binding the breast. If you are not breast-feeding or expressing your milk for feedings, your breasts will begin to slow down producing milk and in a relatively short time will stop milk production. Always follow the manufacturer's instructions carefully when making up formula, as a feeding that is too concentrated is harmful to your baby.

EQUIPMENT FOR BOTTLE-FEEDING

For a fully bottle-fed baby you will need at least eight full size (250ml/8oz) bottles. Buy extra nipples, and keep them ready for use in a clean jar in case a nipple gives an inadequate flow of milk (see page 106). Some bottles are used with throw-away plastic liners, which can reduce the amount of air your baby swallows with his milk: the bag collapses as he sucks milk out, so the nipple doesn't flatten and halt the flow.

BOTTLES AND OTHER EQUIPMENT

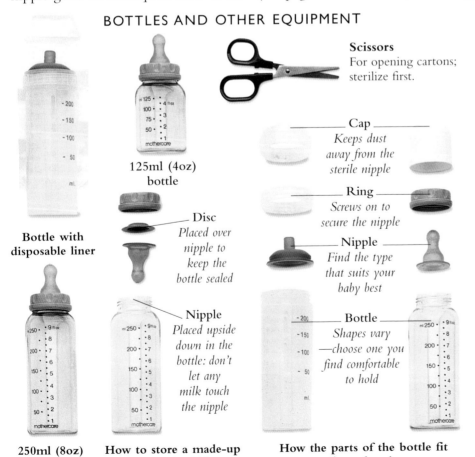

125ml (4oz) bottle

Bottle with disposable liner

Disc *Placed over nipple to keep the bottle sealed*

Nipple *Placed upside down in the bottle: don't let any milk touch the nipple*

250ml (8oz) bottle

How to store a made-up feed in the fridge

Scissors For opening cartons; sterilize first.

Cap *Keeps dust away from the sterile nipple*

Ring *Screws on to secure the nipple*

Nipple *Find the type that suits your baby best*

Bottle *Shapes vary —choose one you find comfortable to hold*

How the parts of the bottle fit together when in use

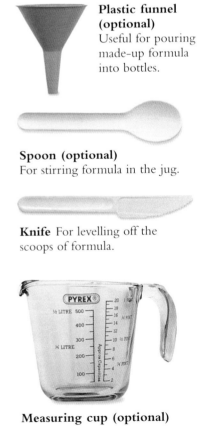

Plastic funnel (optional) Useful for pouring made-up formula into bottles.

Spoon (optional) For stirring formula in the jug.

Knife For levelling off the scoops of formula.

Measuring cup (optional)

NIPPLES

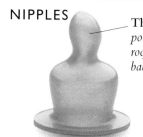

The holes must point toward the roof of your baby's mouth

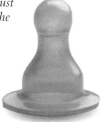

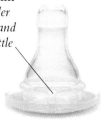

Valve in rim *lets air under the nipple and into the bottle*

Nipples for young babies *have a short nipple*

Natural-shaped nipple
The nipple must go into your baby's mouth with the holes facing upward, so that the milk sprays over the roof of his mouth.

Universal nipple
The standard shape of nipple gives a sucking action that is not really like sucking from your breast. Nipples are sold with different rates of flow, but check at each feed: there should be two or three drops of milk a second. A cross-cut hole gives a better flow of milk than a pinhole.

Anti-colic nipple
An anti-colic nipple lets air into the bottle as your baby sucks milk out. This stops the nipple collapsing, so enabling him to get a steady stream of milk.

Wide-based nipple
This type is not interchangeable among different makes of bottle. As your baby sucks, his lips push against the squashy base and the nipple moves in and out in his mouth. Fit nipple and ring together before assembling the bottle ready for filling.

"There are so many different types of formula—how do I know which one to buy?"

A milk-based, iron-fortified formula is the most acceptable alternative to breast milk. A few babies will have problems with standard formula. If you think that your baby is having a problem with a milk-based formula, ask your doctor or public health nurse for advice. If your healthcare provider identifies a problem you may be advised to buy an alternative formula that is not milk-based, but do not do this without seeking professional advice.

"The rest of my family uses low-fat milk products—when can my baby use these?"

Low-fat milk products (skim, 1% fat and 2% fat) should not be used until your child is at least 2 years old. Low-fat milk products have excessive amounts of minerals and protein, are low in fat content and lack essential fatty acids. Although popular with adults, they are not appropriate for very young children.

"Can I prop up the bottle for my baby to feed from? She always seems hungry when I am busy doing something else!"

Do not leave your baby to feed on a propped-up bottle! Besides the choking hazard, you are missing out on a natural time to be close to your baby and cuddle her.

"Formula is expensive. When can I switch to regular milk?"

Cow's milk is very different in composition from breast milk and a poor source of iron. It should only be introduced when your baby is eating a wide source of other foods, which is usually at 10–12 months of age.

"How do I know when to "burp" my baby?"

There is actually no reason to "burp" your baby. Burping your baby does not reduce crying or spitting up. Stopping half way through feedings to rub your baby's back will not harm your baby, and your baby may burp with the change in position and stimulation. However, if your baby does not burp, there is no reason not to resume feeding.

"Is bottle-feeding harmful to my baby's teeth?"

Bottle-feeding itself is not harmful to your baby's teeth. However, "baby bottle tooth decay" refers to severe tooth decay that can occur in infants or toddlers who go to sleep with a bottle. The milk or juice in the bottle tends to lie in the baby's mouth when he goes to sleep. This causes the new teeth to decay, and the teeth have to be removed. It is therefore very important to always remove a bottle from your child's mouth before he goes to sleep.

KEEPING YOUR BOTTLES CLEAN

Formula, when it is warm or held too long at room temperature, is an ideal breeding ground for the bacteria that cause gastroenteritis, a disease that can be life-threatening in a young baby. There are a few guidelines that you must follow to keep your baby healthy when bottle-feeding. Make sure that your hands are absolutely clean, then wash everything else that comes in contact with your baby's bottle before filling it. Always keep bottles of formula refrigerated, and use them within 24–48 hours of their being made up (check the label). Check with your doctor for recommendations about sterilization.

WASHING

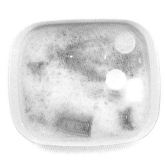
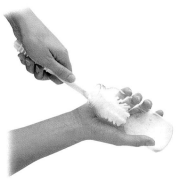
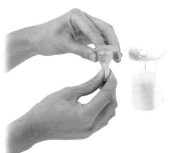
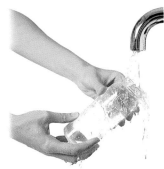

1 Put all the rinsed out bottles, nipples, caps, rings, discs, funnel, spoon, and knife directly into hot soapy water. Wash each of the individual items extremely thoroughly.

2 Scrub inside the bottles with the bottle brush to remove all traces of formula. Scrub around their necks, and scrub the screw thread, where bacteria can grow, too.

3 Make sure you clean the nipples thoroughly. Formula can get caked on and be hard to clean.

4 Rinse the bottles, nipples, and other items of equipment thoroughly under running water. Use a pin that has been heated in a flame to clear the holes in the nipples.

USING A DISHWASHER

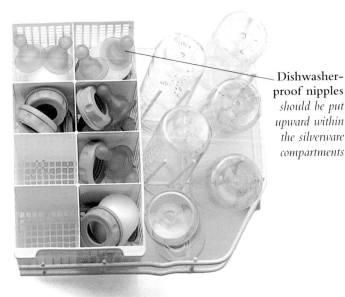

Dishwasher-proof nipples *should be put upward within the silverware compartments*

An easy way to wash equipment is to put it in your dishwasher and make sure it goes through the hot drying cycle. The high heat is usually sufficient to kill any bacteria. But be careful—nipples may have to be boiled separately on the stovetop because dishwashers can turn them into unusable sticky blobs.

STERILIZING BY BOILING

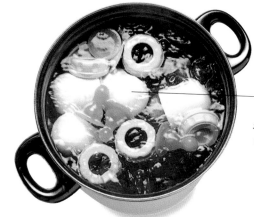

All items *must be fully submerged during the boiling period*

Wash all the feeding equipment and boil it in a deep pan of water for five minutes. When doctors suggest that new mothers sterilize bottles and formula-preparation equipment, this basic boiling method is ordinarily sufficient. Use tongs to remove the hot bottles and fill them when they cool slightly. Don't let the sterile equipment sit around too long on your kitchen counter gathering dust or germs. Store it in the refrigerator or a cupboard. The five-minute boil is the usual length of time suggested.

PROTECTING YOUR BABY FROM AN UPSET STOMACH

If you take the precautions below, you should be able to protect your baby from the bacteria that cause stomach upsets or gastroenteritis.

★ Sterilize all feeding equipment before use, even if brand new.

★ If you have no fridge, make up each feed only when you need it.

★ If your baby doesn't finish his bottle at a feeding, throw the milk away: don't save it for next time, because his saliva will have contaminated it.

★ Throw away any milk warmed for your baby, even if he doesn't touch it; the process of warming the milk encourages bacteria to grow.

★ Store bottles of made-up feeds in the main part of the fridge, not in the door compartment, which is at a lower temperature. Don't keep for longer than 48 hours.

★ Don't drain sterilized equipment in your dishdrainer, or dry it on a dishtowel. Drain on paper towels, and dry the knife only, using paper towels.

★ Wash your hands before preparing baby bottles.

TAKING CARE OF NIPPLES

Your baby can only feed happily if the nipple allows him to suck out formula at the right rate. When you tip the bottle up you should see one drop a second: too small a hole will mean that your baby gets frustrated in his efforts to suck out enough formula; too large and the formula will gush out. Nipples do deteriorate and the holes clog up. Have some spare sterile nipples stored in a jar, so you can just swap an imperfect nipple for a fresh one. Throw away nipples if the holes are too large; holes that are too small can be enlarged with a needle. Check the flow again afterward.

When away from home

If you're going out for more than a couple of hours, make up a batch of bottles for your baby as

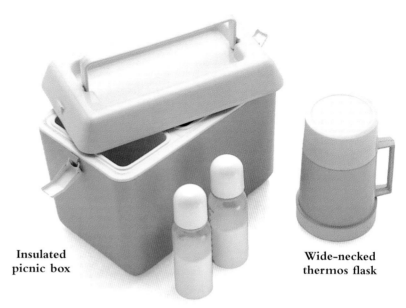

Insulated picnic box

Wide-necked thermos flask

normal and chill them in the fridge. Pack the ice-cold bottles into an insulated picnic box with some ice packs. Then take a thermos filled with hot water, and warm your baby's bottle in this when needed. Never carry warm formula in a thermos: bacteria will grow and may cause a stomach upset.

Cans of made-up formula are also available. These are more expensive than powdered formula, but they are more convenient to use than powder when you are away from home. The

cans of formula should be stored in a cool place to stay safe. When you go out, take sterile bottles and nipples with you in a plastic bag, and simply pour out the formula as your baby asks for it.

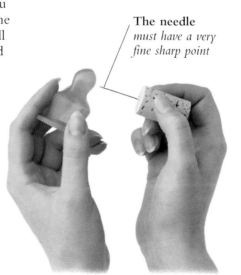

The needle *must have a very fine sharp point*

Enlarging a hole that is too small
Push the eye of a needle into a cork. Heat the point in a flame until hot, then push into the hole.

FORMULA: WHAT'S IN IT?

Cow's milk is not well suited to your baby's needs; it doesn't contain all the nutrients she must have for growth at this stage in her life, and it can also be difficult for her to digest because of the concentrations of protein and fat. Most infant formulas are adapted from a cow's milk base but they are supplemented with other ingredients to make them suitable for young babies. Vegetable oils are added to replace cow's butter fat, and lactose is used to sweeten the mixture. Some formulas provide your baby with additional iron; this is clearly marked on the label. Some formulas are based entirely on soy. If your baby vomits after a bottle; has diarrhea, cramps, or excessive gas; wheezes; develops a rash; or is generally irritable, call your doctor immediately and discuss the problem. Babies can dehydrate quickly.

MAKING UP YOUR BABY'S BOTTLE

In the early weeks of your baby's life you need to have a supply of bottles ready in the refrigerator so that whenever your baby cries, wanting to be fed, you can respond quickly and easily. Until your baby is at least ten months old, give him an infant formula. Most are made from modified cow's milk. Your doctor will help you choose a brand that is right for your baby. You can upset your baby by switching brands, so never do so without seeking professional advice.

Making up formula

Infant formula is most commonly and cheaply available as concentrated liquid or powder that can be readily mixed up as required.

The instructions on the cans tell you the correct amount of liquid or number of scoops of powder you need to add to each measure of water. It is very important to maintain these proportions precisely. If you add too much formula, the feeding will be dangerously concentrated: your baby may gain too much weight, and his kidneys could suffer some damage. If you consistently add too little formula, he may gain weight too slowly. Once the milk is made up correctly, let your baby take as much as he wants at each feed.

Always use fresh, cold, tap water to make up your baby's formula, and boil it once only. Some types of water should never be used:
★ water that has been repeatedly boiled, or left standing in the kettle
★ water from a tap with a domestic softener attached—the extra sodium (salt) can damage your baby's kidneys
★ water from a tap with a domestic filter attached—these filters can trap harmful bacteria
★ mineral water—the sodium and minerals may be harmful.

There are two methods of making up your baby's formula: mixing the formula directly in the bottles, or mixing it in a measuring cup first. Use the cup method if you use bottles with disposable liners.

Ready-to-feed formula

Some brands of infant formula are also available ready-mixed in cans. You need add no water to the formula. If the brand of formula you are feeding your baby comes in this form, then you have a very convenient—but expensive—option. The formula in the can has been ultra-heat treated (UHT). Store unopened cans in a cool place, and do not use after the expiration date.

Once opened, the formula can be stored in the fridge for up to 24 hours (48 hours for some brands), either in a sterile, sealed bottle, or in the can. But unless you can be sure that you won't forget when you put the can in the fridge, it's safer to pour all the milk out when your baby wants a feeding, and throw away any he doesn't drink.

How much will my baby want?

Appetites vary from day to day. During the first weeks of life put 125ml (4floz) of feed into each of six bottles, and see how that matches his appetite. As he gains weight, he will often cry for more at the end of a feeding, so gradually increase the amount in each bottle. By the time he is six months old you will be making up bottles of 200ml (7fl oz). As a rough guide, your baby needs about 150ml of milk per kilogram of body weight (2½floz per 1lb) every 24 hours.

Should I give anything else?

Most bottle-fed babies don't need anything but formula for the first six months of life. Some doctors recommend vitamin and mineral supplements or additional fluoride, but do check first. Too many vitamins can make your baby sick.

The majority of doctors generally suggest holding off on solid foods until a baby is six months of age. You may be tempted to try some cereal in your baby's diet if he appears not to be satisfied with just formula. However, until he can let you know that he wants to take more or less food, pushing solids can amount to force-feeding, so be patient.

THE RIGHT MILK TO GIVE YOUR BABY		Birth	6m	9m	12m	18m
Infant formula	Cow's milk modified to resemble human breast milk. Standard product for bottle-fed healthy term baby, with no family history of allergy.			→———————————→		
Whole cow's milk	Introduce as main milk drink from 10–12 months.				→————————→	

USING CONCENTRATED LIQUID FORMULA

YOU WILL NEED
Can of concentrated liquid formula
Bottles and nipples
Punch-type can opener

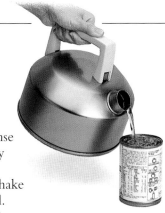

1 Boil water in a kettle or pot. Rinse the top of the can by pouring the boiling water over the lid. Shake the formula can well.

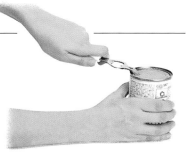

2 Pierce two holes using a clean can opener. Refill the kettle or pot with fresh water from the tap, boil it, then let it cool for five minutes.

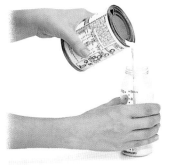

3 Pour the concentrate into a clean bottle until you have half the total feeding amount. Check the amount at eye level.

4 Fill up with an equal quantity of cooled boiled water. With the bottle at eye level, make sure you have doubled the amount of concentrate.

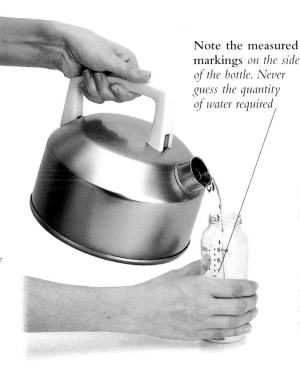

Note the measured markings *on the side of the bottle. Never guess the quantity of water required*

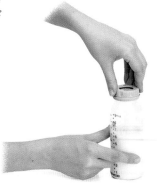

5 Attach the disc and ring to the bottle. Shake the mixture, leaving out the nipple to avoid coating it in milk. Store in the refrigerator.

USING READY-TO-FEED FORMULA

YOU WILL NEED
Can of ready-to-feed formula
Bottles and nipples
Punch-type can opener

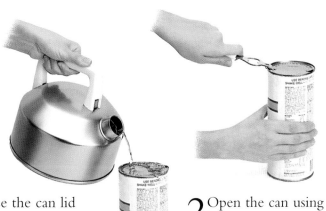

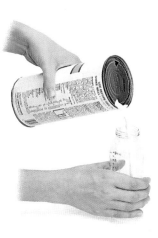

1 Rinse the can lid by pouring boiling water over it. Shake the formula can well to ensure the contents are evenly mixed.

2 Open the can using a clean punch-type opener. Then make a second opening very carefully so the formula does not spill.

3 Pour the formula into a bottle. Attach the nipple and ring. Shake the bottle, test the temperature, and feed.

MAKING UP POWDER FORMULA IN BOTTLES

YOU WILL NEED
Powder formula
Bottles and nipples
Knife
Kitchen paper

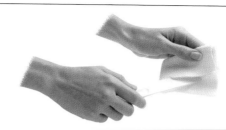

1 Boil water in a pot or a kettle to rinse the freshly washed equipment. Pour the boiled water all over the equipment. Drain everything on paper towels. Dry the knife.

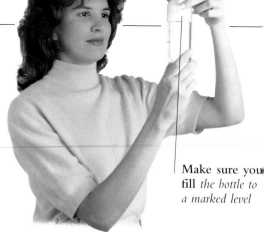

Make sure you fill *the bottle to a marked level*

2 Empty the pot or kettle, fill it with fresh, cold, tap water and re-boil. Pour the boiling water into the bottles, filling them to a suitable measure. Check at eye level: the measure must be exact to mix the formula to the right concentration.

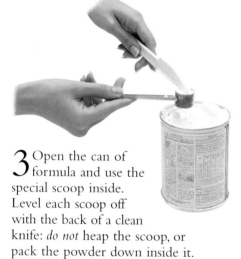

3 Open the can of formula and use the special scoop inside. Level each scoop off with the back of a clean knife: *do not* heap the scoop, or pack the powder down inside it.

4 Drop each scoop of powder into the bottle of water. Add only the number of scoops recommended for that amount of water. The powder will dissolve quickly in the hot water.

5 Put the disc and ring on the bottle—not the nipple at this stage—and screw on tightly to seal. Shake the bottle briskly to mix the formula thoroughly.

MAKING UP FORMULA USING A CUP

YOU WILL NEED
Powder formula or concentrated liquid
Bottles and nipples
Knife
Paper towels
Measuring cup
Spoon
Plastic funnel

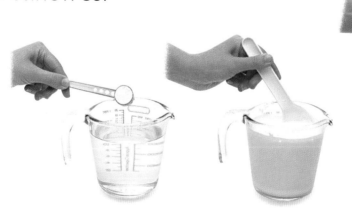

1 Make sure the equipment is clean and dry. Boil fresh, cold, tap water in the kettle. Fill the cup to an exact full measure. Use the scoop inside the formula can. Level each scoop off with the back of a knife.

2 Add scoops of powder or the correct amount of concentrated liquid to the cup. Use only the amount recommended for that measure of water, and never any more.

3 Stir the formula well with a spoon until it is thoroughly mixed. The hot water will dissolve the concentrated liquid.

4 Pour into bottles through the funnel. Put the nipple in upside down. Cover with the disc and ring. Make up more formula until the bottles are full.

USING DISPOSABLE LINERS

YOU WILL NEED
Powder or concentrated liquid formula
Bottles and nipples
Disposable liners
Knife
Paper towels
Measuring cup
Spoon
Plastic funnel

1 Make up the formula in a measuring cup, a pitcher, or any clean container and follow the manufacturer's directions carefully. If you prefer, open a can of ready-to-use formula (see page 103). Wash your hands. Push the nipple into the ring without touching the tip of it. Tear a presterilized disposable liner off its roll.

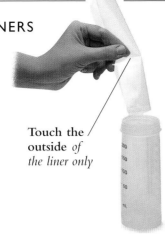

Touch the outside *of the liner only*

2 Fold the liner in half lengthways and place in the "bottle"—it's not a real bottle, but a plastic sleeve that supports the liner, nipple, and ring.

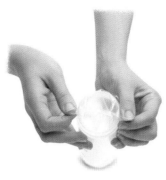

3 Make sure the liner folds well down all around the rim—otherwise formula will spill out.

Touch the plastic ring *only, once the nipple is secure*

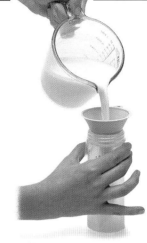

4 Hold the liner firmly in place so the weight of the formula can't pull it down, and pour formula in through the funnel. Add as much as your baby needs.

5 Screw on the ring with the nipple already secured—this will hold the liner. Pull off the perforated tabs and dispose of them immediately. Put the cap over the nipple of each one and store the bottles in the refrigerator.

STORING THE BOTTLES

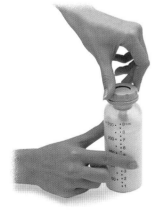

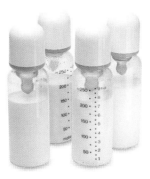

1 To store a batch of bottles, put the nipples in upside down after you've shaken the formula, or insert the nipples later.

2 Cool the bottles under the cold tap and store in the refrigerator with the caps on. Use stored formula within 48 hours.

STORING OPENED CANS

If you prefer to make up bottles as your baby asks for them, you can store the cans of unused formula in the refrigerator for up to 24 hours (48 hours for some brands). Cover the can so bacteria cannot enter. It's easy to forget when you opened the can, so use date labels or mark the date on your calendar. Always throw away any formula opened for longer then 24 hours (48 hours for some brands).

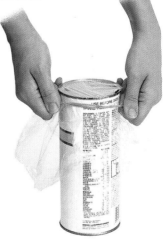

Covering the can
Place plastic wrap over the lid of an opened can and secure with a rubber band.

GIVING YOUR BABY A BOTTLE

Feeding your baby is the most important thing you can do for her—but don't make the mistake of thinking that the formula in the bottle is all she needs, or that "anyone" can feed her. Your love, your cuddling, and attention are just as important to your baby as the formula itself. Always hold her close and cuddle her against you, smile and talk to her. Never leave your baby alone with her bottle, she may choke.

Right from the beginning, give your baby as much control over feeding as you can. Let her set the pace, pausing to look around, touch the bottle, or stroke your breast if she wants to—the bottle may take as long as half an hour if she's feeling playful. Above all, let her decide when she's had enough.

Make yourself comfortable, put a bib on her, and have a cloth diaper to hand.

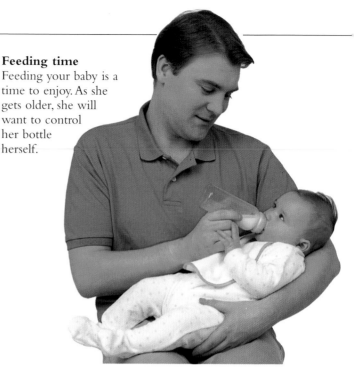

Feeding time
Feeding your baby is a time to enjoy. As she gets older, she will want to control her bottle herself.

FROM BREAST- TO BOTTLE-FEEDING

If you have to change over to bottle-feeding from breast-feeding for any reason, remember that the transition needs a gradual approach and professional help. Replacing one breast-feed every third day is the best method—or you can go more slowly. Start by replacing a lunchtime breast-feed with a bottle. If your baby won't take it, try again at the same feeding the next day— you could offer a different type of nipple, or moisten the nipple with a few drops of breast milk to encourage him. After three days with one bottle-feed, replace a second daytime feeding with a bottle, and wait another three days before tackling a third feeding. Carry on until eventually your baby has a bottle for his nighttime feeding.

GETTING THE BOTTLE READY

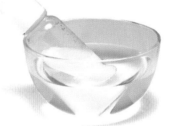

1 Take a bottle from the fridge and turn the nipple the right way up. Warm in warm water. Don't use a microwave oven, because the milk may get very hot although the bottle still feels cool on the outside.

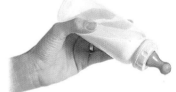

2 Check the flow of milk: it should be about one drop a second. Too small a hole will make sucking hard, too large will let the milk gush out. If the nipple isn't right, swap it for another sterile nipple and test the flow of milk again.

"My baby never seems to finish her bottle: is she getting enough?"

Q & A

Poor feeding could be a sign of illness, or of a serious underlying defect that needs medical attention. Check to see how much formula your baby should have for her weight (see page 102), and see if that matches what she actually takes. If you are at all concerned, talk to your doctor about the problem and make sure your baby is weighed regularly. Your doctor will plot her weight on a growth chart. Poor feeding, if combined with inadequate weight gain, is always a cause for concern.

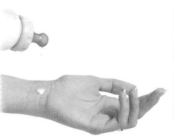

3 Test the temperature by tipping a few drops on to the inside of your wrist—it should feel tepid. Cold milk is safe, but your baby may prefer it warm.

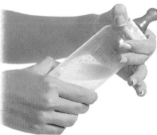

4 Unscrew the ring so that it just stays on the bottle, to let air in as your baby sucks. This will stop the nipple collapsing and halting the flow.

GIVING YOUR BABY HER BOTTLE

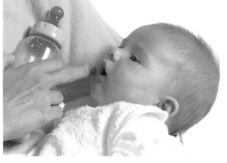

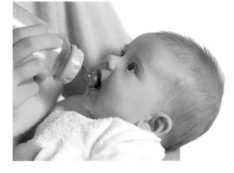

1 For the first ten days or so of life, alert your baby's sucking reflex: stroke the cheek nearest you, and she should turn and open her mouth. If she doesn't, or is older, let some drops of milk form on the nipple, then touch her lips with it to give her the taste.

2 As your baby feeds, hold the bottle firmly so that she can pull against it as she sucks, and tilt it so that the nipple is full of formula, not air. If the nipple collapses, move the bottle around in your baby's mouth to let air back into the bottle.

3 When your baby has finished all the formula, pull the bottle firmly away. If she wants to continue sucking, offer her your clean little finger: she will soon let you know if she wants more.

IF SHE WON'T LET GO

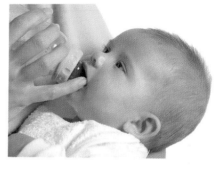

If your baby doesn't want to let go of the bottle even after a long suck, slide your little finger between her gums alongside the nipple.

SLEEPING DURING A FEEDING

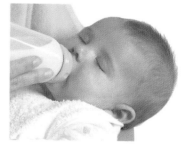

She may doze off during her feeding. Sit her up and gently rub her back for a couple of minutes, then offer her some more formula.

It's easier *for your baby to swallow if she lies in a semi-upright position*

Put a bib *on your baby before you begin*

INTRODUCING SOLID FOOD

Milk is the main source of nutrition for a baby's first six months. Between the age of four to six months, your baby will be ready to sample some solid food. You will notice that even after a full feeding she still seems hungry; she may even demand an extra feeding a day. She will gradually take more and more solid food at each mealtime, until eventually, sometime after her first birthday, she no longer needs the breast or bottle for nourishment. Introduce her to as many new foods as you can, so she is used to a varied diet and not suspicious of unfamiliar tastes and textures. Let her own appetite dictate how much she eats, and avoid confrontations: let her enjoy her food. Mealtimes are an important part of family life, and if you include your baby in family meals from an early age you will be helping her learn essential social skills.

EQUIPMENT FOR FIRST SOLIDS

A clean spoon, a bowl, and a bib are the only essentials for feeding your baby her first tastes. Soon you will need cups for drinks, and once she's sitting up steadily you will need a highchair. You don't need to sterilize equipment for solid food, just wash it well in very hot water, rinse, drain, and dry on paper towels.

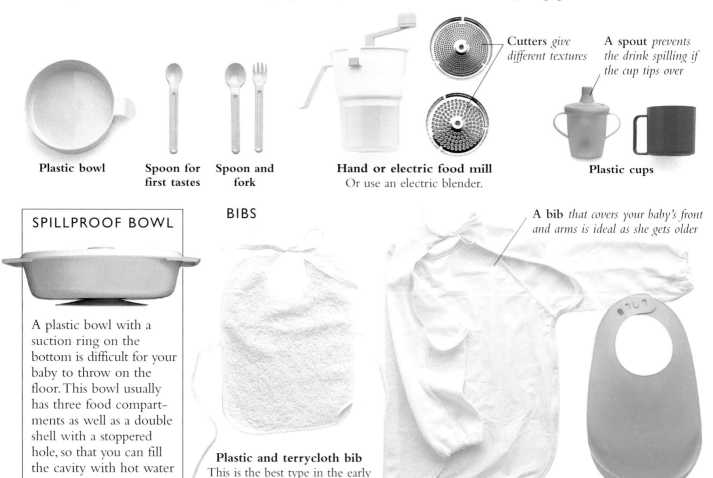

Plastic bowl

Spoon for first tastes

Spoon and fork

Cutters *give different textures*

Hand or electric food mill
Or use an electric blender.

A spout *prevents the drink spilling if the cup tips over*

Plastic cups

SPILLPROOF BOWL

A plastic bowl with a suction ring on the bottom is difficult for your baby to throw on the floor. This bowl usually has three food compartments as well as a double shell with a stoppered hole, so that you can fill the cavity with hot water to keep food warm for a slow eater.

BIBS

A bib *that covers your baby's front and arms is ideal as she gets older*

Plastic and terrycloth bib
This is the best type in the early months. Plastic backing and ties at the sides ensure that your child's clothes are protected.

Bib with sleeves

Plastic bib with crumb-catcher

CHAIRS

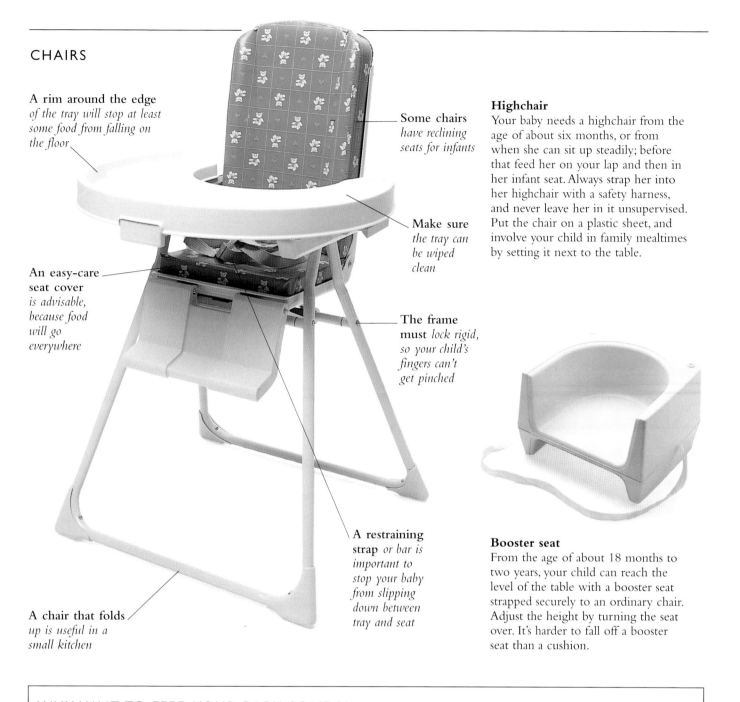

A rim around the edge
*of the tray will stop at least
some food from falling on
the floor*

Some chairs *have reclining
seats for infants*

Make sure
*the tray can
be wiped
clean*

**An easy-care
seat cover**
*is advisable,
because food
will go
everywhere*

**The frame
must** *lock rigid,
so your child's
fingers can't
get pinched*

**A restraining
strap** *or bar is
important to
stop your baby
from slipping
down between
tray and seat*

A chair that folds
*up is useful in a
small kitchen*

Highchair
Your baby needs a highchair from the age of about six months, or from when she can sit up steadily; before that feed her on your lap and then in her infant seat. Always strap her into her highchair with a safety harness, and never leave her in it unsupervised. Put the chair on a plastic sheet, and involve your child in family mealtimes by setting it next to the table.

Booster seat
From the age of about 18 months to two years, your child can reach the level of the table with a booster seat strapped securely to an ordinary chair. Adjust the height by turning the seat over. It's harder to fall off a booster seat than a cushion.

WHY WAIT TO FEED YOUR BABY SOLIDS?

Babies used to be fed puréed foods from a very early age. But we now know that the digestive system of a very young baby isn't ready for solid foods. The gut and kidneys can handle formula or breast milk, but not much else. Allergies, indigestion, constipation, and diarrhea are less likely if you wait till your baby is at least four months old (six months if there is a family history of allergy) before giving solids.

Very young infants cannot easily move food from the front to the back of their mouths, and have such poor head control that it is difficult to hold them in a position where they can be fed and easily swallow semi-solid foods. By four months, most can sit supported in a chair, by five, a baby can easily swallow food from a spoon, and by six, he can chew. A seven-month baby will turn his head away to indicate that he has had enough.

Food tastes and preferences
Food smells, tastes, and feels different from breast or formula milk and it comes in mouthfuls rather than a continuous stream. Don't worry if your baby refuses food or spits it out at first. Let him play with his food, and once he is six months, give finger foods he can hold himself. All this will encourage your baby to experiment with this strange new way of feeding.

WHAT TO FEED YOUR BABY

The average Canadian baby samples a bit of rice cereal mixed with breast milk or formula for her first taste of solid food because rice is less likely to cause an allergic reaction than other forms of food. Introduce puréed vegetables before trying puréed fruit. Try puréed carrots, green or yellow beans, squash, or broccoli. Then introduce fruits such as a little mashed banana, or perhaps some applesauce, puréed apricots, pears, peaches, or plums. Stay away from citrus fruits (including orange juice), tomatoes, fish, berries, egg whites, and spinach; many babies either don't digest these easily or end up with a diaper rash. The key to introducing solid foods is to start with one food at a time and to wait three to four days (especially if there is a family history of allergies) before adding a new one to your baby's diet. If your baby is going to react adversely to a particular food, you'll know by that time. You may want to make your own baby food using fresh fruits, vegetables, and meats, or you can buy specially prepared foods in jars at the grocery store, but be sure you select from the correct age range for your baby. Always check labels before buying. Avoid foods with starches and fillers.

4–6 MONTHS

Texture Give semi-liquid purées, bland and smooth and without any lumps.
Preparation
★ peel carefully
★ cook: steam or boil
★ remove ends and stems
★ purée or sieve
Other good foods
Peas, well-cooked green beans, cauliflower.

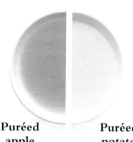

Baby rice **Puréed carrot** **Puréed apple** **Puréed potato**

6–8 MONTHS

Texture Foods can be minced or mashed to the texture of cottage cheese, adding liquid or yogurt. Give plenty of finger foods that are easy for her to pick up herself, for example pieces of peeled fruit.
Preparation, fruit/vegetables
★ peel carefully
★ remove ends and stems
★ purée or sieve.
Preparation, meat/fish
★ trim fat and skin off
★ cook: grill or poach
★ remove all bones
★ mince finely.
Other good foods
Wheat cereals, parsnip, tomato (remove skin first, and sieve), sweet corn, soaked, dried apricots.
Foods to avoid Biscuits, cake, ice cream, pastry, fried foods. Don't give whole egg before one year.

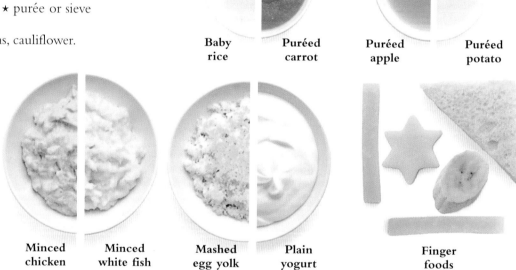

Minced chicken **Minced white fish** **Mashed egg yolk** **Plain yogurt** **Finger foods**

HOW TO STORE YOUR BABY'S FOOD

Have nutritious, home-cooked food for your baby always on hand by making up batches of purées and freezing them. Purée fruits and vegetables separately, and cool them quickly by standing the bowl in cold water. Pour the purée into ice-cube trays, cover with plastic wrap, and freeze. When frozen, empty the cubes out and store in sealed freezer bags, one type of food per bag. Label with the name and date, and don't keep for longer than one month.

Half an hour before a mealtime, put some cubes in a bowl to thaw—one or two will be enough at first. Stand the bowl in hot water to heat the purée, then transfer the purée to your baby's bowl.

You can keep a prepared food for your baby in the fridge for up to 24 hours; always cover it first. After your baby has finished her meal, throw away any food that your baby's spoon has been dipped into, including commercial baby foods if you have fed her straight from the jar.

8–9 MONTHS

Texture Introduce your child to chunkier textures now, so chop food rather than mashing it. Give plenty of finger foods to encourage feeding skills. Stay nearby when she is eating finger foods in case she chokes.

Preparation, fruit/vegetables
★ peel carefully
★ remove ends and stems
★ give in slices or sticks or grate, if raw
★ chop or mash, if cooked: leave plenty of lumps.

Preparation, meat/fish
★ trim fat and skin off
★ cook: grill, stew, or poach
★ mince lumpily.

Other good foods Toast, red meat, home-cooked dishes, e.g. lasagne, soup, or shepherd's pie (cooked without salt).

10–12 MONTHS

Texture Your child is eating almost everything the family eats, chopped into bite-sized pieces. Continue to avoid salt in your cooking; you can salt your own food at the table.

Preparation, fruit/vegetables
★ peel carefully
★ remove ends and stems
★ if cooked, steam whenever possible.

Preparation, meat/fish
★ trim fat and skin off
★ cook: grill, stew, or poach
★ chop up small.

Other good foods Pork (if thoroughly cooked), stronger-flavored foods, for example, cabbage, green pepper, whole peeled tomato.

Foods to avoid Fatty or salty foods, sugary foods, soft unpasteurized cheeses.

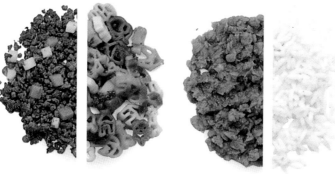

Lean ground beef or lamb   **Pasta**   **Mashed lentils**   **Brown rice**

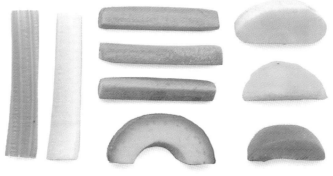

Finger foods

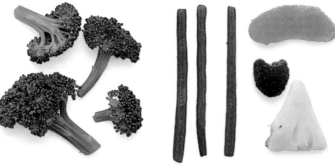

Steamed broccoli   **Green beans**   **Fruits**

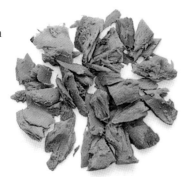

Canned tuna

DEVELOP A WATER HABIT

Many children never drink plain water, but have fruit juices instead. Some derive as much as a third of their daily calorie requirements from these drinks, which reduce their appetite for other foods. They may contribute to tooth decay too. Offer water when your child is thirsty between meals so she doesn't develop a "fruit juice habit." Colas and similar fizzy drinks aren't suitable for young children, neither are "diet" soft drinks, which may contain high levels of artificial sweeteners.

IRON AND VITAMINS

The best way to make sure your baby gets the nourishment she needs is to offer her a wide range of foods. The store of iron she was born with will begin to run out when she is about six months old. Good sources of iron include: red meat, liver, dried fruit, breakfast cereals, lentils and egg yolk. Your baby will be able to absorb more iron if she eats foods containing vitamin C (found in fruit and vegetables) at the same time. Don't give your baby tea—it will reduce the amount of iron she absorbs from her food.

WARNING

Never give a preschool child peanuts. It's easy for a small child to inhale a fragment accidentally, and if this happens the oil in the peanuts can cause severe irritation in the lungs.

INTRODUCING FIRST TASTES

Between four to six months your baby is probably ready to sample small amounts of solid food. There is no rush—you can wait until six months if she seems happy and content on milk alone. For the first weeks you're simply introducing her to the idea of eating solid food from a spoon; breast or formula milk is still providing her with all the nourishment that she needs. Start at the breakfast or lunchtime feeding, avoiding dinnertime because of the possibility of a food upsetting her and giving you both a disturbed night's sleep. She will most likely be more cooperative if you let her partially satisfy her hunger first, so "sandwich" a teaspoon of baby cereal or fruit purée between two halves of her normal breast- or bottle-feed. The whole process might take as long as an hour.

YOU WILL NEED
Bib
Small plastic bowl or eggcup
Small plastic spoon
About a dessertspoonful of fresh apple or pear purée, or baby rice
Damp tissue or washcloth

FEED HER FIRST

Sit down comfortably with your baby's bowl of food within reach. Put a bib on her, then give her half her usual breast- or bottle-feed: let her empty one breast, or give her half her bottle. Don't rush her. She will go on needing her milk feeds for several months to come.

FOLLOW YOUR BABY'S CUES

Infant feeding can be divided into three stages: (1) the nursing period when only formula or human breast milk is given, (2) a transitional period when solids are added, and (3) a modified adult phase during which the bulk of your child's caloric intake comes from the table and less and less from bottle or breast. Most children reach the third stage after their first birthday. Be spontaneous and creative at mealtimes. If your child detests cereal for breakfast and loves sweet potatoes, listen to him. He may not be able to talk but he's speaking his mind loudly and clearly.

GIVING YOUR BABY HER FIRST TASTES

1 With her still on your lap, scoop a little food on to the spoon – enough to coat the tip. Put the spoon between your baby's lips so that she can suck the food off. Don't try to push the spoon in, she will gag if she feels food at the back of her tongue. She may be surprised at the taste and sensation at first, so be patient and talk to her encouragingly.

2 She may quickly discover that she enjoys this new experience. If she pushes the food out, scrape it up and put the spoon between her lips again. When she's had about a teaspoonful of purée or cereal, wipe her mouth and chin and resume her milk feeding.

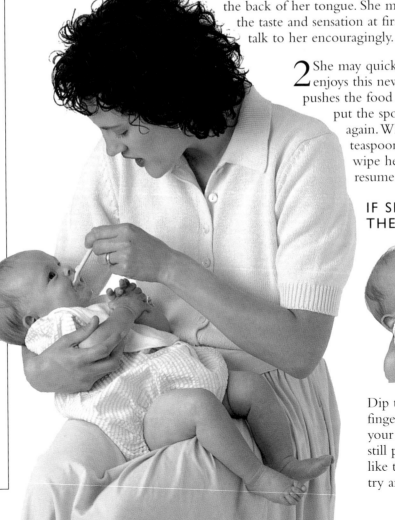

IF SHE FUSSES AT THE SPOON

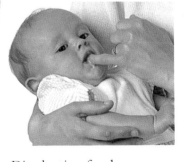

Dip the tip of a clean finger into the food and let your baby suck that. If she still protests, she may not like the taste of that food; try another next time.

YOUR BABY'S NUTRITIONAL NEEDS

How you balance breast- or bottle-feedings with solid foods will depend very much on your baby's temperament and your own lifestyle. The most important thing is not to rush her. Take one step at a time, and let her adjust before taking the next. The chart below is just one way you might approach feeding: it assumes you start at about six months.

Discuss with your doctor the best time for your baby to start solids. Remember that if you are breast-feeding, your milk production system needs to wind down gradually. Drop one feeding at a time, and leave at least three days before dropping another. If your baby will not eat a certain food she may just not like the taste—like adults babies dislike some foods.

A STAGE-BY-STAGE GUIDE TO INFANT FEEDING							
Stage/age	**What to do**	**Drinks**	**Meals and feedings**				
			EARLY AM	BREAK-FAST	LUNCH	DINNER	BED-TIME
Weeks 1 and 2 Age 6 months (ages are guidelines only)	Give small tastes of baby cereal or fruit or vegetable purée at lunchtime, halfway through the breast- or bottle-feeding. Give the same food for three days to accustom your baby to it.	If you are bottle-feeding, offer your baby occasional drinks of cooled boiled water.	▪	▪	▪ ▪ ▪	▪	▪
Weeks 3 and 4 Age 6½ months	Introduce solid food at breakfast, halfway through the feeding: baby cereal or other single-grain cereal is ideal. Increase the amount of solid food at lunchtime to 3–4 teaspoonfuls.	Offer cooled boiled water or diluted fruit juice in a bottle. Don't worry if she doesn't want any.	▪	▪ ▪ ▪	▪ ▪ ▪	▪	▪
Weeks 5 and 6 Age 7 months	Introduce solid food at dinner, halfway through the feeding. A week later, offer two courses at lunch: follow a vegetable purée with a fruit one, giving 2–3 teaspoonfuls of each.	Introduce a trainer cup, but don't expect her to be able to drink from it yet— it's just a toy.		▪ ▪ ▪	▪ ▪ ▪ ▪	▪ ▪ ▪	▪
Weeks 7 and 8 Age 7½ months	Offer solid food as the first part of lunch, then give breast or bottle to top up. She can have two courses at dinner now, a vegetable and a piece of banana, for example. At breakfast and dinner, continue giving the feeding first. She may eat 5–6 teaspoonfuls of solid food at each meal now.	You can start to give your baby drinks in her cup, but hold it for her as she drinks from it.		▪ ▪ ▪	▪ ▪ ▪	▪ ▪ ▪ ▪	▪
Weeks 9 and 10 Age 8 months	After lunch solids, offer a drink of formula or breast milk from a cup. After a few days with no lunchtime breast or bottle, offer solid food as the first part of dinner.	Offer formula or breast milk in a cup at each meal and water or diluted juice at other times.		▪ ▪ ▪	▪ ▪	▪ ▪ ▪	▪
Weeks 11 and 12 Age 8½ months	Offer your baby a drink of breast or formula milk in a cup instead of a full feeding after her dinner. You may find she often refuses her breast or bottle feeding after her breakfast solids now.	As before.		▪ ▪	▪ ▪	▪ ▪	▪
Week 13 onwards Age 9 months	Offer a drink in a cup instead of the feeding before breakfast: now your baby is having solids at three meals a day. Breast or formula milk should be the main milk drink until one year. She can have cow's milk from 12 months.	As before. Your baby may possibly be able to manage her own trainer cup now.		▪	▪ ▪	▪ ▪	▪
			Key	▫ feeding	▪ solid food		

HOW YOUR BABY LEARNS TO FEED HERSELF

Your baby will be keen to try and feed herself long before she's able to do so efficiently. However messy an experience this is—be prepared for food to end up all over her face and clothes, in her hair (and yours!) and on the floor—and however long-drawn-out it makes mealtimes, try to encourage her as much as you can, it is her first real step toward independence. Try to keep a calm and relaxed attitude at meal times and don't rush your baby: if your baby finds them interesting and enjoyable occasions, you are less likely to encounter problems over food and eating in the future.

AT SEVEN MONTHS

Your baby may be making determined efforts to feed herself by this age, but she won't be coordinated enough to get all the food she needs into her mouth. Feed her yourself, but don't stop her from playing with her food. Smearing it over her face may be messy, but it's the first step in learning to feed herself; have a clean washcloth to wipe her with when she's finished. Give her plenty of different finger foods, too. They're easy to handle, so she will gain in confidence and dexterity.

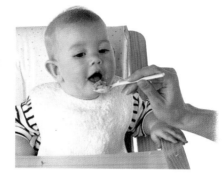

1 She will be hungry at the start of the meal. Keep the bowl out of her reach and spoon-feed her.

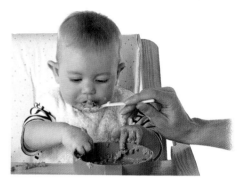

2 Once you've satisfied her initial hunger, let her join in but continue feeding her yourself.

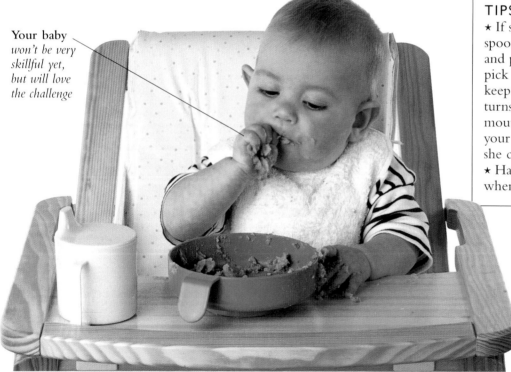

Your baby *won't be very skillful yet, but will love the challenge*

3 Your baby may get so absorbed in the pleasure of dabbling her fingers in her bowl and pushing the food into her mouth that she will lose interest in you feeding her with a spoon. If she's still hungry, she may cry and wriggle out of frustration because she can't get the food in quickly enough, so offer some more spoonfuls. Otherwise let her practice her feeding skills: feeling "I can do it myself" is important to her. She knows when she's had enough.

TIPS TO HELP
★ If she grabs your spoon, use two spoons at the same meal. Fill one and put it in her bowl so she can pick it up. Fill the other one and keep it ready for when her spoon turns over on the way to her mouth. When this happens, pop your full spoon in, and fill hers so she can try again.
★ Have clean spoons ready for when she drops hers on the floor.

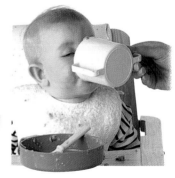

4 Eating solid food may make her thirsty, so offer her formula or breast milk at mealtimes and tip the cup for her—she won't be able to hold it herself yet.

"How much food should I offer my baby?"

Let your baby decide how much food she wants at each meal. At six months, start with no more than four tablespoons of food in her bowl, and offer more if she eats it all. With cereal, start with about two tablespoons. Some days she will eat voraciously, others hardly anything. If she is gaining weight normally, there's no need to worry that she's not getting enough.

"My child will only eat fruits and no meats. What can I do?"

Food fads are extremely common in young children, and thankfully usually don't last more than a couple of weeks. Don't stop offering your child other things at mealtimes, but don't worry or get frustrated with him if he won't eat them; he won't suffer if he is getting vital nutrients from other sources. If you are concerned that he is missing vital nutrients, ask your doctor for advice.

"Should I make him eat things he doesn't seem to like?"

Respect your child's opinions. If he doesn't like something, don't mix it with something he does like—he will only end up disliking both. Try varying the form in which you give a particular food. Young babies are often wary of certain textures, so try making his food less lumpy. For example, if he doesn't like vegetables, he might eat them raw or liquidized in soup.

FIFTEEN MONTHS

Your child will be making a good attempt to feed himself with a spoon or fork with rounded prongs, so cut his food into bite-sized pieces. He may need your help on some days.

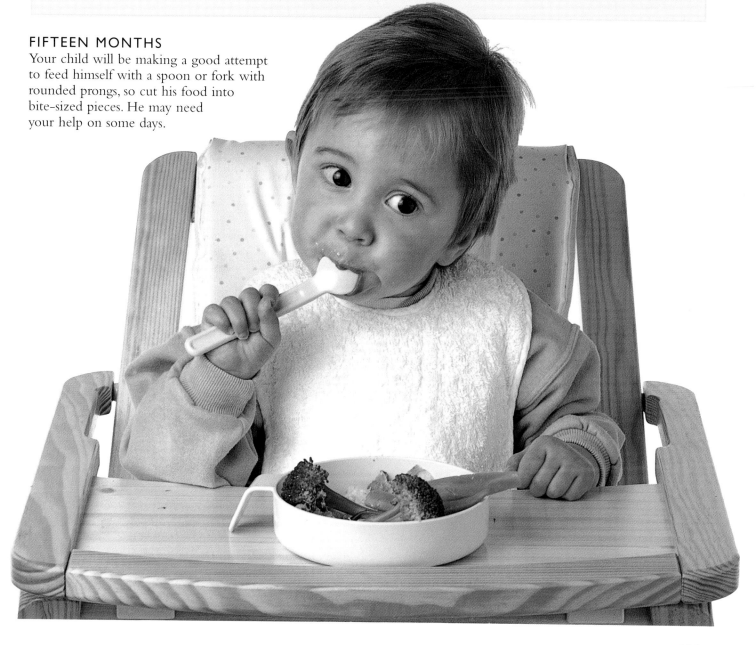

EATING AND YOUR OLDER CHILD

By the age of two your child will probably be ready to graduate out of his high chair and join you at the table. Mealtimes are important social occasions, and learning how to participate as a member of the family is a vital part of your child's social development. What he eats is important too; it's your job to offer enough good food and it's up to him to eat it. Don't force-feed or hover over him worrying about every bite he does or doesn't take. He won't starve, and he knows best how much food he wants.

A healthy snack
An apple is always a good source of fiber and vitamins. Wash it well first, or peel it.

Avoiding mealtime problems

The secret to avoiding mealtime problems is to keep your own attitude relaxed and friendly. From the beginning, make your child feel that eating is a pleasurable way to satisfy his hunger. It is always a mistake to battle over eating—you will end up more upset than your child, and he may refuse more vehemently next time. Instead, keep the eating issue in perspective for both of you, for it should be an enjoyable experience:
★ Offer your toddler a varied diet, and let him choose what he wants to eat. He will soon make his likes and dislikes clear.
★ Don't punish him for not eating a particular food, and don't reward him for eating something either. Saying "if you finish your carrots you can ride your tricycle" will make any child think there must be something terrible about carrots if he has to be rewarded for eating them.
★ Don't spend a great deal of time preparing food especially for him: you will only feel doubly resentful if he doesn't eat it.
★ If he dawdles over his food, don't rush him to finish it. He's bound to be slower than you. If you would expect him to stay at the table while you finish your meal, then you must do the same and wait for him to finish when he's slow.
★ Don't force him to eat more than he wants. Let him decide when he has had enough. He won't starve, and if he's growing normally, you know he's eating enough.

The right diet

Variety is the keynote of a good diet: if you offer many different foods throughout the week, you can be reasonably sure that your child is getting the nutrients he needs. His diet will only be unhealthy if for long periods he eats too much of some kinds of food. For instance, a diet based entirely on crackers, cakes, cookies, highly processed snack foods, or hot dogs and take-out hamburgers is a terrible idea.

Snacks and sweets

Your child will often need a snack to give him energy between meals. Rather than cookies or crackers, offer him healthy, nutritious snacks such as a piece of wholegrain bread, an apple, a carrot, or a banana. If he's not very hungry at the next meal, he won't have missed out nutritionally. Sweets can be a battleground, but it's not fair or realistic to ban them altogether; your child may learn to covet them even more. But sweets provide few nutrients, and they are very bad for your child's teeth.

Control your child's love of anything sweet by keeping sugary and sweetened foods to a minimum:
★ Provide fruit or unsweetened yogurt for dessert at meals. Cheese is excellent too, because it neutralizes the acid that forms in the mouth and attacks tooth enamel.
★ When you do let your child have sweets, offer them at the end of the meal, not between meals.
★ Choose sweets that can be eaten quickly, rather than sucked or chewed for a long time.
★ Give pure fruit juices rather than presweetened or carbonated beverages, and provide them only at meals; offer milk or water at other times.
★ Don't use sweets to reward or punish your child: they will become intensely valuable to him, and thus harder to control.
★ Make brushing with fluoride toothpaste a routine at least after breakfast and before bed (see pages 144–45).

WAYS TO IMPROVE YOUR FAMILY'S DIET

★ Use vegetable margarine and olive oil instead of butter for spreading and cooking.
★ Keep red meat to a minimum: once or twice a week is enough.
★ Cook chicken or fish at least three times a week.
★ Grill or broil rather than fry.
★ Use fresh rather than processed foods—they will contain more nutrients and less salt and sugar.
★ Buy wholegrain bread and avoid presweetened cereals.
★ Serve vegetables raw as often as possible, or cook them only lightly. Any cooking destroys nutrients, but steaming is best.

CRYING AND YOUR BABY

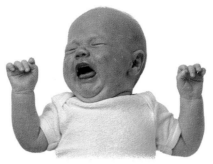

Your baby is bound to cry a lot in his first year. It's his only means of communicating his need for food and comfort, but from around three months you will see a change. Instead of spending much of his waking time crying, he will use that time to learn about the world around him. The crying spells will lessen, and you will become more adept at knowing what he wants. When your baby cries, your instinct will be to cuddle him; don't worry that by doing so you are spoiling him. Your baby needs to know that he can rely on you. Nevertheless, constant bouts of crying are exhausting for you. If you find that your baby cries so much that you are losing patience, talk to your doctor.

WAYS TO SOOTHE YOUR NEWBORN

When your baby cries, it is important to respond quickly, without making a fuss: letting him cry for a long time will agitate him more.

SEVEN WAYS TO SOOTHE YOUR CRYING BABY

Feed her In the first months hunger is the most likely reason for your baby crying, and offering a breast or bottle is the most effective way to soothe her—even if that means frequent feedings day and night. If your baby is bottle-fed and sucks hungrily at her bottle with short gaps between bottles, try offering cool water: she may be thirsty.

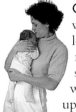

Cuddle her Very often this will be just the sort of loving contact your baby needs to calm down and stop crying. If she quiets when you hold her upright against your shoulder, or face down in your arms (see page 83), it may have been gas that was making her cry. If she has been passed around for relatives and friends to hold, she may just want a few quiet moments of being cuddled by a familiar parent.

Rock her rhythmically Movement often comforts a cranky baby, and may put her to sleep. Rock her in your arms, and if she doesn't quiet down, try rocking faster—perhaps 60 to 70 rocks per minute. Alternatively, jiggle her up and down by shifting from foot to foot, perhaps with your baby in an infant carrier on your chest (see page 85). Or rock with her in a rocking chair, if you have one. You can also put her in her carriage and push her back and forth; if you can take her around the block, the gentle bumping over the pavement will soothe her.

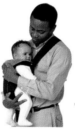

Carry her Very often you will be able to soothe your baby simply by putting him in the carrier and carrying him around with you. This leaves your hands free, and your baby will be soothed both by the close physical contact with you and the motion as you move around. If your baby is crying because of something you've had to do to him —changing his diaper, bathing, or dressing him, for example—using a carrier may be the best way to calm him, and probably may even send him off to sleep.

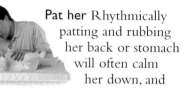

Pat her Rhythmically patting and rubbing her back or stomach will often calm her down, and may help her to bring up gas. The feel of your hand will often comfort her when you first put her down to change her diaper, too.

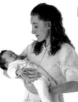

Give him something to suck Almost all babies are soothed by sucking, and nowadays mothers are often sent home from the hospital with a soother for their newborn. You might also offer your cranky baby your own clean little finger. Some newborns suck their own thumbs or fists.

Distract your baby Something to look at may make your baby forget why he was crying, at least for a while. Bright, colorful patterns may fascinate him: he will often gaze intently at postcards, wallpaper, or your clothes. Faces and mirrors are also excellent distractions, and a walk around the house to look at photographs or to peer into a mirror at his own reflection may calm him.

SEVEN REASONS YOUR BABY MIGHT BE CRYING

Often you won't really know why your young baby is crying or why he stopped. There may be times he is crying for no reason at all. If you've tried the simple remedies such as feeding and cuddling, and you've tried the soothing tactics that usually work (see previous page), all without success, there may be another reason. Listed below are other possible causes.

Illness may be making your baby cry, particularly if his crying sounds different from normal. Always call your doctor if your baby shows any symptoms that are unusual for him. A blocked nose from a cold may prevent him from feeding or sucking his soother or thumb, so he can't comfort himself even though he may not be very ill. Your doctor can prescribe medication to help him breathe easily. (See pages 180–81.)

Diaper rash or a sore bottom may make your baby cry. If he has a sore bottom, take off his diaper, clean him thoroughly, and, if possible, don't put a diaper back on for the rest of the day: just lay him on a towel. Try to stop the rash from getting worse (see page 150).

Colic, often called three-month or evening colic, is characterized by a pattern of regular, intense, inconsolable screaming at a particular time each day, usually the late afternoon or evening. The pattern appears at about three weeks, and continues until 12 or 14 weeks. The crying spell may last as long as three hours. Always ask for medical advice the first time your baby screams inconsolably. Colic isn't harmful, but you might misdiagnose it and miss other, serious symptoms.

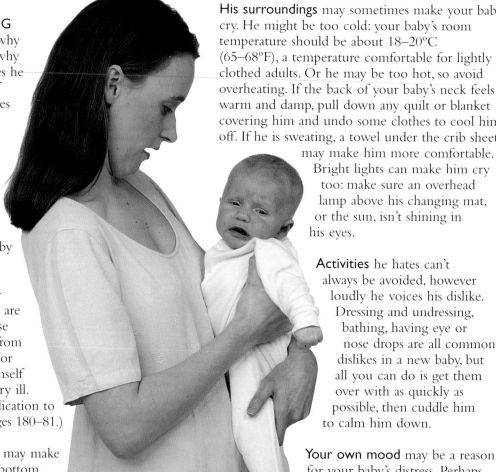

His surroundings may sometimes make your baby cry. He might be too cold: your baby's room temperature should be about 18–20°C (65–68°F), a temperature comfortable for lightly clothed adults. Or he may be too hot, so avoid overheating. If the back of your baby's neck feels warm and damp, pull down any quilt or blanket covering him and undo some clothes to cool him off. If he is sweating, a towel under the crib sheet may make him more comfortable. Bright lights can make him cry too: make sure an overhead lamp above his changing mat, or the sun, isn't shining in his eyes.

Activities he hates can't always be avoided, however loudly he voices his dislike. Dressing and undressing, bathing, having eye or nose drops are all common dislikes in a new baby, but all you can do is get them over with as quickly as possible, then cuddle him to calm him down.

Your own mood may be a reason for your baby's distress. Perhaps it's evening and you are feeling tired; perhaps his crankiness is making you feel irritable. Knowing that your baby is often just reacting to your own emotions may help you to be calmer with him.

Too much fussing can sometimes make an upset baby cry all the more. Passing him between you, changing a diaper that doesn't need to be changed, offering to feed him again and again, discussing his crying in anxious voices, may all make him even more agitated, so he cries all the harder. If there seems to be no obvious reason for his crying, don't keep trying to find one: he probably just wants to be held.

COPING WITH COLIC

All you can do if your baby has colic is learn to live with it, in the certain knowledge that he isn't ill or abnormal, and that the colic won't last. Don't suffer alone: this will be a difficult three months for you, your partner, and your baby. Try to remember these three points:

★ Do whatever you can to try to soothe your baby. Keeping him in motion, feeding him frequently, rubbing his stomach rhythmically, or just cuddling him, may all soothe him for a short while.

★ Don't resort to medications. You can't cure his colic, so you will be giving your baby large doses of medication for no real purpose.

★ Try to have an occasional evening out. You can leave your partner or a competent, trusted relative in charge.

YOUR CRYING OLDER BABY

From the age of about three months, you may notice a real change in your baby. She's now much more aware of what goes on around her, she's responsive and interested in everything —more of a person altogether. She'll still cry a lot, and will continue to do so for many months to come, but by now you may have a much better idea of why.

SIX REASONS WHY YOUR OLDER BABY MIGHT BE CRYING

Hunger is still an obvious reason for your baby to cry. As her first year progresses and she becomes mobile and moves on to solid food, she will often get tired and cranky between meals— her life is a busy one. A snack and a drink may restore her energy and cheer her up.

Anxiety will be a new reason for crying from the age of seven or eight months, because by then she's discovered her unshakable attachment to you. You are her "safe base;" she'll be happy to explore the world, provided that she can keep you in sight. She may cry if you leave her, or if she loses sight of you. Be patient with her, and let her get used to new people and situations gradually.

Pain, from bumps as she becomes mobile, will be a frequent cause of tears. Often it will be the shock that makes her cry, rather than any injury, so a sympathetic cuddle and a distracting toy will usually help her forget it quickly.

Wanting to get her own way will often be a cause of friction and tears, particularly from the age of two. It's worth asking yourself if you're frustrating her unnecessarily, or perhaps trying to assert your own will; but sometimes she will need to be held back for her safety. If she gets so angry that she throws a tantrum, don't shout at her, or try reasoning with her, or punish her afterward. It's best to ignore the tantrum completely. Wait until the fit of temper has passed, then continue with whatever you were going to do (see also page 176).

Frustration, as your baby tries to do things that are beyond her capabilities, will be a more and more common reason for crying. You can't avoid this although you can make life easier for her. For example, put her toys where she can reach them. Distraction is the best cure: introduce a new game or toy and her tears may soon be forgotten. Or help her if she's struggling, but don't take over completely.

"Every new tooth my toddler cuts is preceded by days of crying. What can I do to help him?"

The first teeth shouldn't cause any trouble, but the back teeth, cut during the second year, can be painful. Your child will probably dribble a lot and have a red cheek for a couple of days. There are ways you can help him:
■ Rub his gums with your little finger.
■ Give him something firm to chew on: a teething ring is fine and is even more soothing if you chill it in the refrigerator first.
■ If you use a gel- or water-filled teething ring, put it in the refrigerator, not the freezer: frozen ones can cause frostbite.
■ Check for sharp edges on his smaller toys.
■ Avoid giving him repeated doses of medications or teething gels.

Overtiredness will show itself in whininess, irritability, and finally tears. By the end of her first year your child's life is so full of new experiences that she can run out of energy before she's run out of enthusiasm. She needs you to help her relax enough to get the sleep she needs. A quiet time sitting on your lap listening to a story may work, and a calming, enjoyable bedtime routine (see pages 124–25) that you all stick to every evening will help, too.

SLEEP AND YOUR BABY

Broken nights and lack of sleep for you will be a fact of life for many weeks until your baby settles into a routine that coincides more closely with yours. At around nine months, new problems may develop. She may be very reluctant to let you leave her, or she may settle into a pattern of night waking. Careful handling at bedtime from around the middle of your baby's first year can

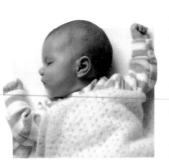

help avoid problems later: a relaxing bedtime routine that takes place in exactly the same way every night will give her the sense of security she needs. Until at least the age of two-and-a-half, and probably much longer, some daytime sleep will be essential. Your toddler's life is an active, exciting one, and she will need a reviving nap to prevent her from getting overtired and irritable.

EQUIPMENT FOR SLEEP

What you buy for your baby to sleep in will be a significant investment, so shop around. If you buy a secondhand crib, make sure it was manufactured after September 1986, when regulations on lead paint, spaces between bars, and mattress support systems were consolidated. You will need machine-washable bedding—a comforter is light and warm, but a restless child may sleep better tucked in with a sheet and blankets.

Crib Your baby will be sleeping in this for some time, so invest in a sturdy, well-made one. Safety is paramount: a new crib should conform to the 1986 Cribs and Cradles Regulations of the Hazardous Products Act, which is enforced by Health Canada.

WHAT TO SLEEP IN

Cradle A cradle may be used in the first months of your baby's life, until she can sit up—then you should use a crib. Discontinue using a crib, however, as soon as your child can climb out unaided or when she reaches 90cm (35in).

Infant carrier For your young baby, a carrier that you clip to a wheeled chassis is very handy. Make sure it conforms to safety standards: it provides somewhere for her to sleep day or night, and a good way to transport her outdoors.

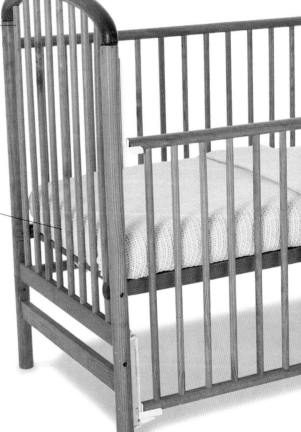

Watch for _any sharp edges: sand them down if necessary_

A fitted sheet _in 100% cotton is easy to put on and comfortable for your baby_

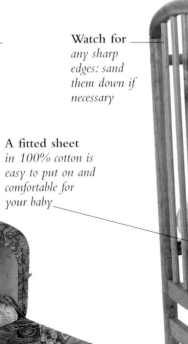

Handles _enable you to transport your baby easily while she's asleep_

YOUR BABY'S BEDDING

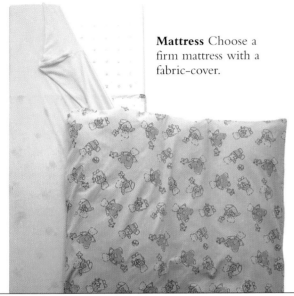

Mattress Choose a firm mattress with a fabric-cover.

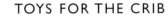

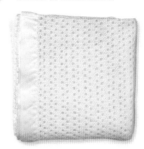

Bumper pad Bumper pads are not recommended for young babies, as they interfere with air circulation. As well, older babies may be able to climb up on the pads, which is hazardous.

Fitted sheet and comforter Light and warm, a comforter is suitable for a baby over a year old. For your newborn baby, however, choose a brushed cotton sheet and cellular blankets so you can regulate her temperature and avoid overheating.

Cellular blanket Cellular cotton blankets are best for very young babies.

TOYS FOR THE CRIB

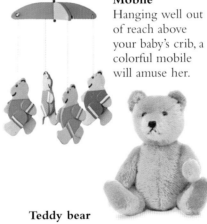

Mobile Hanging well out of reach above your baby's crib, a colorful mobile will amuse her.

Teddy bear

YOUR BABY'S ROOM

★ Keep the room warm: 16–20°C (61–68°F) is ideal. At this temperature a sheet plus up to three layers of blankets is enough for her.

★ Install a dimmer switch or nightlight, so you can check on your baby while she's asleep without disturbing her.

★ A baby monitor is useful to have in your baby's room, unless you live in a small flat. The type that can be plugged in wherever you are is the most flexible.

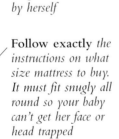

The dropside mechanism *should be one that your baby can't release by herself*

Follow exactly *the instructions on what size mattress to buy. It must fit snugly all round so your baby can't get her face or head trapped*

The mattress base *should be at least 59.5cm (2ft) from the top edge of the cot, so your baby cannot climb out. You should be able to lower the base*

The spaces *between the bars should not be less than 2.5cm (1in), so she can't get an arm or leg stuck; and not more than 6cm (2½in), so she can't slip out feet first*

BABY MONITORS

Baby monitors have two separate units —one part is left close to the baby and the other goes with whoever is listening. A microphone means you can sit anywhere in the house and know your baby isn't crying. Many monitors now come with additional features such as adjustable volume on the parent unit, integrated nightlight, and remote digital room temperature display. As with any electrical equipment sold or used in Canada, look for the certification mark (CSA, ULC, or $_c$UL) to indicate the product is certified to Canadian Standards.

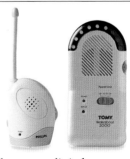

DAYTIME AND NIGHTTIME SLEEP

Your newborn baby will sleep as much as she needs to; the only trouble is she may not take her sleep when you would like her to. In the early days she will sleep in short bursts randomly throughout the day and night. The chart below shows how her sleep pattern might develop: as the months pass, her longest period of sleep coincides more and more with the hours of night, and her wakeful times become longer. However, babies vary. Don't worry if yours takes longer than you expected (or hoped) to sleep through the night.

Emphasizing day and night

Right from the newborn stage, make a clear distinction between how you treat daytime and nighttime sleep, to help your baby learn which time is for play, and which for sleep. During the day put her to sleep in a carriage, cradle, or bassinet: if you're using a crib already, save it for nighttime only. A carriage can go outside with you, in a shady spot. Always cover the carriage with an insect net and have the brakes on. Indoors, make sure pets can't get into the room where your baby is, but there is no need to keep the house especially quiet for her. When your baby cries, pick her up and make the most of her waking time: help her to associate daylight hours with play and wakefulness.

At night, cover your baby lightly in her carriage, or crib if you're already using one. Keep the room dark. When she wakes and cries for a feeding, pick her up and feed her quietly, talking as little as possible and only changing her diaper if she's very wet or messy. She'll start to learn that nighttime feedings are business only, not social times, and her sleep pattern will become more like yours as the weeks go by.

Your toddler's naps

From the age of about six months, bedtime will become a more important ritual in your baby's day, and she needs to be tired and ready for bed if she is to sleep through the night. She needs some daytime sleep to give her energy for her active life, and will go on needing it throughout toddlerhood, but don't let her nap for too long. Allow two hours for each nap (she may wake earlier), then wake her. She may be grumpy and confused if she was deeply asleep, so give her plenty of time before introducing the next activity.

"My ten-month-old wakes up at 6am and will not go back to sleep again. Is there anything we can do about this?"

Early-morning waking probably just means your baby has had enough sleep. Put a few toys in his crib each night to occupy him for a while when he wakes. When he tires of his toys and calls for you, try changing his diaper and offering him some new toys in his crib to see if it gains you an extra hour's sleep.

If early waking is a regular pattern for your baby, you could try adjusting his sleep times throughout the day so that he has a later bedtime. Put up thick curtains in his bedroom so that the sun won't wake him. Don't worry, as he gets older he will probably waken later.

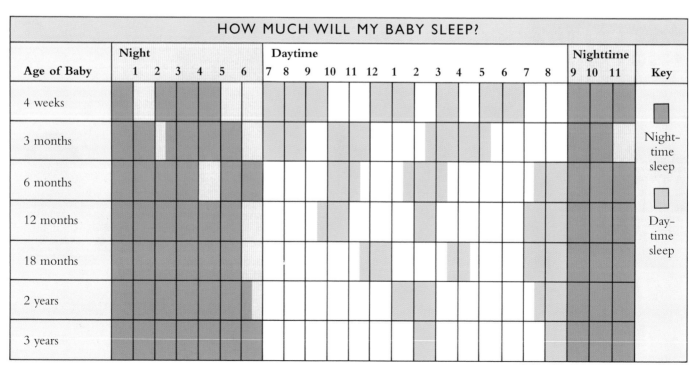

HOW MUCH WILL MY BABY SLEEP?

Age of Baby	Night						Daytime													Nighttime			Key
	1	2	3	4	5	6	7	8	9	10	11	12	1	2	3	4	5	6	7	8	9	10	11	
4 weeks																								
3 months																								
6 months																								
12 months																								
18 months																								
2 years																								
3 years																								

Key: ■ Nighttime sleep □ Daytime sleep

GETTING THE TEMPERATURE RIGHT

The risk of crib death is increased when a baby is overwrapped or overheated, especially if he is feverish or unwell. And yet it is important not to let your baby become chilled. The ideal room temperature for the room where your baby sleeps is about 18°C (65°F)—a comfortable temperature for a lightly clothed adult. If the room is at this temperature, a baby who is wearing a sleep suit and an undershirt will also need to be covered by a sheet and three layers of blankets. Wrapping a very young baby snugly in a blanket stops his limbs jerking as he drops off to sleep and often helps him settle more easily. But there is a risk of overheating unless you remember that a baby who is wrapped like this will need fewer blankets to cover him. Comforters should not be used for babies under a year. Don't add extra bedding if your baby is unwell or feverish, or expose the baby to direct heat from a hot water bottle, electric blanket, or radiant heater.

Lay your baby
half way down the bed

SLEEPTIME SAFETY

★ Never let your baby sleep with a pillow until at least two: it could smother her.
★ Put your baby to sleep on her back. Doctors believe this is the safest position. Babies who sleep on their front seem to run an increased risk of crib death.
★ Remove any plastic packaging from the mattress and don't use a plastic sheet.
★ Don't let your baby get too hot or too cold.
★ Don't smoke, and keep your baby in a smoke-free atmosphere.
★ Place your baby in the feet to foot position so he can't slip down beneath the covers.

Crib death A few babies each year die unexpectedly in their cribs. There is no explanation for crib death, or Sudden Infant Death Syndrome, but doctors have suggested some safety precautions (see left) that can help minimize the risk of crib death occurring. If you always put your baby to sleep on his back, make sure that he is not exposed to cigarette smoke, and are careful to see that he does not become overheated, you can greatly reduce the risk of crib death.

If you think your baby is unwell, consult your doctor straight away.

PUTTING YOUR BABY IN THE "FEET TO FOOT" POSITION

Place your baby's feet at the foot of the crib and tuck in the covers securely so they reach no higher than his shoulders and cannot slip up and cover his head. Babies whose heads are accidentally covered with bedding get too hot and run a greater risk of crib death.

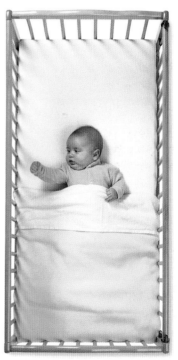

Putting a baby to bed
Babies regulate their body temperature by losing heat from their face and head. If a baby slips beneath the bedclothes so that his face and head are covered, heat can't be lost as easily. Make sure the bedding is arranged so that this can't happen. Unless the room is very cold, infants over one month should not wear hats indoors for sleeping.

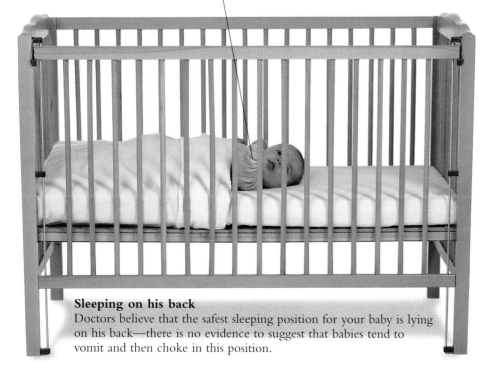

Sleeping on his back
Doctors believe that the safest sleeping position for your baby is lying on his back—there is no evidence to suggest that babies tend to vomit and then choke in this position.

SETTLING FOR SLEEP

There will be times when your baby won't settle contentedly off to sleep after a feeding. Gentle rocking, or a quiet period in your arms may help to relax her and send her off to sleep. But eventually you want her to learn to fall asleep on her own, so try to keep these soothing methods for times when she is really fretful so she does not become too dependent on them.

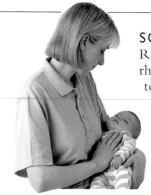

SOOTHING CONTACT
Rubbing your baby's stomach rhythmically may soothe her enough to send her to sleep. Don't alter the rhythm or you will disturb her, and don't stop until her eyelids have closed.

ROCKING
Rock your baby to and fro in your arms to lull her to sleep. You may have to keep it up for some time, and she may wake every time you stop to put her in her crib, but it's still a tried and true way to send her to sleep.

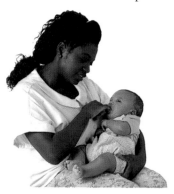

SUCKING
Your baby will be soothed by sucking, and your clean little finger is ideal. He may suck his own fist. If you don't mind him having a soother, use a natural-shaped one. Ask your doctor for advice.

Ensure adequate *support for his head*

AN INFANT CARRIER
If your baby wakes every time you put him down, try carrying him around in an infant carrier: the motion of your body will keep him asleep (see page 85).

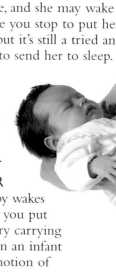

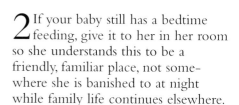

YOUR OLDER BABY'S BEDTIME ROUTINE

From about six months, your baby will settle down to sleep more happily if the whole process of going to bed takes place in exactly the same way—babies love routine and rituals. From now on she won't be quite so ready to go to sleep in strange surroundings, and her sleep patterns will be easily upset by a change in daily life, so try to impose the normal routine even if you're away from home. Make getting ready for bed as much fun as you can, so it's a pleasurable, but undemanding, part of your baby's day.

WHAT TIME IS BEDTIME?
It's up to you and your partner to choose a time that fits in with your own routine—and one that you can stick to more or less every day. Make sure it's late enough that you're both home, and not so late that the routine takes up all your evening. Any time between 6 pm and 8 pm is suitable.

THE BEDTIME ROUTINE
1 Start the routine in the same way every evening. A bath is ideal, because it's both fun and relaxing. If she doesn't like being bathed, 20 minutes spent playing a gentle game together might help her unwind.

2 If your baby still has a bedtime feeding, give it to her in her room so she understands this to be a friendly, familiar place, not somewhere she is banished to at night while family life continues elsewhere.

3 Put your baby into her crib with her favorite teddy bear or soft toys and her security blanket if she has one.

4 Now perhaps your partner could take over, so you're both involved in the bedtime routine. This last half hour or so needs to be always the same, to mark it clearly as the end of the day.

RHYTHMIC MOVEMENTS

Pushing your baby to and fro in her buggy will often soothe her to sleep, although she may keep trying to look at you. When she does drop off, don't lift her out right away to put her in her crib, even if it is nighttime.

A CAR RIDE

If you get desperate, try putting your baby in his car seat and going for a drive round the block: the motion will probably put him to sleep automatically. When you get home again, leave him undisturbed in his seat and carry both indoors. Cover him with a blanket to keep him warm.

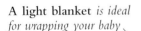

*A **light blanket** is ideal for wrapping your baby*

WRAPPING

Some babies sleep more peacefully with their arms tucked in to their covers. Others will always work their arms loose from the covers. If your baby prefers to sleep this way, don't worry if his arms are left free; he won't catch cold.

OTHER METHODS

Lullabies, as you rock your baby to and fro, are an age-old method of soothing her to sleep. Your baby won't mind if you can't sing in tune.
Taped music playing softly in her room may help your baby to drop off to sleep. For difficult sleepers, a **soothing tape** of the sounds she heard in the womb may work.

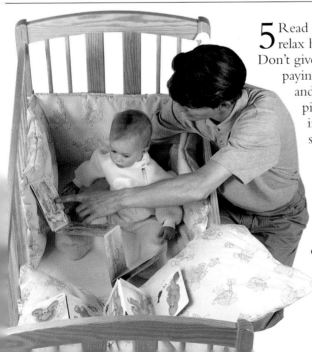

5 Read a story with your baby to relax her and help her wind down. Don't give up if you think she isn't paying attention: she will be tired and won't respond to the pictures with her usual lively interest, but that doesn't mean she isn't listening.

6 Tuck your baby up with her favorite toy or security blanket and kiss her good night. Turn the light down, or switch a nightlight on. Spend a moment or two lingering in the room before you go.

Q&A "Is it a good idea to take my baby into bed with me?"

Night feedings can be easier if you take your baby into bed, and provided neither you nor your partner has taken drugs or drunk alcohol, there's no risk of lying on him. Put him in the middle so you can't push him out. As he gets older, it's up to you to set the rules, although you will all sleep better in your own beds. Sleeping with you can become a habit, which may later be hard to break.

125

OVERCOMING SLEEPING PROBLEMS

NIGHT FEEDINGS	NIGHT WAKING	UNSETTLED BEDTIME

By the time your baby is six months old, she can go until morning without food; but she may well settle into a pattern of waking to be fed. If you want to wean her off these nighttime feedings, start by reducing the feedings gradually, then stop them but go in to see her and offer reassurance for as long as she cries.

The tactics below are a way of reassuring your older baby when she wakes at night that you have not abandoned her, while giving the message that she is going to get only the minimum of attention from you during these hours. If she is not sleeping through within a week, ask your doctor's advice.

From the age of about nine months, establish a method of handling bedtime, then stick to it. If your baby gets into a pattern of not settling when you put her to bed, a week of following the tactics below may break it. She'll soon get the message that you'll always come to her if she cries, but you won't pick her up.

At her bedtime feeding, do not let your baby fall asleep with a bottle in her mouth: this can lead to tooth decay. As soon as her eyelids droop, ease her off the bottle (or breast). Continue to hold her for a few more minutes and then tuck her into bed.

If your baby whimpers at night, wait a few minutes to see if she goes back to sleep again.

Keep to a bedtime routine, making it fun for your baby but relaxing and loving as well. If she cries when you leave her after tucking her in for the night, go back and give her a reassuring kiss, but *don't* pick her up, and *don't* stay more than a moment or two.

For a few nights, feed her when she wakes, but reduce the amount. Put her back in her crib, asleep or not, kiss her, and *leave*.

If she cries loudly, go in to make sure that nothing is wrong. Soothe her and calm her down: rubbing her back may be enough, but you may need to pick her up and cuddle her. When the crying has subsided into sniffles, put her back into her crib, tuck her in so she is snug, and kiss her goodnight. Then go back to bed yourself.

If she cries again, call out to her reassuringly, but wait five minutes before going in again.

If you are breast-feeding, your partner will have to take over at this point because your baby will smell your milk and want to be nursed. If she continues to cry, wait five minutes, then go back in to give her a pat and rub her back to reassure her. Then go back to bed, even if she's still crying.

If the crying continues, call out reassuringly from your own bed if you are near enough to be heard, but wait five minutes before going in to her.

When you do go in, make sure that nothing's wrong, such as a wet diaper or something chafing. Pat her back to soothe her, kiss her goodnight again, and tuck her in. Be cheerful but firm, and then go. Don't hesitate—your baby's will is stronger than yours at this point, and you'll be only too easily persuaded to stay.

Continue to go back every five minutes. Pick her up only if she is beside herself with crying; when her sobs subside put her back in her crib and leave her for a few minutes. You may have a couple of hours of this, but persevere.

When you do go back, just reassure her by patting and rubbing her back—don't pick her up unless she's really upset—then tuck her in and leave her.

If she keeps on crying, continue going in for a brief look at five-minute intervals. After half an hour, start to increase the intervals between visits, but never let your baby cry for longer than 15 minutes.

For the next few nights, stop offering the feeding; instead, adopt the tactics for night waking (see right) for as long as it takes to teach your baby to sleep through.

Continue going back in this way at five-minute intervals for as long as it takes her to fall back to sleep. After half an hour, increase the intervals between visits to 10 minutes, but never let her cry for more than 15. A week of gentle firmness on your part should be enough to establish a more sociable sleeping pattern.

Eventually she will realize that the brief reward of you coming in at intervals isn't worth all the effort that she's putting in, and she will drop off to sleep.

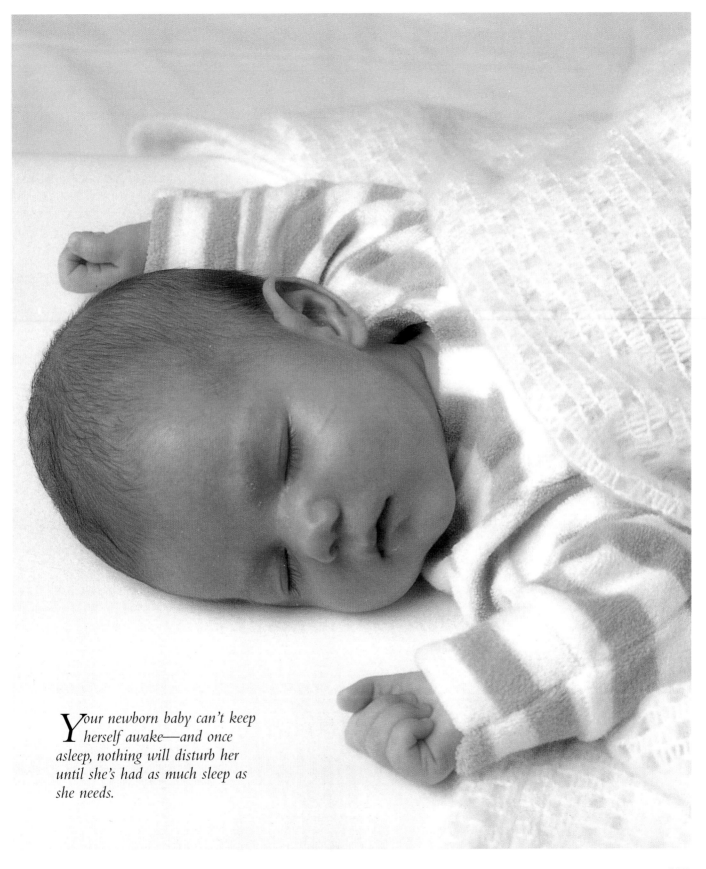

*Y*our newborn baby can't keep herself awake—and once asleep, nothing will disturb her until she's had as much sleep as she needs.

CLOTHES AND DRESSING

In the early weeks, your baby may need clean clothes as often as he needs a clean diaper, so you will need plenty of newborn clothes. Ask your friends or relatives with children if they have any to lend you. As your child turns into an active toddler, you will need to have clothes that are comfortable and unrestricting—and you'll need far fewer. Your child is growing so fast that an extensive wardrobe or shoes and clothes "for best" don't make sense—his clothes will be outgrown long before they are outworn. Choose them carefully: easy-to-manage fastenings and elasticated trousers, for example, will all help him as he learns to dress and undress himself. Choose clothes that are easy to care for, and machine-washable—keeping neat, still, and clean shouldn't have to figure in your child's life. He shouldn't have to worry about his clothes, and nor should you.

BUYING CLOTHES FOR YOUR BABY

Clothes for a young baby should be easy to put-on, machine-washable, and if possible made from natural fibers, which allow your baby to regulate his own temperature as well as he can. Don't use harsh detergents or fabric conditioners to wash your baby's clothes, they may irritate his skin. The basic item of clothing now and throughout the first six months is the all-in-one stretchsuit.

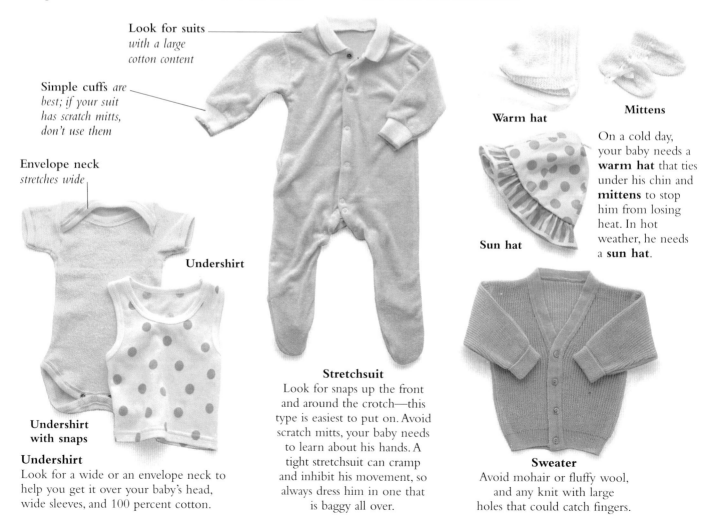

Look for suits *with a large cotton content*

Simple cuffs *are best; if your suit has scratch mitts, don't use them*

Envelope neck *stretches wide*

Undershirt

Undershirt with snaps

Undershirt
Look for a wide or an envelope neck to help you get it over your baby's head, wide sleeves, and 100 percent cotton.

Stretchsuit
Look for snaps up the front and around the crotch—this type is easiest to put on. Avoid scratch mitts, your baby needs to learn about his hands. A tight stretchsuit can cramp and inhibit his movement, so always dress him in one that is baggy all over.

Warm hat

Mittens

Sun hat

On a cold day, your baby needs a **warm hat** that ties under his chin and **mittens** to stop him from losing heat. In hot weather, he needs a **sun hat**.

Sweater
Avoid mohair or fluffy wool, and any knit with large holes that could catch fingers.

For your newborn, a **nightgown** or stretchsuit is ideal sleepwear. For an older baby, a **sleepsuit** with integral feet will keep him warmest, but ensure there is plenty of room for growth in the legs.

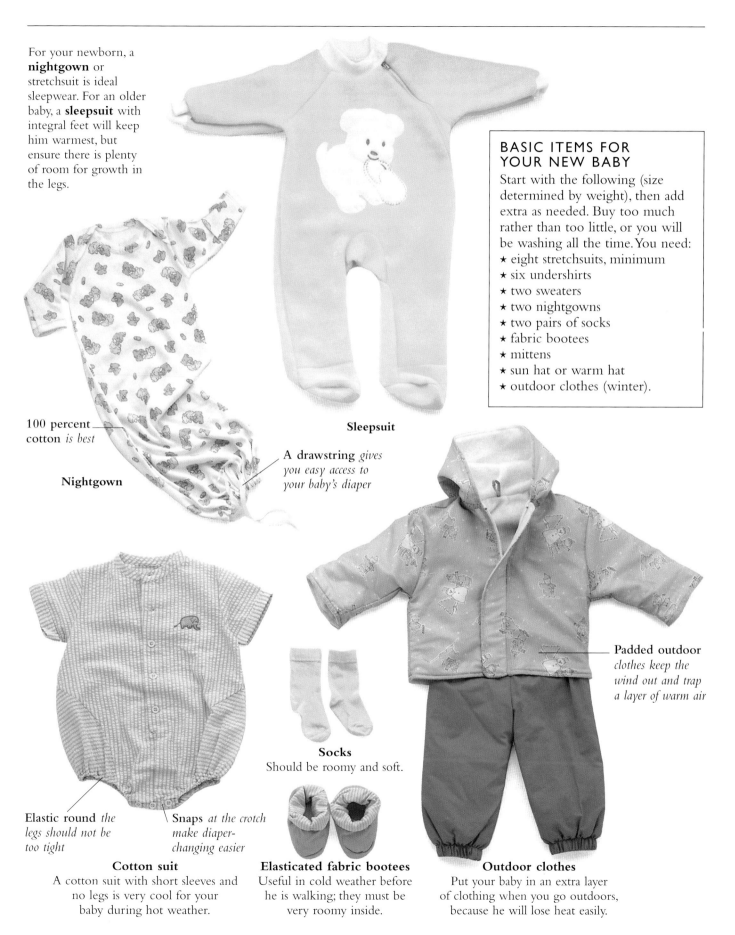

BASIC ITEMS FOR YOUR NEW BABY

Start with the following (size determined by weight), then add extra as needed. Buy too much rather than too little, or you will be washing all the time. You need:
- ★ eight stretchsuits, minimum
- ★ six undershirts
- ★ two sweaters
- ★ two nightgowns
- ★ two pairs of socks
- ★ fabric bootees
- ★ mittens
- ★ sun hat or warm hat
- ★ outdoor clothes (winter).

Sleepsuit

100 percent cotton *is best*

Nightgown

A drawstring *gives you easy access to your baby's diaper*

Padded outdoor *clothes keep the wind out and trap a layer of warm air*

Socks
Should be roomy and soft.

Elastic round *the legs should not be too tight*

Snaps *at the crotch make diaper-changing easier*

Cotton suit
A cotton suit with short sleeves and no legs is very cool for your baby during hot weather.

Elasticated fabric bootees
Useful in cold weather before he is walking; they must be very roomy inside.

Outdoor clothes
Put your baby in an extra layer of clothing when you go outdoors, because he will lose heat easily.

HOW TO DRESS YOUR BABY

Dressing and undressing your baby is a lovely opportunity to let him learn about his own body by stroking and caressing his soft skin. He may hate being dressed, but you can make it pleasurable with lots of nuzzling, cuddles, kisses, and chat; be especially gentle, too. Gather up the clothes you need and undo all the snaps. Lay your baby on his changing mat.

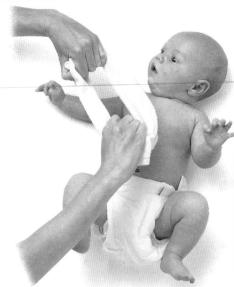

PUTTING ON AN UNDERSHIRT

1 Hold the shirt with the front facing you and gather it into your hands. Put the back edge at your baby's crown.

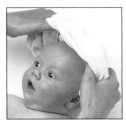

Position the back edge at the top of his head

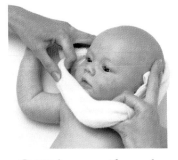

2 With one swift, gentle movement bring the front edge of the shirt down to your baby's chin. Hold all the fabric gathered up together and stretch it as wide as you can, so that none of it drags on his face and upsets him.

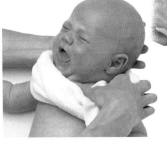

3 Gently lift your baby's head and upper body and pull the back of the shirt down so it is round his neck and lying behind his shoulders. Lower him to the mat without jolting or letting his head flop.

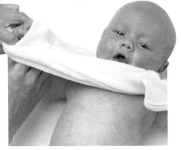

4 If your baby's shirt has sleeves, put the fingers of one hand down through the first sleeve and stretch it wide, then with the other hand guide his fist into your fingers.

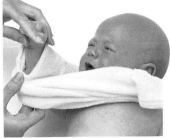

5 Hold your baby's hand with your first hand, and ease the sleeve over his arm with the other. Pull the shirt down below his arm. Do the same with the other sleeve, pulling the shirt, not your baby.

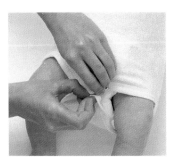

6 Pull the shirt over his stomach. Lift his lower body by his ankles and pull the back down. Fasten the snaps at the crotch.

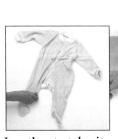

Lay the stretchsuit out flat

PUTTING ON A STRETCHSUIT

1 Pick your baby up while you lay the clean stretchsuit out flat on the changing mat, the front upward and all the snaps undone. Lay your baby on top, his neck in line with the stretchsuit's.

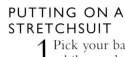

A shirt underneath the stretchsuit is essential in anything but the hottest weather

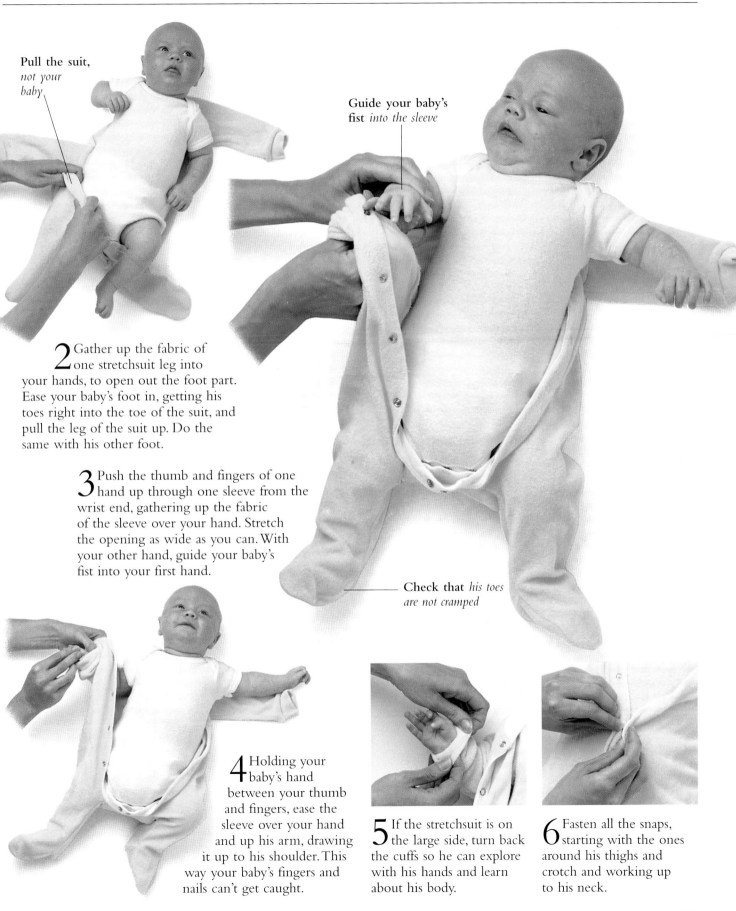

Pull the suit, *not your baby*

Guide your baby's fist *into the sleeve*

2 Gather up the fabric of one stretchsuit leg into your hands, to open out the foot part. Ease your baby's foot in, getting his toes right into the toe of the suit, and pull the leg of the suit up. Do the same with his other foot.

3 Push the thumb and fingers of one hand up through one sleeve from the wrist end, gathering up the fabric of the sleeve over your hand. Stretch the opening as wide as you can. With your other hand, guide your baby's fist into your first hand.

Check that *his toes are not cramped*

4 Holding your baby's hand between your thumb and fingers, ease the sleeve over your hand and up his arm, drawing it up to his shoulder. This way your baby's fingers and nails can't get caught.

5 If the stretchsuit is on the large side, turn back the cuffs so he can explore with his hands and learn about his body.

6 Fasten all the snaps, starting with the ones around his thighs and crotch and working up to his neck.

UNDRESSING YOUR BABY

Your baby may be un-nerved by the feel of cold air against his skin as you undress him, so nuzzle his bare stomach, and make the most of this opportunity for skin-to-skin contact. Have a towel on hand to wrap your baby in when you've undressed him, or dress him again quickly. Lay your baby on his changing mat.

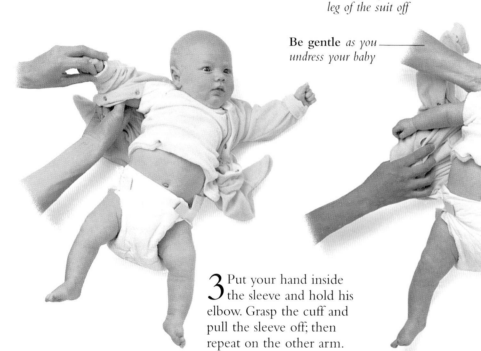

TAKING OFF A STRETCHSUIT

1 Undo the stretchsuit snaps. Hold one ankle inside the suit and pull the suit leg off. Do the same with the other.

Hold his ankle *while you pull the leg of the suit off*

2 Undo the snaps on his shirt, then lift his lower body by his ankles and slide the shirt and stretchsuit up underneath him as far as you can.

Be gentle *as you undress your baby*

Support *your baby's head*

3 Put your hand inside the sleeve and hold his elbow. Grasp the cuff and pull the sleeve off; then repeat on the other arm.

4 Slide your hand underneath your baby's head and neck and lift his upper body so you can remove the stretchsuit.

TAKING OFF AN UNDERSHIRT

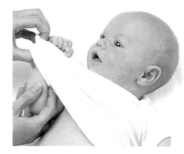

1 Hold his elbow inside the shirt with one hand and ease all the fabric over his fist. Do the same on the other side.

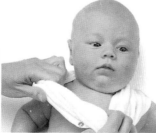

2 Gather up all the shirt in your hands, so there is no spare fabric that might drag over your baby's face as you take it off.

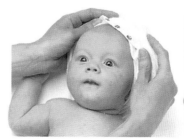

3 Stretch the opening as wide as you can, then with one swift movement take it up and over your baby's face to his crown.

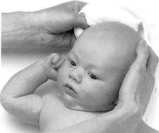

4 Slide your hand underneath your baby's head and neck and lift his upper body so you can slide out the shirt.

HOW YOUR CHILD LEARNS TO DRESS HIMSELF

By about two years your child will probably manage to pull off his own socks or T-shirt, and the majority of children will begin to dress themselves by the age of about three. You can encourage this new independence by buying clothes that are easy for your child to manage, and by letting him dress and undress as much as he can himself.

WAYS TO HELP

★ Allow plenty of time—if you're not in a rush, you won't get too irritated by his slowness.

★ Lay out his clothes in the order he needs to put them on.

★ Buy pants or skirts with elasticated waistbands. Avoid pants with zippers for a pre-school boy in case he gets his penis caught.

★ Look for clothes with large buttons, snaps, or Velcro fastenings.

★ Teach him to start doing buttons up from the bottom upward.

★ Let him choose his "favorite" foot, then mark his shoe so he can get it on the correct foot.

★ Avoid jackets with difficult zippers.

★ When you have to help, make a game of getting dressed, playing "peek-a-boo" as you put garments over his head.

★ Once he's dressed, let him stay dressed—even if he gets dirty.

CHOOSING SHOES

Bare feet are best for babies who are learning to walk. They make it easier to balance, and walking barefoot makes for healthy feet. Once your child is ready to walk outdoors he will need shoes, but even then, let him go barefoot as much as possible. Shoes are necessary only to protect feet, not to "support" them—the muscles give all the support the foot needs. Buy shoes from a store where children's feet are carefully measured for length *and* width. Have the fit checked every three months. Buy new socks at the same time as new shoes: too-small socks can be just as constricting as shoes.

What sort of shoes should I buy?

Any leather or canvas shoe is suitable *provided* your child's feet have been properly measured and the shoes fit in length *and* width. Sneakers are fine and come in a wide variety of sizes and designs. Rubber boots aren't usually available in half-sizes, but they're still essential for wet weather walks. Buy them on the large side, and fit an insole.

Avoid buying any shoes made from plastic, because plastic doesn't mold itself to the shape of your child's foot like leather, or canvas.

What to look for in your child's shoes

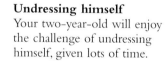

The space between *your child's longest toe and the end of the shoe should be 1.25cm (¼in)*

Wide toes *are important to give your child's toes room to splay out inside*

T-bar with buckle

Open-toed sandal

The fastening *should hold your child's foot snugly: buckles or Velcro are easiest for your child to manage*

The seams *must be smoothly finished, so nothing can rub your child's skin*

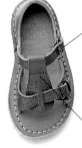

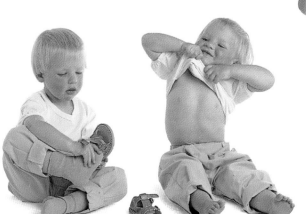

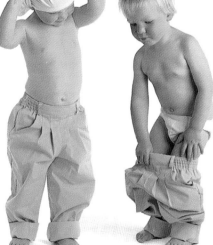

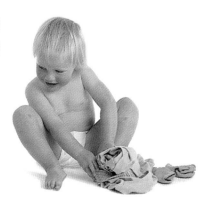

Undressing himself
Your two-year-old will enjoy the challenge of undressing himself, given lots of time.

BATHING AND WASHING YOUR BABY

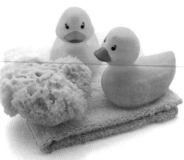

Alarge part of taking care of your new baby day-to-day will be keeping him clean. His skin is delicate and soft, and even his own bodily functions —sweating, urinating, dribbling— will irritate it and make it sore. As your baby grows, his bathing needs change: he will be pushing food into his hair, exploring the world with his hands, helping you with his diaper changes, and generally getting himself dirty. So from a hygiene point of view, be vigilant about washing off urine, feces, and sweat as well as milk and food. You don't have to give your baby a daily bath: sponge bathing is quite adequate to keep him clean. But in all likelihood your baby will quickly come to love being bathed, and it will become an important part of your daily routine together.

EQUIPMENT FOR BATHING AND WASHING

There are plenty of products available designed to make bathtime easier for you, but make sure that you only buy products intended for use on babies. Adult shampoos, soaps, lotions, and creams contain too many additives and chemicals to be safe for your baby's delicate skin.

EQUIPMENT FOR BATHING

Baby bath
Until your baby is ready to go into an adult bath (between three and six months), a proper baby bath will make bathtime easy for you. Place it at a convenient height on a worktop, or put it on the floor. If you buy a special bath stand, make sure it puts the bath at the right height for you.

Small bowl of clean water　**Cotton balls**

You will need clean water and plenty of cotton balls to wash your baby's eyes, ears, and face.

A rubber bath mat *stops your baby from slipping down*

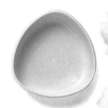

Waterproof apron
A cotton fabric with waterproof backing will feel softer to your baby than plastic.

Rubber bath mat
Once your baby moves into the big bath, a suctioned rubber bath mat is a must to stop him from sliding on the bottom of the tub.

BABY TOILETRIES

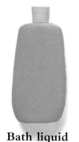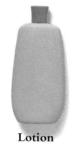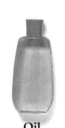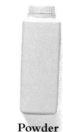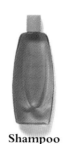

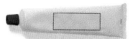

Soap **Cotton swabs**

Bath liquid **Lotion** **Oil** **Moisturizer** **Powder** **Shampoo** **Fluoride toothpaste**

Baby bath liquid is an excellent alternative to soap since it is mild.
Baby lotion is useful for cleaning your baby's diaper area, particularly if his skin is very dry.
Baby oil is a good moisturizer when your baby's skin is dry or scaly.

Baby moisturizer can be used instead of baby oil.
Baby powder will absorb any dampness left on your baby's skin. Use only a little, putting the talc on your hands and then rubbing it on the baby. Don't shake it over the baby; he might inhale it.

Baby shampoo may be needed once a week.
Baby soap need only be used if you don't use bath liquid. With a young baby, soap him all over on your lap, then rinse the soap off in the baby bath—but remember his body will be very slippery, so hold him firmly.

Cotton swabs are useful for cleaning between your baby's fingers and toes, but never push them into his ears, nose, eyes, or bottom.
Toothpaste can be an adult brand. Try not to let your child eat it—if he does, avoid using it until he's old enough not to eat it (see page 144).

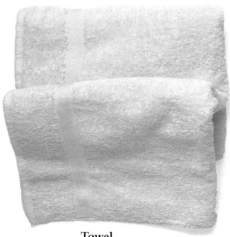

Towel

Keep a large, very soft towel for your baby's use only. Some towels have a corner piece that makes a hood.

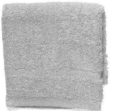

Natural sponge

Washcloth

Keep a new washcloth or sponge for your baby's use only, and wash the cloth regularly. Don't let an older baby eat the sponge.

HAIR, NAILS, AND TEETH

Hairbrush This should have soft bristles and be small enough for your child to brush his own hair from about eighteen months.
Comb Choose a small comb with rounded teeth.
Baby nail scissors These have rounded ends and short blades, so there's no danger of jabbing your baby.

Baby hairbrush and comb

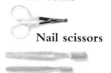

Nail scissors

Toothbrush

Toothbrush This must have a small head so it can reach into the corners of his mouth, and soft, rounded bristles. Nylon or bristle is equally good. Let your baby play with a baby size brush, but use a child's size brush to clean his teeth. Change his brush regularly, and check with your dentist that it is cleaning adequately.

TIPS FOR WASHING YOUR YOUNG BABY

★ Until your baby is six months old, always use separate, clean water to wash his eyes, ears, mouth, and face.
★ Only clean the parts you can see—do not try to clean right inside your baby's nose or ears, just wipe away any visible mucus or wax with damp cotton balls. Otherwise you may push the dirt back up into the nose or ear.
★ With a baby girl, never try to separate her vaginal lips to clean inside them. You will hinder the natural flow of mucus that washes bacteria out.
★ With a baby boy, never try to

push back his foreskin to clean under it: you may hurt him, or tear or damage the foreskin.
★ Always wipe from front to back when you are cleaning a baby girl's diaper area. This prevents germs from spreading from the anus into the vagina and causing infection.
★ When wiping your baby's eyes and ears, use a fresh cotton ball for each one, or you may spread minor infections.
★ Always leave cleaning your baby's bottom until last, and use a fresh cotton ball for each wipe. Dip in warm tap water.

SPONGE BATHING A YOUNG BABY

Sponge bathing simply means cleaning only the parts of your baby that really need cleaning —her hands, face, neck, and diaper area. Sponge bathe your baby as part of your morning or bedtime routine—it's an excellent alternative to a bath, particularly during the first six weeks, when neither you nor your baby will feel very sure of bathing in the baby bath. Make sure that the room is warm and you have all that you need. Pour some clean water into a small bowl to cool. Wash your hands. Lay your baby on her changing mat and undress her down to her undershirt.

YOU WILL NEED
Small bowl of clean, warm water for your baby's face
Bowl of warm water
Cotton balls
Tissues
Warm towel
Diaper-changing equipment
Clean clothes

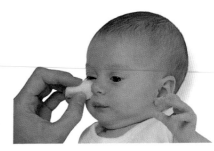

1 Wipe each eye from the nose outward with cotton wool dipped in clean water. Use a fresh piece for each wipe, and for each eye. Dry gently with a tissue.

Wipe away *dirt and fluff behind her ears*

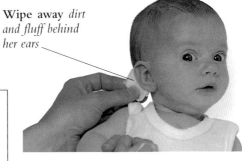

5 Uncurl her fingers *gently to wipe her hands*

2 With fresh moist cotton ball, wipe each ear. Don't try to wipe inside: just wipe over and behind it. Use a fresh cotton ball for each ear, and dry with the towel.

CLEANING YOUR BABY'S CORD STUMP

The shrivelled-up stump of your baby's umbilical cord will probably have dropped off by the time he is a week old. Until it drops off, you must clean it every day. Careful cleaning makes sure infection cannot set in, and helps the cord separate. Dry the stump with a cotton swab dipped in rubbing alcohol.

Once the stump of cord has dropped off, you will need to clean the navel every day as part of your routine until it is fully healed.

Consult your doctor as soon as possible if your baby's navel starts to look red, swollen, inflamed, or starts to ooze fluid of any kind. A small amount of bleeding is normal, and usually nothing to worry about.

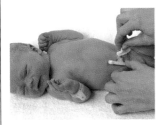

1 Using cotton ball moistened with rubbing alcohol, wipe carefully in the skin creases around the stump. (After two weeks you can use clean water.)

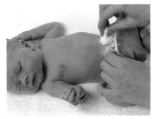

2 Dry with a fresh cotton ball. Dust a little baby powder on a piece of cotton ball and dab it over the navel like a powder puff to absorb remaining moisture.

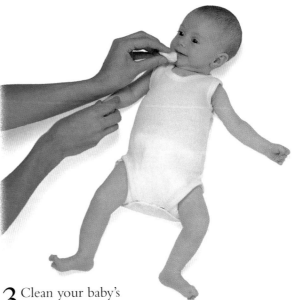

3 Clean your baby's face of milk and drool by wiping around her mouth and nose, then, wipe over her cheeks and forehead. Dry with the towel.

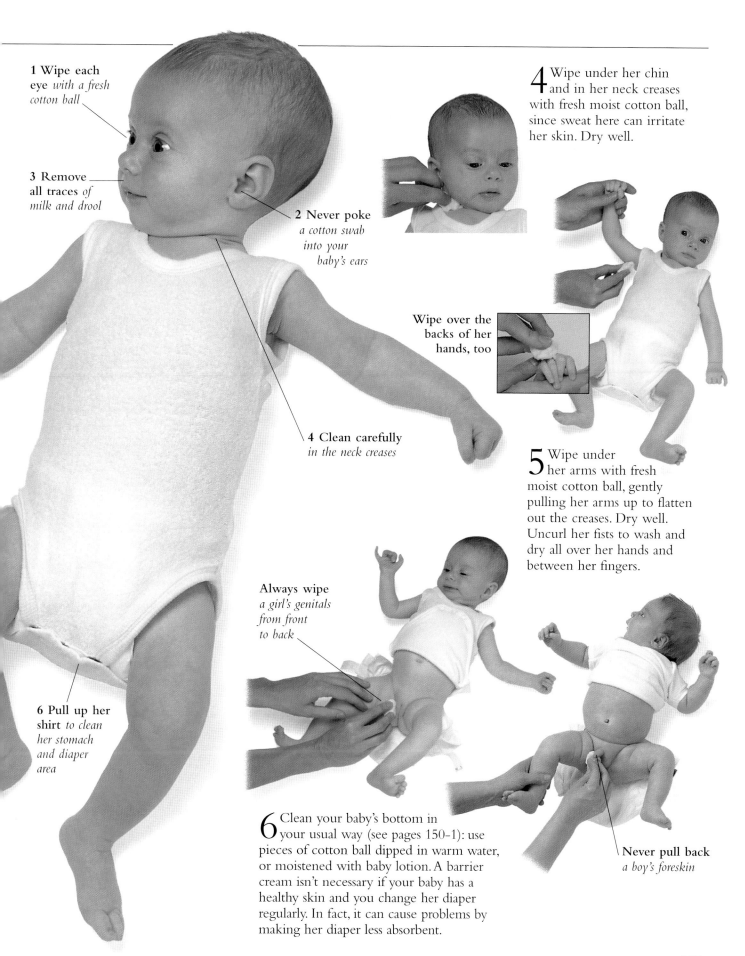

1 Wipe each eye *with a fresh cotton ball*

3 Remove all traces *of milk and drool*

2 Never poke *a cotton swab into your baby's ears*

4 Clean carefully *in the neck creases*

6 Pull up her shirt *to clean her stomach and diaper area*

Always wipe *a girl's genitals from front to back*

4 Wipe under her chin and in her neck creases with fresh moist cotton ball, since sweat here can irritate her skin. Dry well.

Wipe over the backs of her hands, too

5 Wipe under her arms with fresh moist cotton ball, gently pulling her arms up to flatten out the creases. Dry well. Uncurl her fists to wash and dry all over her hands and between her fingers.

6 Clean your baby's bottom in your usual way (see pages 150–1): use pieces of cotton ball dipped in warm water, or moistened with baby lotion. A barrier cream isn't necessary if your baby has a healthy skin and you change her diaper regularly. In fact, it can cause problems by making her diaper less absorbent.

Never pull back *a boy's foreskin*

BATHING YOUR YOUNG BABY

Most babies come to love the sensation of being bathed; but in the early days you and your baby will probably both have mixed feelings. A new baby often dislikes the feeling of being "unwrapped", and you may feel nervous of holding your baby's small, slippery body. In the first weeks, you can simply sponge bathe your baby to keep her fresh and clean; practice with a full bath once a week, and a hair wash every two weeks. Make sure the room is warm enough. You can kneel, sit, or stand to bath your baby, but make sure your back doesn't start to ache.

YOU WILL NEED
Baby bath
Changing mat
Your baby's bath towel
Hairwashing towel, if you're washing her hair
Waterproof apron
Bowl of clean water for washing her face
Cotton balls
Baby bath liquid (optional)
Diaper-changing equipment
Baby powder (optional)
Clean clothes

GETTING READY FOR THE BATH

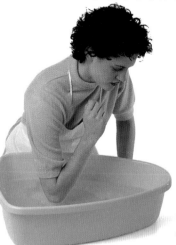

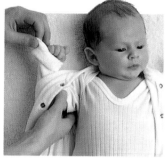

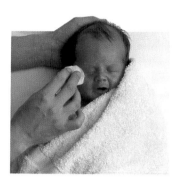

1 Put in cold water, add hot and mix. Test with your elbow: the water should feel just warm, and be 10cm (4in) deep.

2 Lay the bath towel on the changing mat and undress your baby on it down to her diaper.

3 Wrap her up snugly and wipe her eyes and face in cotton balls dipped in clean water.

WASHING YOUR BABY'S HAIR

1 Cradle her head in one hand, her back along your forearm, and tuck her legs under your elbow. Gently pour water from the bath over her head with a cupped hand. Don't splash her face and keep smiling.

"My four-week-old baby has ugly crusty patches on his scalp. What should I do about them?"

This is a harmless form of dandruff known as cradle cap. Rub your baby's scalp with baby oil and leave for 24 hours. Comb very gently, then wash the crusts off. If the cradle cap doesn't improve, ask your doctor for advice.

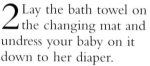

Avoid splashing *water over her face*

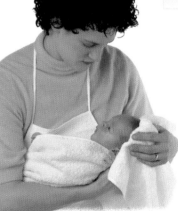

2 Bring your baby back to your lap to pat her head dry gently with a second towel.

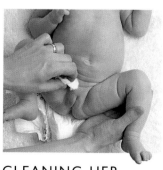

CLEANING HER BOTTOM

Lay her on her mat. Take off her diaper and clean her bottom (see pages 150–51).

PUTTING YOUR BABY IN THE BATH

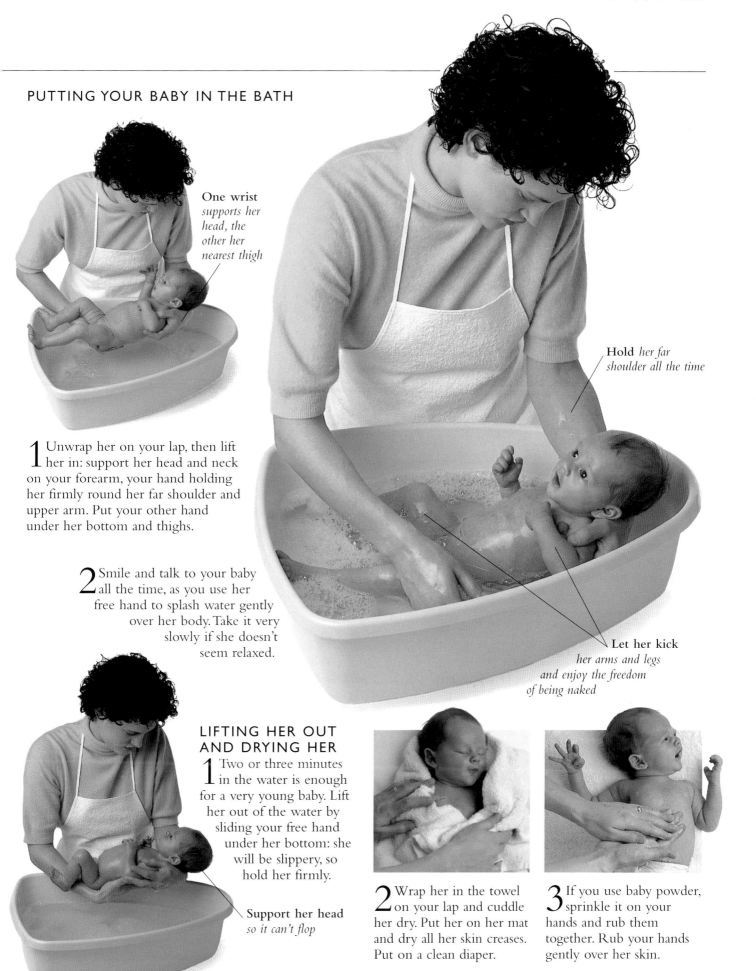

One wrist *supports her head, the other her nearest thigh*

1 Unwrap her on your lap, then lift her in: support her head and neck on your forearm, your hand holding her firmly round her far shoulder and upper arm. Put your other hand under her bottom and thighs.

2 Smile and talk to your baby all the time, as you use her free hand to splash water gently over her body. Take it very slowly if she doesn't seem relaxed.

Hold *her far shoulder all the time*

Let her kick *her arms and legs and enjoy the freedom of being naked*

LIFTING HER OUT AND DRYING HER

1 Two or three minutes in the water is enough for a very young baby. Lift her out of the water by sliding your free hand under her bottom: she will be slippery, so hold her firmly.

Support her head *so it can't flop*

2 Wrap her in the towel on your lap and cuddle her dry. Put her on her mat and dry all her skin creases. Put on a clean diaper.

3 If you use baby powder, sprinkle it on your hands and rub them together. Rub your hands gently over her skin.

BATHING IN THE BIG BATH

Your baby will probably be ready to graduate to the exciting territory of the big bath at the age of three or four months—and some babies are ready for the experience even earlier. If your baby hasn't yet learned to enjoy bathtime, don't rush the change—give him a few more weeks of being bathed in his baby bath, until he really is too big for it, or is more confident. To bathe your three-month-old, arrange everything you will need beside the bath. Make sure the room is warm. Put the rubber mat on the floor of the bath and run in cold water, then hot, so that the water is just warm. Put your baby on his changing mat to wash his face, eyes, and ears, using clean water. Then, undress him carefully and clean his bottom thoroughly before placing him gently in the bath.

YOU WILL NEED
Rubber bath mat
Waterproof apron
Baby bath liquid cleanser and baby shampoo
Large soft towel
Baby's own sponge or washcloth
Equipment for washing your baby's face
Diaper-changing equipment
Pouring and other toys for an older baby
Toothbrush for an older child
Clean clothes

WASHING YOUR BABY

1 Lay your baby in the bath on a rubber mat. Keep his head and shoulders supported on your arm, his ears clear of the water.

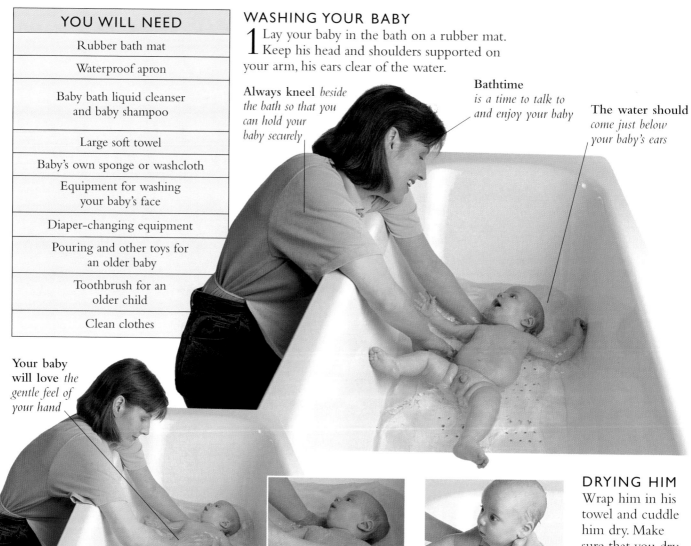

Always kneel *beside the bath so that you can hold your baby securely*

Bathtime *is a time to talk to and enjoy your baby*

The water should *come just below your baby's ears*

Your baby will love *the gentle feel of your hand*

2 Scoop up a little of the soapy water in your free hand, then run your hand gently over his body, particularly around all his creases. There's no need to scrub him!

3 Rinse off the lather by splashing water gently over him, avoiding his face. Smile and talk to him all the time.

LIFTING HIM OUT
Put your hands under your baby's armpits to lift him out. Take care, he will be slippery.

DRYING HIM
Wrap him in his towel and cuddle him dry. Make sure that you dry him thoroughly, especially in the creases under his armpits, at the top of his thighs, and around the neck region. Between the fingers and toes also need careful attention.

WASHING YOUR BABY'S HAIR

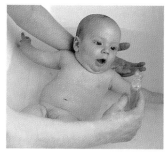 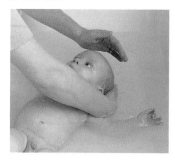 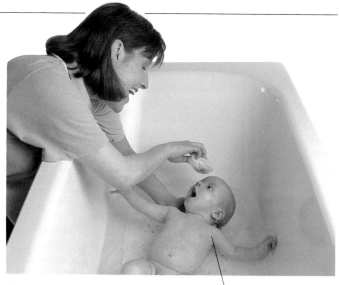

1 It is only necessary to wash your baby's hair about once a week. Wet the hair first. Using a baby shampoo, slide your supporting hand forward and pour a small amount into the palm.

2 Support your baby's head with your free hand, and with the other hand rub the shampoo gently over his hair. Be careful not to get the shampoo in his eyes. Rinse your hand.

3 Swap hands again and rinse the shampoo off with a wet, well squeezed out sponge or washcloth.

Take your cue *from him—he might enjoy a teasing game*

BATHTIME SAFETY

Always follow these few rules:
★ Never leave a baby or small child alone in the bath, or move out of easy reach, even for a second. It takes no time for a child to slip and drown, even in very shallow water.
★ Never let your child pull himself to standing in the bath even when he can stand steadily, and even though you have a rubber mat in the bath.
★ Even when your baby can sit steadily, keep a hand ready to support him if he slips.
★ A rubber mat in the bottom of the bath is essential.
★ Never top up with hot water while your child is in the bath. If any topping up is necessary, mix hot and cold water in a jug so it's just warm, then pour it in.
★ Make sure the thermostat on your water heater is not set too high.
★ If the tap gets hot, tie a wash-cloth around it so your child can't burn himself on it.
★ If you bathe with your baby, have the water cooler than you would usually have it.

MAKING BATHTIME FUN

Once your baby can sit steadily, bathtime becomes a wonderful play-time—not just a way of getting him clean. Search out some bath toys: things that pour, like plastic jugs and funnels, sandcastle buckets with holes in them, even plastic colanders, will fascinate him; and floating toys like boats or ducks are ideal, too. About once a week, use a pouring toy to wash his hair, but don't let water run over his face—he will probably hate it.

Always supervise bathtime, *and never leave your child alone in the bath*

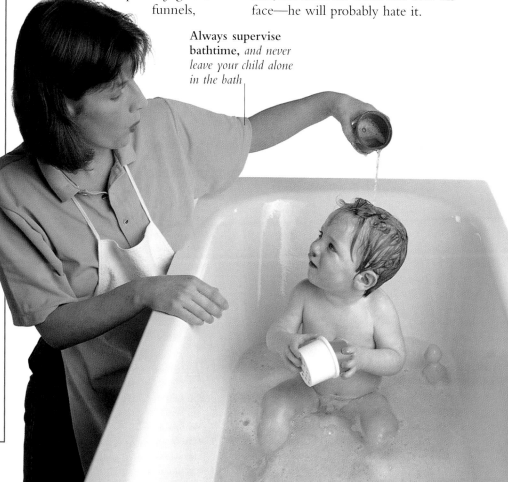

BABIES WHO HATE WATER AND WASHING

BABIES WHO HATE BATHING

Some babies are frightened by bathtime—and often a baby or toddler may suddenly take a dislike to bathing. If this happens, give up baths for a short time: daily sponge baths will keep a small baby clean, though a mobile baby will need an all-over sponge bath on your lap (see below). After two or three weeks, try having a bath with your baby to help him overcome his fear of the water.

Playing with water
Sit your baby beside a bowl of water on the kitchen floor and let him splash and play. Pouring jugs and floating toys can often persuade a child that water can be fun.

BABIES WHO HATE WASHING

Even if your child hates having his hands washed, it's important to do so before and after every meal. Make it more fun by wash-ing his hands between your own wet and soapy ones.

BABIES WHO HATE HAIRWASHING

Babies and young children often particularly dislike having their hair washed, even if they love bathtime —around two-and-a-half to three years is often the most difficult time. If your child doesn't like having his hair washed, abandon it for a couple of weeks. Respect his dislike, but help him be more reasonable about it: for example, go out together in the rain and show him how pleasurable raindrops feel on his face.

Reintroduce hair-washing at bathtime gradually. It may help to give him a washcloth to hold over his eyes and face: often it's the feel of water on their faces that children hate most. If your child will wear one, you could try putting a plastic "halo" round his hairline to keep the water off his face.

Sponging her hair
You can keep your child's hair clean by sponging out any bits of food and dirt with a damp washcloth or sponge.

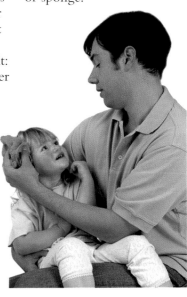

GIVING YOUR BABY A SPONGE BATH

If your baby doesn't like water, there is no need to bath him: once he can hold his head up, a daily sponge bath on your lap is enough. First, lay him on his mat and wipe his eyes, face, and ears with clean cotton balls. Sit him on your lap with everything you need within reach.

YOU WILL NEED
Large bowl of warm water, with a little baby bath liquid added
Small bowl of cooled boiled water and cotton wool for your baby's face
Waterproof apron
Your baby's own sponge or washcloth
Warm towel
Diaper-changing equipment

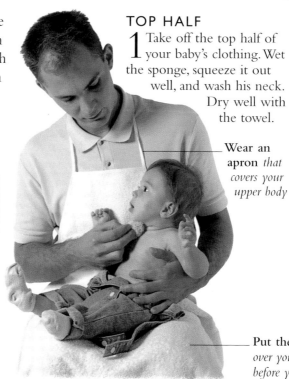

TOP HALF
1 Take off the top half of your baby's clothing. Wet the sponge, squeeze it out well, and wash his neck. Dry well with the towel.

Wear an apron *that covers your upper body*

2 Dip the sponge in the water again, squeeze it out so it doesn't dribble, then wash all over his chest and stomach. Dry him well with the towel.

Put the towel *over your lap before you begin*

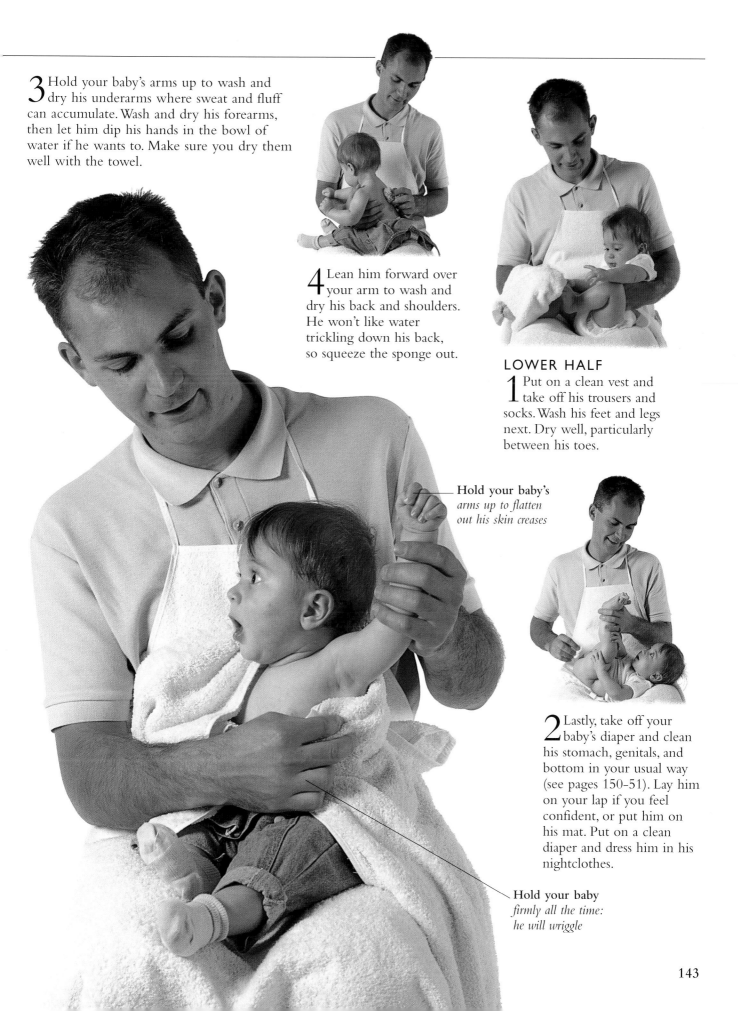

3 Hold your baby's arms up to wash and dry his underarms where sweat and fluff can accumulate. Wash and dry his forearms, then let him dip his hands in the bowl of water if he wants to. Make sure you dry them well with the towel.

4 Lean him forward over your arm to wash and dry his back and shoulders. He won't like water trickling down his back, so squeeze the sponge out.

LOWER HALF

1 Put on a clean vest and take off his trousers and socks. Wash his feet and legs next. Dry well, particularly between his toes.

Hold your baby's *arms up to flatten out his skin creases*

2 Lastly, take off your baby's diaper and clean his stomach, genitals, and bottom in your usual way (see pages 150–51). Lay him on your lap if you feel confident, or put him on his mat. Put on a clean diaper and dress him in his nightclothes.

Hold your baby *firmly all the time: he will wriggle*

143

CARING FOR YOUR CHILD'S TEETH

It's never too early to start cleaning your child's teeth. Once your baby has one or more, wipe his teeth and gums each evening with a wet handkerchief (see below). When he has a few more teeth, clean them for him after breakfast and at bedtime, but let him play with a brush himself at bathtime too, to get him used to the feel of it. Taking care of the primary teeth helps ensure that when the permanent teeth come in around age five or six, they will be correctly positioned and in healthy gums—and you will be establishing good, lifelong habits in your child.

If your baby or toddler falls asleep sucking on a bottle, always remove the bottle once the infant is fast asleep. Otherwise the milk or juice in her mouth will rot her teeth, a common and preventable problem.

CLEANING YOUR BABY'S TEETH

1 Wet a clean handkerchief. Sit your baby on your lap. Wrap the handkerchief around your finger and spread on a small amount of toothpaste. Bear in mind that toothpaste should be used sparingly in very young children.

2 Rub your finger over your child's gums and teeth.

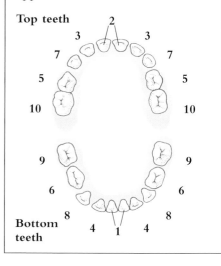

HOW THE TEETH COME IN

Your baby might cut his first tooth at any time during the first year, and he will be teething into his third year. Babies' teeth usually appear in the same order.

Top teeth

Bottom teeth

WHY DO TEETH DECAY?

Teeth decay because bacteria in the mouth react with sugar to form acid, which eats through the enamel covering the teeth. Candy and sugary foods increase the risk of tooth decay, particularly if they're eaten between meals because the teeth are bathed in sugar most of the time. Try to confine candy to mealtimes, always brush your child's teeth afterward, and give him snacks that are low in sugar (see page 116).

Fluoride

Children can have their teeth protected with fluoride, a chemical which hardens tooth enamel, and even heals small breaches in it. Brushing twice daily with fluoride toothpaste will help protect your child's teeth from decay, particularly if you let it linger in his mouth. Fluoride is present in some water supplies, or is given in drops or tablets. Ask your doctor for advice.

Too much fluoride?

You needn't worry if your child swallows a little toothpaste as you brush his teeth, but he might love the taste so much that he wants to eat it from the tube. Don't let him. If he's getting fluoride from water or supplements, the extra in the toothpaste might be excessive.

VISITING THE DENTIST

From the time your child has a full first set of teeth (at around two and a half) you should arrange regular dental check-ups every six months. Children under two and a half should see the dentist as well if you are concerned that there is a problem. Your dentist will have treatments available to prevent tooth decay, and will be able to advise you about fluoride supplements—so keep up the visits even if you are sure your child's teeth are healthy. If there are any cavities, it's important that they are spotted in good time. Get your child used to the idea of going to the dentist before he has any treatment.

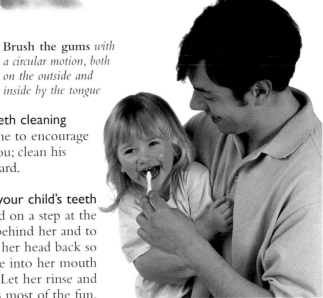

CLEANING YOUR CHILD'S TEETH

Start cleaning your child's teeth for him with a wetted toothbrush. Brush them for him for as long as he will let you; he will probably want to brush them himself from the age of about two. Always supervise—he needs to brush correctly. Teach him by standing behind him in front of a mirror, and holding his hand, showing him the correct movements.

Top teeth: *brush downward, away from the gums*

All biting surfaces: *brush back and forth along the flat tops of the teeth, all around the mouth*

Bottom teeth: *brush upward, away from the gums*

Get the brush *right to the back of your child's mouth*

Brush the gums *with a circular motion, both on the outside and inside by the tongue*

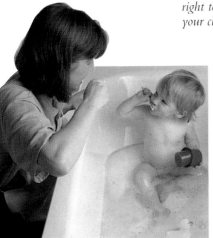

Making a game of teeth cleaning
Play games at bathtime to encourage your child to copy you; clean his teeth properly afterward.

Cleaning your child's teeth
Stand your child on a step at the sink, with you behind her and to one side. Hold her head back so you can see into her mouth as you brush. Let her rinse and spit out—that's most of the fun.

CUTTING NAILS

YOUR NEWBORN BABY

Even newborn babies can have fingernails that are quite long. Keep your baby's fingernails short so that there's no chance of her scratching herself.

The best time to cut your baby's nails is after a bath, when her nails are soft. Don't feel tempted to trim them by biting them off yourself. Instead, use special baby scissors, designed for this purpose. They have blunt ends and are safest for cutting your baby's nails. Follow the shape of the fingernails. Always cut your baby's toenails straight across. When you have finished, check for any sharp points.

If your baby wriggles, don't try to fight her. Instead, trim her nails while she is sleeping. You may find that your baby's nails grow very fast, especially during the summer months.

YOUR OLDER BABY

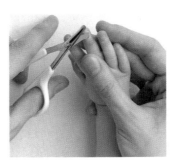

Sit your baby on your lap, facing forward. Hold one finger at a time and cut her nails with baby scissors.

CUTTING TOENAILS

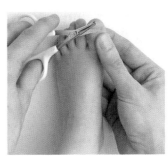

Lay a young baby on a mat; sit an older baby on your lap. Hold her foot firmly since she will kick.

DIAPERS AND DIAPER CHANGING

The first few weeks of your newborn's life may seem like a constant round of diaper changing. Because your baby's bladder is small, she wets often, so at the very least you need to change her after a feeding, after she wakes, before she goes to bed, and in the early weeks often after night feedings, too. In fact, change her whenever her diaper is wet or soiled, to help prevent diaper rash. Changing her isn't always your first priority: when she wakes in the morning she'll be hungry, so try taking off her wet diaper, wrapping her in a towel, and feeding her before you change her. Diaper changing need not be a chore: it's a time for games, and an important way to show your baby that you love her. Keep a set of all you need in one place; in a two-storey house, put a duplicate set downstairs. As the months go by, you'll notice that her diaper needs changing less. By around two years, your child will start to recognize the feeling of a full bladder, and may be ready for potty-training.

THE CONTENTS OF YOUR BABY'S DIAPER

All these are common sights on a baby's diaper:

★ **greenish-black, sticky tar (first two or three days only):** this is meconium, which fills the bowels before birth and must be passed before digestion begins

★ **greenish-brown or bright green semifluid stools, full of curds (first week only):** "changing stools" show that your baby is adapting to feeding through her digestive system

★ **orange-yellow, mustard-like stools, watery with bits of milk curd in them, often very copious:** the settled stools of a breast-fed baby

★ **pale brown, solid, formed, and smelly stools:** the settled stools of a bottle-fed baby

★ **green, or green-streaked, stools:** quite normal, but small green stools over several days may be a sign of under-feeding.

Consult your doctor if:
★ the stools are very watery and smelly, your baby is vomiting and not eating: diarrhea is life-threatening in a young baby
★ you see blood on the diaper
★ anything at all worries you.

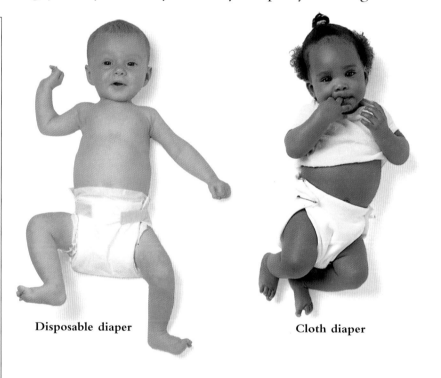

Disposable diaper

Cloth diaper

TYPES OF DIAPER

Your baby won't mind whether you use disposable or cloth diapers, provided the diaper is comfortable and she's not left in a wet or dirty one. Disposables tend to fit snugly. Cloth diapers are bulkier, and the clothes you buy your baby may need to be a few sizes larger to accommodate the diaper. Using a diaper service, especially in the newborn stage, is a good idea.

A mat with a raised edge *won't stop your baby from rolling off*

CHANGING YOUR BABY'S DIAPER

Since you will be changing your baby's diaper frequently, make your changing area a pleasant place for both of you: a mobile above your baby's head, a teddy bear nearby, bright decals on the walls or furniture alongside will all amuse your baby—and may encourage her to lie still for you. A changing mat is cheap and very convenient, and your baby will be safe if you put the mat on a reasonably clean and dry floor. A specially designed changing table may be useful for storing clean diapers and toiletries, but your baby can fall off unless she is buckled on with a restraining belt, and she will soon outgrow it. If you do buy one or use a countertop, chest of drawers, or your bed to change the baby, never turn your back on her even for a second.

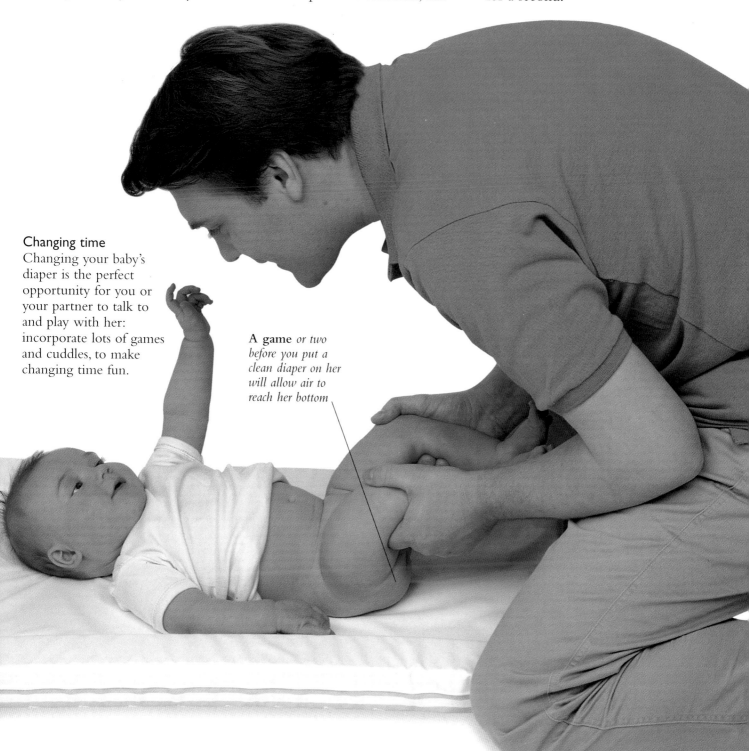

Changing time
Changing your baby's diaper is the perfect opportunity for you or your partner to talk to and play with her: incorporate lots of games and cuddles, to make changing time fun.

A game *or two before you put a clean diaper on her will allow air to reach her bottom*

EQUIPMENT FOR CHANGING YOUR BABY'S DIAPER

Such an extensive array of equipment can seem daunting to a new parent, but it need not be. You will not need everything shown on this page: the cotton balls, washcloths, and baby wipes, for example, are alternatives. The cotton balls or washcloths can be moistened with water, baby lotion, or baby oil. Never use lotions or creams that are not especially designed for use on young babies. You may be able to flush used tissues, diaper liners, and wipes down the toilet, but put disposable diapers into a pail lined with a plastic bag. Drop dirty cloth diapers into a special pail, too, so you can launder them separately or send them out with the regular diaper delivery service.

EQUIPMENT FOR CLEANING YOUR BABY'S BOTTOM

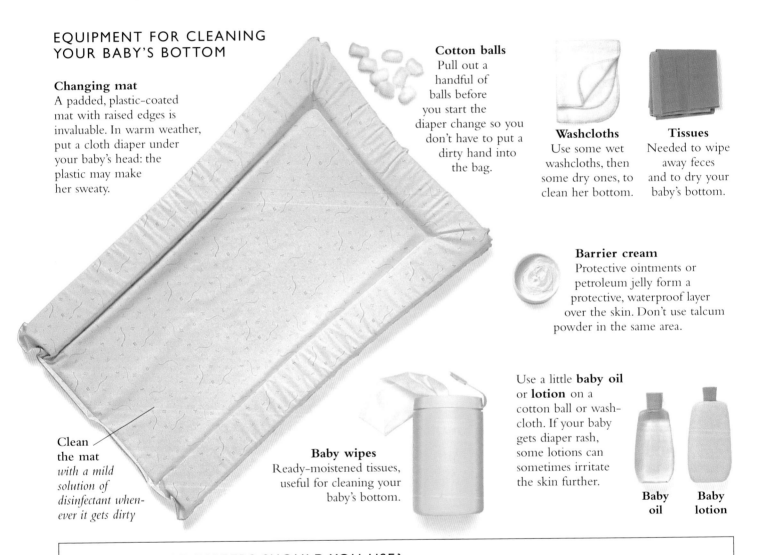

Changing mat
A padded, plastic-coated mat with raised edges is invaluable. In warm weather, put a cloth diaper under your baby's head: the plastic may make her sweaty.

Cotton balls
Pull out a handful of balls before you start the diaper change so you don't have to put a dirty hand into the bag.

Washcloths
Use some wet washcloths, then some dry ones, to clean her bottom.

Tissues
Needed to wipe away feces and to dry your baby's bottom.

Barrier cream
Protective ointments or petroleum jelly form a protective, waterproof layer over the skin. Don't use talcum powder in the same area.

Use a little **baby oil** or **lotion** on a cotton ball or wash-cloth. If your baby gets diaper rash, some lotions can sometimes irritate the skin further.

Baby oil

Baby lotion

Clean the mat *with a mild solution of disinfectant when-ever it gets dirty*

Baby wipes
Ready-moistened tissues, useful for cleaning your baby's bottom.

WHAT KIND OF DIAPERS SHOULD YOU USE?

You really have three choices when it comes to diapering your baby: use disposables, hire a service, or buy and wash your own cloth diapers. Cotton cloth diapers, shaped or squares, that you'll be washing at home really are the cheapest option, but don't forget to consider your time and labor when it comes to cost. You'll also be buying more laundry detergent and using more water to run the diapers through the washing machine rinse cycle several times to help get rid of the detergent. A good diaper service provides up to 90 diapers a week, picks up the dirty ones and returns a properly washed and dried supply. You may still need to buy rubber pants and diaper pins, however. Disposable diapers, which are the most extensively used type, are clearly the most convenient. Initially at least, you may want to use both cloth and disposable diapers. Having some cloth diapers handy for emergencies is always a good idea. You'll need to buy up to 70 disposables every week, so plan shopping trips ahead.

DISPOSABLE DIAPERS

Disposable diapers are absorbent paper pads and plastic pants all in one. When you're happy with a brand, buy in large quantities: in the first weeks you may be changing your baby 10 or 12 times a day, so 70 diapers will only be one week's supply. A diaper that is too small might be uncomfortable, so buy the next size up if it looks tight. "Ultra" brands are slim and very absorbent; those labeled "standard" are cheaper and bulkier, but you will have to change your baby more often.

You will also need:
Plastic bag or pail with a liner inside: Drop the used diaper into this, then when the bag is full, put it with your garbage. Disposable diapers are guaranteed to plug up your toilet.
A dozen cloth diapers: Use for general mopping up around your baby.

Elastic around the legs protects against leaks

Experiment until you find a brand with reliable adhesive tapes and good absorbency

Disposable diapers

Sticky tape or diaper pins
For when the tapes won't stick, or you need to reseal the diaper.

CLOTH DIAPERS AND RUBBER PANTS

Buy the best quality **100 percent cotton cloth diapers** you can find; you need 24 to begin with and rubber pants to go over the top. They are bulkier than disposables so the smallest baby clothes may not fit for long. Shaped cloth diapers have Velcro closures, and are as easy to put on as disposables.

ALL-IN-ONE REUSABLE DIAPER

The all-in-one reusable diaper has convenient Velcro fastenings, a soft cotton lining with an inner absorbent pad, and a built-in outer waterproof layer that makes for very easy changing, just like a disposable.

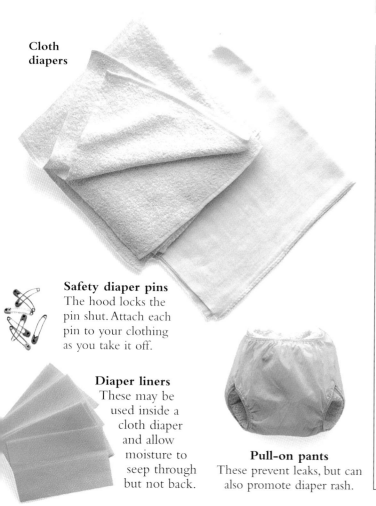

Cloth diapers

Safety diaper pins
The hood locks the pin shut. Attach each pin to your clothing as you take it off.

Diaper liners
These may be used inside a cloth diaper and allow moisture to seep through but not back.

Pull-on pants
These prevent leaks, but can also promote diaper rash.

DIAPER-WASHING EQUIPMENT

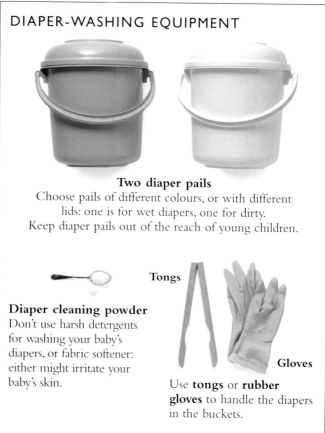

Two diaper pails
Choose pails of different colours, or with different lids: one is for wet diapers, one for dirty. Keep diaper pails out of the reach of young children.

Tongs

Diaper cleaning powder
Don't use harsh detergents for washing your baby's diapers, or fabric softener: either might irritate your baby's skin.

Gloves

Use **tongs** or **rubber gloves** to handle the diapers in the buckets.

CLEANING A GIRL

Clean your baby's bottom thoroughly at every diaper change, otherwise she will soon get red and sore. Wash your hands first. Put your baby on her mat, and undo her clothing and diaper. If she's wearing a cloth diaper, use a clean corner to wipe off most of any mess. With a disposable, open the diaper out: wipe off the worst of the mess with tissues and drop them into the diaper. Then lift your baby's legs and fold the diaper down under her.

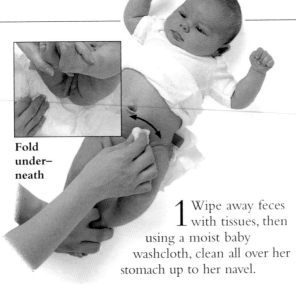

Fold under-neath

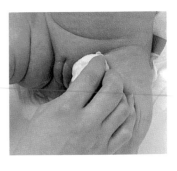

1 Wipe away feces with tissues, then using a moist baby washcloth, clean all over her stomach up to her navel.

2 Using a fresh washcloth clean inside all the creases at the tops of your baby's legs, wiping downward and away from her body.

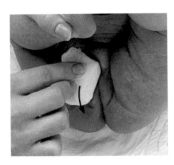

3 Lift her legs up with a finger between her ankles and clean her genitals next: always wipe from front to back to prevent germs from the anus entering the vagina. Do *not* try to clean inside the vaginal lips.

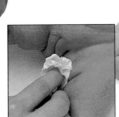

4 With a fresh washcloth, clean her anus, then her buttocks and thighs, working inward toward the anus. When she's clean, remove the disposable diaper, seal the tapes over the front, and drop in the pail. Wipe your hands.

Dry the skin creases well

5 Dry her diaper area with tissues, then let her kick for a while without a diaper so her bottom is open to the air.

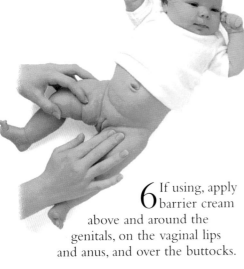

6 If using, apply barrier cream above and around the genitals, on the vaginal lips and anus, and over the buttocks.

DIAPER RASH

All babies get a red or sore bottom from time to time. Consult your doctor if the rash won't clear up.

To avoid diaper rash:

★ change the diaper frequently
★ clean and dry her bottom and skin creases thoroughly, using warm water
★ leave your baby without a diaper as often as possible
★ if using cloth diapers, buy snap-on rubber pants, as these allow air to circulate
★ wash and rinse all cloth diapers thoroughly.

At the first signs of redness:

★ change diapers more frequently
★ use a healing diaper rash cream
★ leave your baby without a diaper for as much of the day as possible
★ if using cloth diapers, try a more absorbent type of liner
★ stop using rubber pants: they make diaper rash worse because they help keep urine close to the skin. If you don't like the leaks, switch to using disposable diapers for a while.

CLEANING A BOY

Your baby boy's urine will go everywhere, so you need to clean his bottom very thoroughly at every diaper change to guard against a sore bottom. Wash your hands. Put your baby on his mat and undo his clothing and his diaper. If he's wearing a cloth diaper, wipe off the worst of any mess with a clean corner. With a disposable, undo the tapes, then pause (see right).

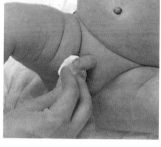

1 Your boy baby will often urinate just as you take his diaper off, so wait a couple of seconds with the diaper held over his penis to avoid urine going everywhere.

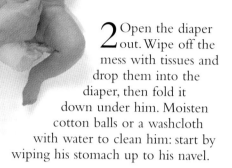

2 Open the diaper out. Wipe off the mess with tissues and drop them into the diaper, then fold it down under him. Moisten cotton balls or a washcloth with water to clean him: start by wiping his stomach up to his navel.

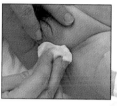

Clean carefully under his testicles

3 With fresh cotton balls, clean thoroughly in the creases at the tops of his legs and at the base of his genitals, wiping away from his body. Hold his testicles out of the way while you wipe underneath them.

4 With fresh cotton balls or washcloth, wipe all over your baby's testicles, including under his penis, as there may be traces of urine or feces here. Hold his penis out of the way if necessary, but take care not to drag the skin.

5 Clean his penis, wiping away from the body: do not pull the foreskin back to clean underneath, this will keep itself clean.

Put barrier cream *over his lower stomach to protect against diaper rash*

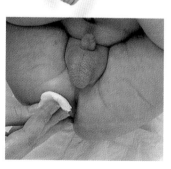

6 Lift your baby's legs to clean his anus and buttocks, keeping a finger between his ankles. Wipe over the back of his thighs too. When he's clean, remove the diaper.

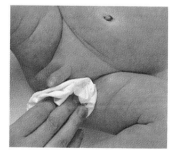

7 Wipe your hands, then dry his diaper area with tissues. Let him kick for a while, with tissues at hand just in case he urinates.

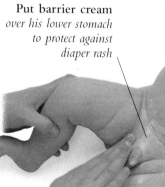

8 If using, apply barrier cream sparingly above the penis (but not on it), around the testicles and anus, and over the buttocks.

PUTTING ON AN ALL-IN-ONE DISPOSABLE DIAPER

Before you put on a new diaper, make sure that you clean your baby's bottom thoroughly and if using, apply a barrier cream. Wipe your hands well on a tissue, as the diaper's adhesive tapes won't stick very well if you get grease on them or on the front of the diaper.

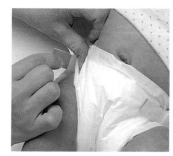

1 Open up the diaper with the tapes at the top. Lift your baby by her ankles with one finger between them and slide the diaper under her, until the top edge lines up with her waist.

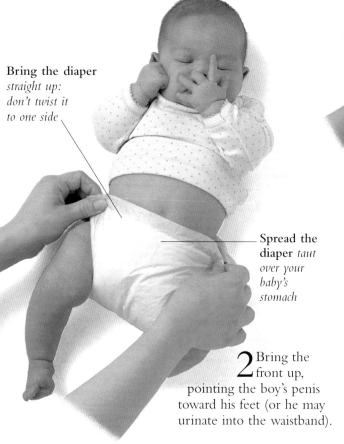

Bring the diaper *straight up: don't twist it to one side*

Spread the diaper *taut over your baby's stomach*

2 Bring the front up, pointing the boy's penis toward his feet (or he may urinate into the waistband).

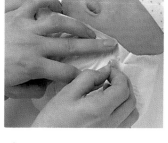

3 Hold one corner in position and, with the other hand, unpeel the tape and pull it forward to stick to the front, parallel with the top edge of the diaper.

4 Do the same with the other side, making sure the diaper is snug round your baby's legs, and not twisted around to one side.

"How can I make my 15-month-old son lie still while I change his diaper? He wriggles so much I can't clean him properly or pin the diaper on".

No self-respecting toddler will lie patiently and quietly while you change his diaper—but you must still be able to get his bottom thoroughly cleaned. Use diapers that are quick and easy to put on. Remember to make changing time fun, with games. You can also try giving him some interesting toys to hold. If he's very dirty, it will be easier to clean him by standing him in the bath on a non-slip mat and washing his bottom down with warm water. Always dry him well.

Fold the waistband *over if it is so high it could chafe your baby's navel*

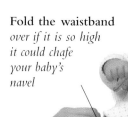

5 The diaper should fit snugly round your baby's waist—just room enough for one of your fingers. Check the fit, and if it's too loose unpeel the tapes and reposition them.

FOLDING CLOTH DIAPERS

TRIPLE ABSORBENT FOLD

The triple absorbent fold is very useful for newborn or small babies: it is small and neat when on, and gives several layers of fabric between your baby's legs, making it extra absorbent.

1 Fold a diaper in four. Put the folded edges nearest you and to the left.

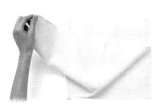

2 Pick up the top layer by the right-hand corner, and pull it out.

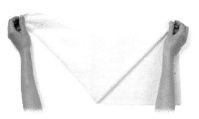

3 Make a triangle, with all the edges meeting neatly at the top.

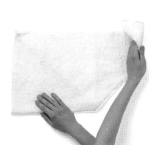

4 Turn the diaper over carefully, and straighten the edges again.

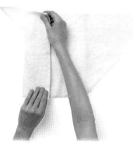

5 Pick up the vertical edge and fold into the middle by one third.

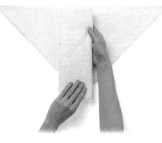

6 Fold these layers over again to make a thick central panel.

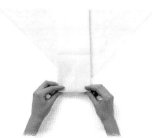

7 Put a diaper liner in position, folding one end up if necessary.

KITE FOLD

This way of folding the diaper is good for your growing baby: you can use it from the age of two or three months until your baby is out of diapers completely. As your baby gets bigger, adjust the size by varying the depth of your fold at step 3.

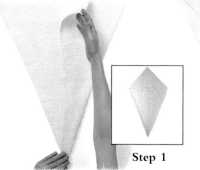

Step 1

1 Lay the diaper out flat. Fold the two edges into the middle until they meet.

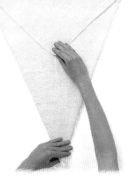

2 Fold the top point down, adjusting to make neat top corners.

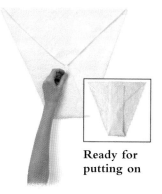

Ready for putting on

3 Fold the bottom point up and put a diaper liner in position.

YOUR DIAPER-WASHING ROUTINE

Cloth diapers must be washed and rinsed very thoroughly, so they don't irritate your baby's delicate skin and cause diaper rash. The following is a common diaper-washing routine:

★ Keep a covered plastic bucket beside your changing table, ready for used diapers

★ Soiled diapers can be dipped in toilet water, so that feces are then flushed down the toilet

★ Wash the diapers in a hot water wash, using a mild laundry soap

★ Rinse the diapers well—a common recommendation is three rinse cycles

★ Do not use any commercial laundry softeners in the rinse cycle or dryer.

★ To soften the diapers, you can add 1 cup of vinegar to the rinse cycle.

★ Wash rubber pants in warm water with a mild laundry soap added. Pat dry and leave to air.

Your local public health unit is a good source of information on cloth diapers.

Many areas have diaper services. These are commercial businesses that deliver clean diapers and pick up dirty diapers on a regular basis.

PUTTING ON A TRIPLE ABSORBENT FOLD CLOTH DIAPER

Have all your clean cloth diapers ready-folded with liners in position, so you don't have to fold one every time. Clean your baby's bottom thoroughly and, if using, apply barrier cream. Always put the soiled diaper well out of your baby's inquisitive reach, and deal with it when you've finished changing your baby.

1 Lift your baby's legs by the ankles and slide the diaper under her. Align the top edge with her waist.

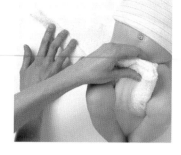

2 Bring the diaper up between her legs (tuck a boy's penis downward to prevent leakage around the waist), and hold it there while you turn up one long edge a short way.

Position the thick central panel under her bottom

3 Bring that corner up around your baby's waist, pulling slightly on the diaper to get it taut. Hold it in position while you fold up the other long edge.

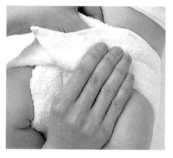

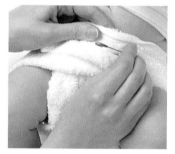

4 Still holding the first corner, bring the second corner forward, pulling the diaper quite tight: it will loosen when you pin it.

Fold up the long edge by about 4cm (1½in) first to give a good fit around her legs.

5 Slide your fingers between the diaper and her stomach so you can't jab her, then pin all layers together. Put the pin in horizontally, and clip it shut.

Tuck the rubber pants in around her waist and legs to protect her clothes from leaks

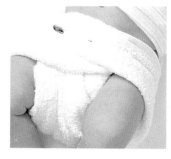

6 A good diaper will fit snugly round waist and legs: test with your finger. Cloth diapers always loosen as your baby wriggles, so if the diaper is baggy already, take the pin out and start again.

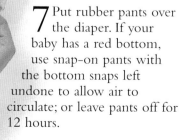

7 Put rubber pants over the diaper. If your baby has a red bottom, use snap-on pants with the bottom snaps left undone to allow air to circulate; or leave pants off for 12 hours.

PUTTING ON A KITE FOLD CLOTH DIAPER

To make diaper changing more efficient, try to have all your clean cloth diapers ready folded with their liners in position. Thoroughly clean your baby's bottom, and, if using, apply barrier cream. Once your baby is broader around the stomach, the two corners of the diaper will not overlap in the front, so fasten the diaper with two pins.

SMALL BABY

1 Lift your baby's legs gently by the ankles and slide the diaper under her. Then, fold the two long edges in by approximately 4cm (1½in).

2 Bring the short edge up between your baby's legs as far as it will go; tuck a boy's penis downward. Hold the diaper there with one hand while you bring one side corner forward and over the top.

Use one hand *to hold the two long edges folded down*

Hold the diaper *tightly—don't let it loosen*

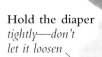
Align the top edge *of the diaper with her waist*

Pull the diaper taut *as you bring each corner forward*

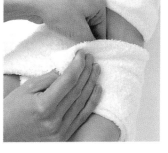

3 Bring the other corner forward and over the first, pulling on the cloth as you do so to get a snug fit.

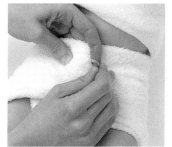

4 Without letting the diaper loosen, put your fingers inside the diaper and pin horizontally.

LARGE BABY

Repeat step 1, then bring the diaper up between your baby's legs as far as it will go, tucking a boy's penis downward. Take one front corner round his waist, pull the back corner of the diaper forward tightly, and pin horizontally. Do the same on the other side, pulling the diaper firmly round your baby's waist. Put the second pin in. Check for bagginess around his legs, tucking excess cloth in, then put rubber pants on.

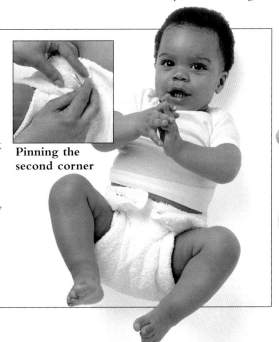
Pinning the second corner

A good fit *around the legs is essential to avoid leaks*

5 Check you have a good fit—re-pin the diaper if it looks baggy—then put rubber pants on your baby.

GIVING UP DIAPERS

Becoming toilet-trained is a big, complicated step in your toddler's life. You can't force him to use a potty chair any more than you can force him to walk. It's all part of his natural development and it may take a day, a week, a month, or half a year. All you need to do is wait until he's ready and then provide encouragement while you help him understand what's happening. Until your child turns two, he's probably physically incapable of recognizing the signs of a full bladder or bowel, or of using his muscles to control them. Be patient and nonjudgmental when he has an accident. Bowel control usually comes first, in the second year, followed by daytime bladder control, and staying dry at night is last.

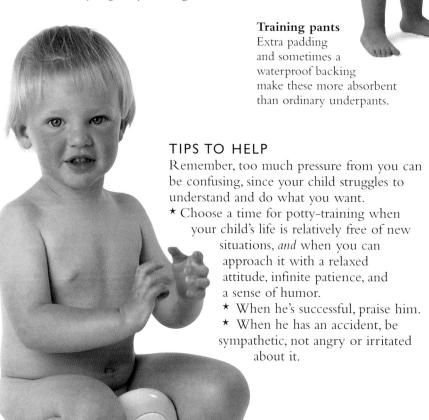

Training pants
Extra padding and sometimes a waterproof backing make these more absorbent than ordinary underpants.

TIPS TO HELP
Remember, too much pressure from you can be confusing, since your child struggles to understand and do what you want.
★ Choose a time for potty-training when your child's life is relatively free of new situations, *and* when you can approach it with a relaxed attitude, infinite patience, and a sense of humor.
★ When he's successful, praise him.
★ When he has an accident, be sympathetic, not angry or irritated about it.

Your child and his potty chair
Let him play with it and on it. He will soon understand what it's for.

ACHIEVING DAYTIME CONTROL

1

Wait until your child is ready
Your child can learn to use the potty chair only if he:
★ is two to two and a half (some boys may not be ready to do so until age three)
★ recognizes that he's done something in his diaper, perhaps by pointing and shouting, or by telling you that it's wet
★ is often dry after a nap.

2

Introduce the potty chair
Show him a potty chair and tell him what it's for. Put it in the bathroom for a few days or even months, so he gets used to it. Show him how to sit on it, with or without his diaper on at first.

3

Set aside a suitable time
The ideal time to start potty-training is in the summer when your child can wear training pants while playing outside in the yard. Accidents won't be as disastrous on the grass and you won't have to worry about outer clothing. Set up his potty chair where he can see it outside. It's important he can access his potty easily. Don't start when your routines are upset for any reason or when away from home.

4

Buy or borrow a pile of training pants
Make sure you keep a stack of clean training pants in the bathroom so when he has an accident, he can quickly discard one pair for another. Buy or borrow a dozen. Avoid overalls with complicated straps, zippers, or buttons. Time is of the essence when he has to go.

5

Help him to use the potty chair
Be encouraging about sitting on the potty chair, but don't put pressure on him. Buy him pants he can pull down by himself but help him sit down on the chair. If he's managed to tell you he needs the potty, thank him.

If your child jumps up immediately
Suggest that he sit a little longer and make it easier by distracting him with a toy or a book. If nothing happens, let him get up and keep on playing.

When he does go in the potty
When he does use the potty chair successfully, praise him and tell him what a good boy he is. Wipe off drips of urine with toilet paper or clean his bottom quickly (wipe a girl from front to back). Hold the potty chair steady as he stands up. Offer to pull up his pants for him. Don't show disgust at the contents, flush it away, wipe the potty chair clean, rinse it, and wash your hands.

6

When your child has an accident, don't scold him
You can't expect him to be able to use the potty every time at this stage. When he wets or dirties his pants, don't scold him. Clean him up and be sympathetic. Have a supply of clean training pants handy in the bathroom.

If he doesn't get the hang of it
If after two weeks your child is showing no signs of understanding, and is not telling you he needs the potty chair on at least some occasions, he's not ready to give up diapers yet. Put him back in them for a few more weeks, then try again—you may have several two-week training stints before he gets himself to the potty chair on most occasions when he needs to.

7

Take the diaper off during naps
Once your child is using the potty chair fairly reliably during the daytime, and his diaper has been dry after a nap for about a week, you can take his diaper off—he may even ask you to remove it. Suggest that he sit on the potty chair after he wakes from his nap.

8

When you go out
Until your child is fairly reliable, put a diaper on him when you go out, but talk to him about it. Try to ensure, without forcing him, that he uses his potty chair before you go. For car trips, a diaper might be essential unless you can stop easily. Take a potty chair, spare clothes, and an old towel in case of accidents.

9

Suggest using the toilet
After a few weeks or months of using the potty chair during the day, suggest that he might try using the toilet. Clip a child's seat on it to give him confidence that he won't fall in, and put a step in front so he can climb up. Help him the first few times, until he gets the hang of it. If he just wants to urinate, lift the seat and lid and show him how to aim his penis. Otherwise help him pull his pants down and climb up to sit on the seat; do the same for a girl. Stay nearby until he's finished, wipe his bottom and help him down. Many children aren't able to wipe their own bottoms until at least four. He will probably want to flush the toilet afterward. Then wash his and your hands.

ACHIEVING NIGHTTIME CONTROL

1

Wait until your child is already dry at night
If you have taken a dry diaper off your child in the morning for at least a week, he can start going without one at night.

2

Don't force the issue of staying dry at night
Your child will stay dry at night when his bladder is mature enough and you aren't putting pressure on him. If you make a toddler nervous or anxious about something he has no control over, it will only take longer. If you both feel more at ease when he remains diapered at night, let him wear one. If he wants to wear his training pants, let him.

3

If he wets the bed
If your child starts to wet his bed, don't scold, punish, or blame him. Has he suffered some upheaval in his life? There are numerous explanations for why some children never wet their beds and others are unable to stay dry. Because bedwetting seems to run in families, doctors have looked for physical causes. Is he a deep sleeper, unable to wake when the urge might be extreme? The size of the bladder is also linked to bedwetting. Put a nightlight in his room by the potty chair. Try waking him to use the toilet at 10 or 11 pm. and protect his mattress with plastic garbage bags under the bottom sheet.

Adapted toilet seat
This seat fits on an adult toilet, giving your child more confidence.

TAKING YOUR BABY OUT

S ome form of carriage or stroller and a car seat are essential for your new baby. Other useful items are an infant carrier (see page 85) or a backpack if your baby is older. A diaper bag with detachable changing mat is convenient for parents on the go: pack it with disposable diapers, changing equipment, spare clothes, plastic bags for dirty diapers, and whatever feeding equipment you need (but see page 101 for how to transport formula safely). It's a good idea to take a container of diluted juice or water and a bottle or training beaker, and don't forget her favorite toy or security blanket.

Your older baby will get enormous enjoyment from your adventures—there's always something to see. Whether you're going to the zoo to show her the animals, to the park, or a friend's house, she will enjoy the outing.

WHAT KIND OF CARRIAGE?

While it may not be quite as difficult as buying a car, deciding on what kind of carriage to purchase for your baby can be almost as troublesome. These checklists should help you sort out the pros and cons of baby carriages and strollers. Before you go shopping, however, consider how many months of the year you'll be using your purchase, how old your baby is, and where you'll be walking. You don't want to succumb to a sale on an old-fashioned baby carriage if you'll be able to use it for only a month, for instance.

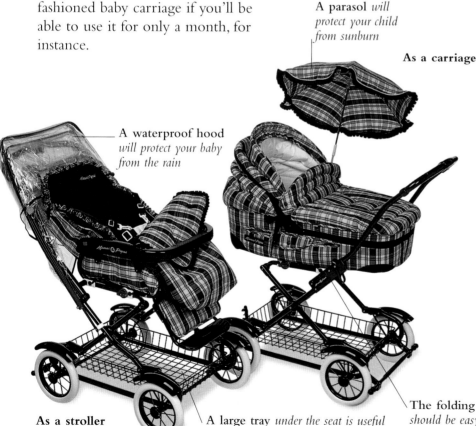

A parasol will protect your child from sunburn

As a carriage

A waterproof hood will protect your baby from the rain

As a stroller

A large tray under the seat is useful for shopping and changing equipment

The folding mechanism should be easy to use

CARRIAGE
Use from birth
☑ Gives your young baby good protection in bad weather.
☑ Gives your baby a comfortable ride.
☑ Can be used up to about one year.
☒ Can't easily be used on public transportation.
☒ Needs ample storage space at home.

CONVERTIBLE CARRIAGE-STROLLER
Use from birth as a carriage
Use from three months as a stroller
☑ Your young baby can face you.
☑ When your baby is older you can convert to the stroller position so she can ride looking forward and see around her.
☑ As a carriage, it gives your young baby good protection in bad weather. Your young baby can be snug under a baby blanket or comforter.
☑ As a stroller, the rigid seatback gives good support.
☑ In either position the carriage is light, and easy to maneuver.
☑ It can be easily stored when folded flat.
☒ It can be awkward to take on public transportation.

UMBRELLA-STYLE FOLDING STROLLER
from six months

☑ Folds up neatly so it's good on public transportation and if storage is limited.
☑ The cheapest option; also the lightest.
☒ Soft seatback offers poor support, so not suitable for babies under six months.

YOUR WALKING CHILD
A harness is an ideal way to keep your child from wandering off when you are out and about, and gives her more freedom than holding your hand. Take the stroller with you, too.

CARRIAGE AND STROLLER SAFETY

★ Check that the safety bakes of a carriage or stroller are set in the locked position before you put the baby in.
★ In a stroller, always strap your child in with the seat belts or stroller harness.
★ In a carriage, fit and always use a harness when your baby starts to sit up.
★ Put the brake on as soon as you stop.
★ Never let your child pull herself up or stand in the carriage: she may tip it over.
★ Never hang heavy shopping bags on the handles: you may tip the stroller over.
★ Never let your child play with a folded stroller.

SAFETY IN THE CAR

Every child must be securely buckled into an approved car seat when traveling in a car. The seat must suit your child's age and weight. The back seat is the safest place for children 12 years of age or under, including babies. Children aged 12 and under must not be in a seating position that has an airbag.

IN-CAR ENTERTAINMENT
Make car trips fun by:
★ bringing along children's cassettes of songs or stories
★ singing songs or reciting nursery rhymes
★ packing a bag full of finger puppets, books, puzzles, teethers, toy cars, and an activity center
★ stopping frequently.

WHAT SEAT FOR WHAT WEIGHT?

Stage 1: Rear-facing infant seat Use a rear-facing infant seat from birth until your baby is around 1 year old. Use an infant seat in the rear-facing position until your baby has reached the height and weight specified by the seat manufacturer. Infant seats will safely restrain your baby until 9-10kg (20-22lb). For heavier babies, use a car seat (infant or infant/child) that allows a higher weight in the rear-facing position.

Stage 2: Forward-facing child seat Use a forward-facing child seat from when your child is about 10kg (22lb) until 18kg (40lb), from about age 1 to 4½ years. Some child seats can be used until your child weighs 22kg (48lb). Always follow the guidelines in the instructions and on the label of your car seat.

Stage 3: Booster seat Use a booster seat from 18kg (40lb), generally from about age 4½ to 8. Children are ready to use a booster seat when they are over the maximum weight and height for their child seat—but no sooner than this. For this age group, booster seats are the safest way to position a seat belt correctly over a child's body.

Stage 4: Seat belt Use an adult seat belt for children who weigh over 27kg (60lb), which is usually from about age 8. Make sure you keep the lap belt low and snug across the hips and the shoulder belt positioned over the shoulder and across the chest.

TRAVELING TIPS

Never travel with a child on your lap or a baby in your arms. In the event of a collision you will not be able to hold on and your child may be killed or injured. Buckle children up properly every time— even for short trips.

You should **always**:
★ Select a child car seat that fits your child and your car.
★ Face infants toward the **rear**.
★ Fasten the car seat with the seat belt, properly routing the belt as directed by the manufacturer.
★ Fasten the child seat harness snugly over her shoulders.
★ Use only child safety seats that conform to Canadian Motor Vehicle Safety Standards. (Seats certified to U.S. standards do not meet Canadian standards.)
★ Never leave your baby or child unattended in your car. If you get out of your car, always take her with you.

WHEN YOU HAVE TO LEAVE YOUR CHILD

During your first few days or weeks with your new baby you may feel that you will never have the time to do anything but care for the baby ever again. So, the first time that you leave your baby, even if it is just for an hour or two's shopping, a trip to the gym, or a visit to the cinema, is a real milestone for you. Leaving your precious new baby in the care of even the most trusted friend, grandparent, or babysitter is a real wrench. You may even feel a bit guilty because it suddenly seems such a relief to be free, albeit briefly, from the feeling of total responsibility that you have for your tiny infant.

GETTING YOUR CHILD USED TO OTHER PEOPLE

BABYSITTERS
Nothing is more important during your baby's early months than your loving closeness. And yet eventually he has to learn to lead a separate existence independently of you. His eventual transition to school will be easier and his confidence will grow if he has opportunities to explore the world outside his immediate family, to be independent of you, and to make close relationships with other people—grandparents, babysitters, and friends.

So it isn't frivolous and it isn't selfish to get your baby used to a regular babysitter when he is very young. And if you plan to go back to work within the next year or so, then it is essential that they get used to the idea that someone else besides you can be relied on to love and care for him. There are several things you can do to make babysitting easier both for the sitter and the baby.

★ Always tell your baby what's going to happen, even if he is too young to understand.

★ If you go out in the evening, make sure he knows the babysitter, so that if he wakes he won't be terrified at seeing a stranger.

★ Don't introduce any new baby-sitting arrangement when your baby is tired, hungry, or sick. Pick a time of day when you think he'll be at his most alert and happiest.

★ If you have a new babysitter, don't rush to go out even if you are in a hurry. Spend some time holding him and letting him size up this new person. Let the baby see that you like the babysitter.

★ Show the babysitter which are his favorite toys and how to play the games he likes to play.

★ If the babysitter has to put your child to bed, make sure they know every detail of his bedtime routine so that your child will go to bed happily.

SEPARATION ANXIETY
At some time, usually between seven months and a year, your baby may start to seem reluctant even to let you out of his sight for a second. He'll cling when you try to put him down, or cry inconsolably if he is left with anyone else. Don't worry about such behavior. This "separation anxiety" is quite normal and means that he recognizes you as separate from him and realizes how essential you are to him. Even the most clingy baby will eventually become independent. But meanwhile, accept his utter dependence on you lovingly and patiently. If you have to go out, always tell him—don't just sneak out to avoid a scene. Tell him where you are going and reassure him that you will be coming back.

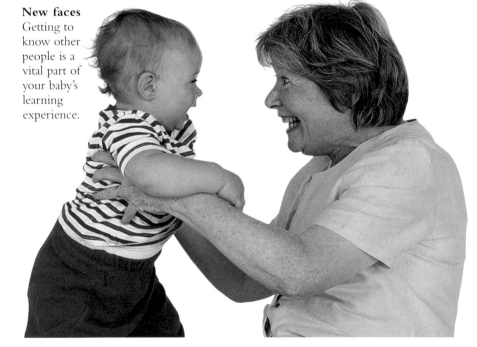
New faces
Getting to know other people is a vital part of your baby's learning experience.

CUDDLIES AND SECURITY BLANKETS

By eight or nine months most children form a strong attachment to a favorite soft toy, blanket, or a special object. This powerful need for something cuddly grows even stronger after the first birthday. The child may carry it around continually during the day, take it to bed at night, cuddling or sucking it for comfort. Eventually it becomes a kind of talisman, something the child turns to for comfort whenever they are sad, frightened, or frustrated. Your child's cuddly will become grubby, shabby, and eventually probably unsanitary, because the child will be reluctant to let you wash it since its smell is part of its comfortable familiarity. Don't try to persuade them to give it up. It fulfills a real need. Keep it handy, make sure babysitters know about it, and try to forestall the disaster of losing it by keeping a duplicate somewhere safe.

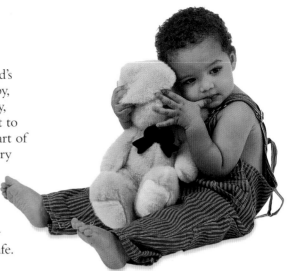

CHILDCARE OPTIONS

GOING BACK TO WORK

Whether you are going back to work because you love your job or whether it is a matter of financial necessity, returning to work is bound to be stressful at first. How smoothly it goes depends almost entirely on the childcare arrangements you make. It will take a little while for everything to settle down, so don't worry too much if the first few days are difficult. Children are pretty adaptable, and most settle down quickly under a new routine. But keep a careful eye on your child during the first few weeks you are back at work. If his behavior deteriorates or if he seems generally unhappy, you may need to re-think your childcare plans.

Grandparent care

This may be an ideal arrangement provided that the grandparent is willing. It is important that they know and respect your views on childcare—and vice versa. Problems may arise if you feel that your baby is being "taken over".

Shared care with a friend or relative

If you intend to work part-time, and have a good friend or close relative who also has small children, this may be a workable solution. It's important to formalize the arrangement and stick to it, so that neither party feels they are being taken advantage of.

Caregiver

Regulations concerning caregivers may vary among provinces. A caregiver may register with a local authority, which ensures that the caregiver follows certain standards. This includes a limit on the number of young children cared for.

But you also need to talk to the caregiver yourself, to make sure that she is the kind of person you want to care for your child. It may be difficult to find a place for a very young baby.

Day care center

Private day care centers offer full day care, usually from around 7:30 am to 6 pm, and usually stay open during holiday periods. There is usually a fairly high ratio of staff to children and a stimulating environment. Staff may have a diploma in Early Childhood Education.

Nanny care

This is the most expensive childcare option. Having a nanny means your child has one to one care in his or her own home. A qualified nanny will have a childcare qualification such as an Early Childhood Development diploma. Always ask to see registration documents and childcare qualification certificates, and always check references before offering a job.

N.B. An au pair is a mother's helper, not a caregiver. Au pairs are untrained and will have little or no childcare experience. He or she may babysit on occasion, but is not trained as a full-time caregiver.

Adapting well
Your child will soon get used to someone else looking after him.

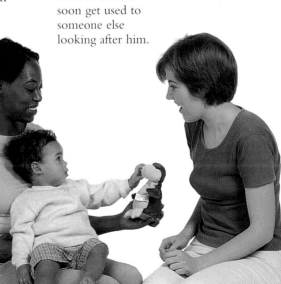

GROWING AND LEARNING

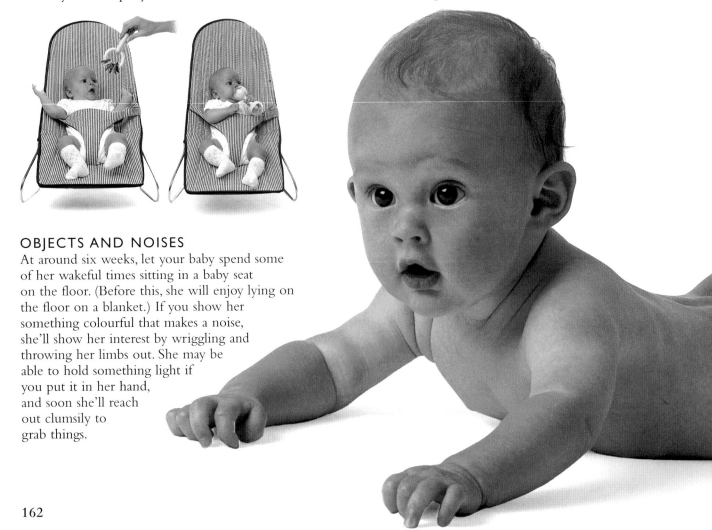

Watching your child grow and learn is a rewarding experience. Every stage brings something new: at first it's rolling over, using his hands, sitting, crawling, walking. Once he's mastered those he will learn to talk, and will refine his coordination and dexterity. Even though you might think there's nothing so thrilling as watching him take his first steps, the next year will bring some subtler achievements that will fill you with pride.

Throughout these pre-school years, your child needs your help. He needs your stimulation and responsiveness, and he needs you to structure his play, too. Everything he knows about the way things behave, colours and shapes, cause and effect, he learns through playing with toys and everyday objects. To your child everything is a wonderful game. Getting dressed, unpacking the shopping, laying the table—it's all a chance to participate and learn.

THE FIRST SIX MONTHS

During these months you will see your baby develop into a real personality, able to reward you with lots of enchanting smiles and gurgles. Although there are a lot of toys aimed at this age group, he needs—and loves—your company most of all. When he's wakeful, take the time to talk and smile to him. Plenty of stimulation in the form of things to look at, sounds to hear, and textures to explore is vital too. You don't need expensive toys: old postcards and photographs, rattles, non-glass mirrors, will all do just as well.

OBJECTS AND NOISES

At around six weeks, let your baby spend some of her wakeful times sitting in a baby seat on the floor. (Before this, she will enjoy lying on the floor on a blanket.) If you show her something colourful that makes a noise, she'll show her interest by wriggling and throwing her limbs out. She may be able to hold something light if you put it in her hand, and soon she'll reach out clumsily to grab things.

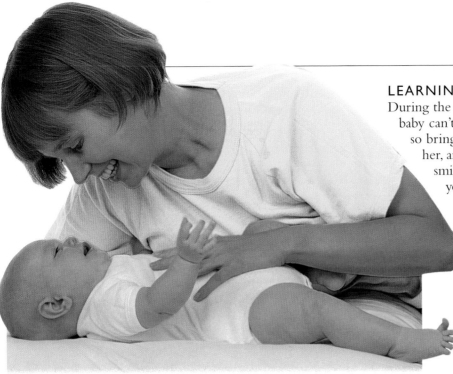

LEARNING ABOUT EACH OTHER

During the first couple of months of life, your baby can't focus beyond about 25cm (10in), so bring your face close when you talk to her, and exaggerate your expressions and smiles. It's this eye contact that helps your baby become a person, and shows her what building a loving relationship is all about.

ROLLING

Sometime during this six months, your baby will learn to roll over, from front to back first, then from back to front. It will give him a great sense of achievement: he's beginning to make his body move for him. Remember that even before he's learnt to roll he can fall off things, so never leave him unattended on a high surface, not even the bed.

LEARNING TO SIT

As your baby gets more control over his body, help him learn to sit by surrounding him with cushions. They will help him balance, and protect him if he topples over.

PREMATURE BABIES

Your premature baby will probably reach all his developmental milestones rather later than other babies. Remember that in reality he has two "birthdays": one is the day he was born, but the more important one for the first few months is the date on which he was expected to be born. If you take those missing weeks in the womb into account, you will almost certainly find that his progress is not slow at all. Take him to your doctor for regular monitoring; he should have caught up with other children born at the same time by the age of two.

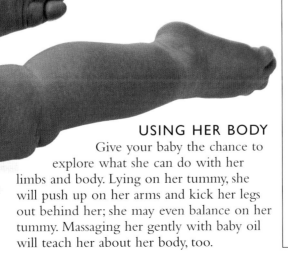

USING HER BODY

Give your baby the chance to explore what she can do with her limbs and body. Lying on her tummy, she will push up on her arms and kick her legs out behind her; she may even balance on her tummy. Massaging her gently with baby oil will teach her about her body, too.

MILESTONES CHART

Babies don't all develop at the same rate, or learn a particular skill at a particular time. But because everything they learn acts as a "milestone" to the next stage of development, they do acquire skills in the same order. The chart below shows the "milestones" in various areas of your child's development—physical skills, manual dexterity, sight, hearing and speech, and social behavior and play. Your child may learn to do something either sooner or later than the average age given in the chart, and he may acquire skills more slowly in one area than another. This is unimportant—all that matters is that he makes steady progress, at his own pace, from one milestone to the next.

MILESTONES IN CHILD DEVELOPMENT

Age	Physical Movements	Manual Dexterity	Hearing, Vision, and Speech	Social Behavior and Play
One Month	Lies on back with head to one side. Held sitting, head falls forward with back in one complete curve. Held standing on hard surface, presses down feet, straightens body, and often makes reflex "stepping" movements.	Hands normally closed, but if open will grasp a finger if it touches his palm.	Startled by loud noises. Turns head and eyes toward light. Eyes will follow a dangling toy held 6–8in (15–20cm) away and moved slowly from side to side.	Stops crying when picked up and spoken to. Looks at mother's face intently when she feeds or talks to him.
Three Months	Lies on back with head in mid-line. Kicks vigorously. Held sitting, can hold head erect and steady for several seconds. Placed face down, lifts head and upper chest well up. Held standing with feet on hard surface, sags at knees.	Watches movements of own hands and begins to clasp and unclasp hands. Holds rattle placed in his hands for a few moments, but can't look at it at the same time.	Very alert. Interested in people's faces. Moves head to look around. Eyes converge as a toy held above his face is moved nearer. Smiles at mother's voice. Vocalizes when spoken to or pleased. Turns head and eyes toward a sound.	Smiles at 5–6 weeks. Recognizes and begins to react to preparations for bath, feeds, etc. by smiles, coos, excited movements. Responds with obvious pleasure to friendly handling, tickling, being talked or sung to.
Six Months	Raises head when lying on back. Sits with support. When hands are grasped, can pull himself up. Rolls over, front to back. Placed face down, lifts head and chest up. Held standing on hard surface, takes his weight and bounces.	Stretches out both hands to grasp interesting object. Usually uses both hands to scoop up an object, occasionally uses just one hand. Shakes rattle deliberately, and often looks at it at the same time. Takes everything to mouth.	"Sings" and chats to himself using single and double syllables, e.g. ka, muh. Turns immediately to mother's voice across room. Screams when annoyed. Recognizes and responds to different emotional tones of mother's voice.	Laughs, chuckles, and squeals aloud in play. Still friendly with strangers, but sometimes shows some anxiety, especially if mother is out of sight. When he drops a toy he'll forget about it.
Nine Months	Sits alone for 10–15 minutes on floor. Progresses on floor by rolling or squirming. Tries to crawl on all fours. Pulls self to standing with support but can't lower himself. Held standing, steps purposefully on alternate feet.	Examines objects by passing them from one hand to the other. Stretches out one hand to grasp small objects. Will hold out toy to adult, but can't yet let go unless pressing against hard surface. Grasps spoon while being fed.	Shouts to attract attention, listens and shouts again. Babbles tunefully, using long strings of syllables e.g. dad-dad. Understands "no" and "bye-bye." Imitates adult noises—cough, brrr etc. Watches people and activities with interest.	Looks after toys falling over edge of stroller or table. Can find partially hidden toy. Plays "peek-a-boo." May be wary of strangers, clinging to known adult and hiding face.

Age	Physical Movements	Manual Dexterity	Hearing, Vision, and Speech	Social Behavior and Play
Twelve Months	Sits well for indefinite time. Crawls rapidly. Can pull self to standing. Walks round furniture stepping sideways. Walks with one or both hands held. May stand alone for a few moments. May walk alone.	Can pick up small objects with thumb and index finger. Points at objects he wants or which interest him. Holds spoon but usually cannot use it alone. Drinks from cup with little assistance.	Knows and responds to own name. Babbles loudly and incessantly. Shows by behavior that he understands several familiar words and also commands associated with gestures "clap hands," etc.	Shows affection to familiar people. Tries to help with dressing. Throws toys deliberately and watches them fall to ground. Waves bye-bye and claps hands in imitation. Puts wooden cubes in and out of box.
Fifteen Months	Walks unsteadily with feet wide apart. Goes from standing to sitting by collapsing backward with a bump, or falling forward on hands. Crawls upstairs. May be able to bend over to pick up toys from floor.	Builds tower of two cubes after being shown. Grasps crayon and imitates scribble. Brings spoon to mouth to lick, but can't stop it turning over. Holds cup when given it, and gives it back.	Speaks 2–6 recognizable words and understands many more. Understands and obeys simple commands, e.g. shut the door, bring me your shoes. Looks with interest at pictures in book and pats page.	Helps more constructively with dressing. May easily get upset or frustrated. Very dependent on mother's reassuring presence. Can push large wheeled toy on level ground.
Eighteen Months	Walks well. Runs stiffly, but can't run around obstacles. Carries large toys while walking. Walks upstairs with helping hand. Creeps backward downstairs. May sit on stairs and bump down a few steps.	Can pick up tiny objects with delicate pincer grasp. Preference for one hand more obvious. Scribbles with crayon, using preferred hand. Builds tower of three cubes after demonstration.	Babbles to himself. Uses 6–20 words and understands many more. Sings and tries to join in nursery rhymes. Enjoys picture books, often recognizing and pointing out colored items. Turns pages two at a time.	Takes off shoes, socks, and hat. No longer takes toys to mouth. Plays contentedly alone, but likes to be near adult. Emotionally still very dependent on familiar adults, especially mother.
Two Years	Runs safely. Walks backward. Pulls wheeled toy. Climbs on and off furniture. Goes up and down stairs holding rail, two feet to a step. Throws small ball. Sits on wheeled toy and moves forward with feet.	Builds tower of six cubes or more. Draws spontaneous circle and dots. Can imitate vertical line. Recognizes familiar adults in photograph after having been shown once. Hand preference becoming obvious.	Turns pages one by one. Uses 50 plus recognizable words. Puts two or more words together to make simple sentences. Refers to himself by name. Constantly asking names of objects. Joins in nursery rhymes and songs.	Follows mother around house and copies what she does. Plays simple make-believe games. Plays near other children but not with them. Tantrums when frustrated, but easily distracted.
Two and a Half Years	Walks upstairs alone, but downstairs holding rail, two feet to a step. Can climb easy climbing frame. Jumps with two feet together. Can kick large ball. Sits on tricycle and steers, but can't yet pedal.	Can build tower of seven or more cubes and line up blocks to form a "train." Can draw a horizontal line and circle when shown how. Eats skillfully with spoon and may use a fork.	Uses 200 plus words. Knows full name. Uses "I", "me" and "you." Always asking questions beginning "what?" and "where?" Can say a few nursery rhymes. Recognizes self in photo, once shown.	Rebellious and throws violent tantrums if frustrated and is less easily distracted. Enjoys make-believe play. Likes to watch other children at play and may join in for a few minutes. Still has little idea of sharing toys.
Three Years	Walks alone upstairs with alternating feet, downstairs with two feet to step. Climbs with agility. Rides tricycle. Can walk on tiptoes. Can stand on one foot for a moment. Sits with feet crossed at ankle.	Eats well with fork and spoon. Can wash hands. Pulls underpants down and up. Can build tower of nine blocks or more. Can draw man with head and some features. Paints "pictures" with large brush. Uses scissors.	Can give full name, sex, and sometimes age. Can carry on simple conversations and talk about past experiences. Listens eagerly to stories and demands favorites over and over. Can match 2–3 primary colors.	Less prone to tantrums. Affectionate. Likes to help with adult's activities. Enjoys floor play with bricks, cars, etc. Plays with other children. Understands about taking turns. Affectionate toward younger siblings.

165

THE SECOND SIX MONTHS

Your baby will cram a great deal into these months. He will sit up unsupported, he may crawl and even stand or walk by his first birthday. It won't be steady progress, and not every child goes through each stage. Don't be surprised if your child never crawls, for example: it won't hinder his walking development. This is the age when he learns to explore every new thing by putting it in his mouth—so finger foods are ideal. From now until around two years old, make sure your child never gets hold of anything sharp or toxic, or so small that he could swallow it.

EXPLORING BOXES
Don't be surprised if the baby finds the boxes her toys arrive in just as fascinating as the toys. Check for and remove any staples.

MAKING NOISES
A wooden spoon and a saucepan make a perfect drum—your baby will love banging away and listening to the loud noise.

SITTING UP
Your baby will lean forward and splay her legs out wide and straight when she first learns to balance sitting up. (Put a cushion behind her until she's really steady.) Now she has both hands free to explore. A board book is easy to handle, and even more fun if you look at it with her and point out the action, objects, and characters.

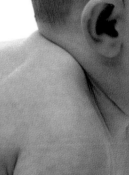

CRAWLING
Getting about on all fours is a great achievement. She may not use each leg in the same way: a lop-sided shuffle with one knee and the other foot are quite normal.

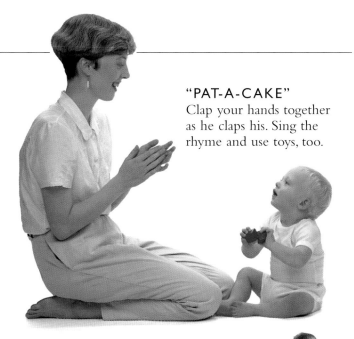

"PAT-A-CAKE"
Clap your hands together as he claps his. Sing the rhyme and use toys, too.

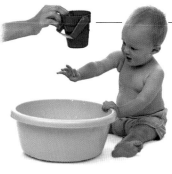

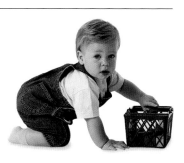

WATER PLAY
Show your baby how water behaves and feels on her hands. Sieves and plastic jugs make good substitutes for toy pails.

BOXES AND OBJECTS
Give your older baby a box and some blocks, and he will happily take them out one by one, then put them back in again.

INTRODUCING A BALL
At seven months your baby may be fascinated to see a ball rolling around, but surprised when she accidentally makes it move. By a year, she may be able to pick it up, throw it, and roll it—she's learned how a ball behaves.

PULLING UP AND CRUISING
At ten months, your child may be able to coordinate his arms and legs well enough to pull himself up on furniture (clear away anything unstable). The next stage is to start shuffling sideways holding on—known as cruising. He will probably sit down with a heavy bump.

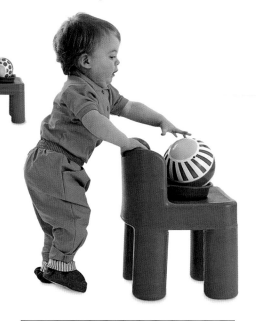

CLIMBING STAIRS
As soon as your child shows interest in the stairs, for his own safety teach him how to go up *and* down on all fours, facing into the stairs. Fit a baby gate for when you're not watching.

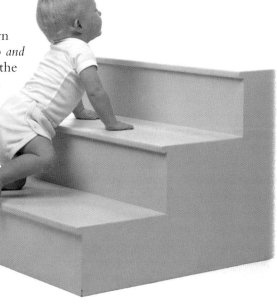

PLAYPENS
A **playpen** can be a useful safe place if you have to leave your mobile child alone for a few moments—to answer the door, for example. However, you should never leave him in it for more than a few minutes, he will simply get frustrated and bored. As well as being a safe place for your baby, a playpen can also serve as a great storage spot for the mountains of toys your baby may have accumulated. The key to a successful playpen is not to overuse it, save it for the times when you really need to leave your baby momentarily.

YOUR ONE-YEAR-OLD

First steps and first words will probably be your child's most exciting and significant achievements during his second year. New worlds open up for him once he can get about as you do, and communicate with you in word. Handedness becomes apparent around the middle of this year: he will show a definite preference for one hand, and once he starts to draw and paint this will become more marked. Although he will amuse himself for short periods, you're still his essential and most-valued playmate, and his most effective teacher too.

First steps will be unsteady

USING STAIRS
Toward the end of this year, your child may grow confident and skillful enough to go up and down stairs upright and facing forward.

LEARNING TO WALK
Once your child has taken her first hesitant steps unsupported, it will only be a few days before she's waddling about enthusiastically, if unsteadily. She'll keep her feet wide apart and her arms out for balance. Let her go barefoot as often as possible: she only needs shoes for walking about out of doors.

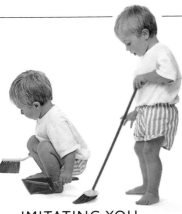

WALKING SKILLS
A pull-along toy will help his sense of balance.

IMITATING YOU
Copying you is how your child learns—and "helping" is always a favorite game. Toy tools make it easy for him to join in.

BUILDING A TOWER
From about 18 months, your child will be able to build a tower of four or even five bricks.

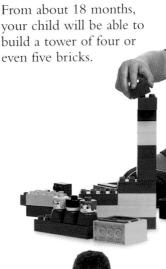

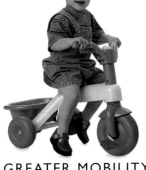

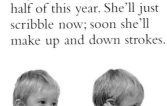

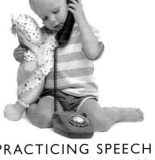

GREATER MOBILITY
At around 18 months, a simple, stable, ride-on toy will improve coordination and confidence, and provide a new challenge.

USING CRAYONS
Introduce non-toxic crayons during the second half of this year. She'll just scribble now; soon she'll make up and down strokes.

LEARNING SHAPES
Sorting shapes into their correct holes is an absorbing and challenging lesson. Give plenty of praise when he gets one right.

PRACTICING SPEECH
A telephone is an invaluable toy for practicing the art of communication by copying what you do.

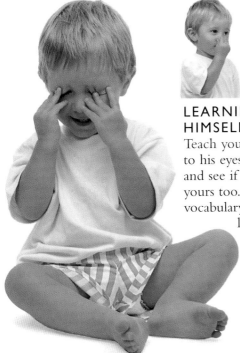

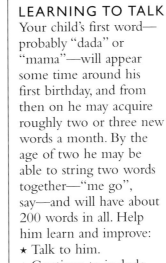

LEARNING ABOUT HIMSELF
Teach your child to point to his eyes, nose, and ears, and see if he can point to yours too. It will expand his vocabulary, and help him learn to see himself as a person in his own right.

LEARNING TO TALK
Your child's first word—probably "dada" or "mama"—will appear some time around his first birthday, and from then on he may acquire roughly two or three new words a month. By the age of two he may be able to string two words together—"me go", say—and will have about 200 words in all. Help him learn and improve:
★ Talk to him.
★ Continue to include picture books and rhymes in your playtimes.

★ Listen to him, be interested in what he's saying, and try to understand.
★ Don't interrupt him to make him repeat things "properly". He won't always get the pronunciation right at first.
★ Use adult language when you talk back to him, so he can hear the words spoken correctly.
★ Be clear and direct: "Put the brick on the top" is less confusing than "Let's see if we can get this nice red brick on top of the other one."

YOUR TWO-YEAR-OLD

This year, your child may surprise you with a burgeoning imagination that can make an absorbing game out of anything. Don't waste money on expensive kits and toys that can only stifle his creativity. A big cardboard box makes a house, a car, a boat, a spaceship—then when it gets battered, you can throw it away and get another one (remove any staples). A sheet draped over two chairs is a haven, a tent, a house—anything he can think of. Toward the end of this year your child might join a playgroup, and start to play with other children in a constructive way; and you'll notice that he's becoming open to suggestion and reason when you want him to do things.

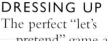
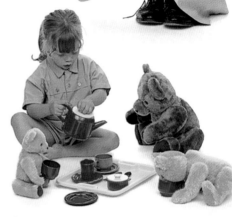

DRESSING UP

The perfect "let's pretend" game at any age. Your old clothes, shoes, purses, and hats are all ideal items for a dressing-up box, and much more fun to play with than the special childsize outfits in the stores.

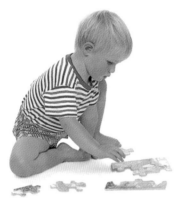

IRREGULAR SHAPES

Jigsaws demand concentration, dexterity, and visual understanding. If he gives up quickly, try giving him a simpler one.

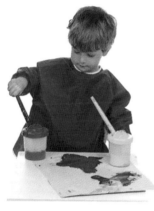

COLOR AND PAINT

Painting is a good way to learn about color and texture. Give him thick brushes and non-spill pots, and protect his clothes.

IMAGINARY FRIENDS

Dolls and teddies will become friends to your girl or boy, and she will want to control their lives in the way you control hers.

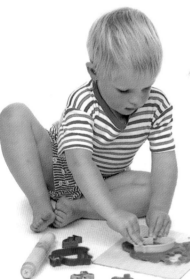

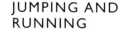

USING HIS HANDS

Help your child refine his hand movements. He can screw and unscrew small objects now, and will enjoy using pastry cutters to make shapes out of play dough or your pastry.

JUMPING AND RUNNING

Learning to jump, run, and balance are new physical challenges. Jump with him to show him how to bend his knees as he lands.

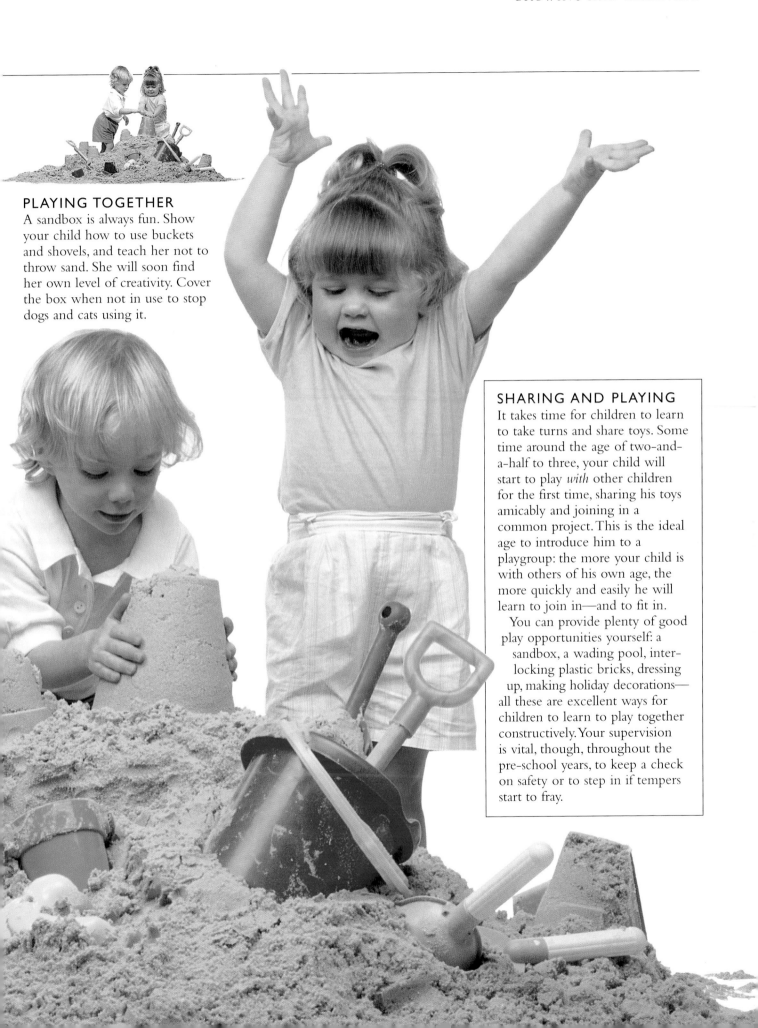

PLAYING TOGETHER

A sandbox is always fun. Show your child how to use buckets and shovels, and teach her not to throw sand. She will soon find her own level of creativity. Cover the box when not in use to stop dogs and cats using it.

SHARING AND PLAYING

It takes time for children to learn to take turns and share toys. Some time around the age of two-and-a-half to three, your child will start to play *with* other children for the first time, sharing his toys amicably and joining in a common project. This is the ideal age to introduce him to a playgroup: the more your child is with others of his own age, the more quickly and easily he will learn to join in—and to fit in.

You can provide plenty of good play opportunities yourself: a sandbox, a wading pool, inter-locking plastic bricks, dressing up, making holiday decorations—all these are excellent ways for children to learn to play together constructively. Your supervision is vital, though, throughout the pre-school years, to keep a check on safety or to step in if tempers start to fray.

GAMES TO PLAY WITH YOUR BABY

Most parents realize how important it is to talk to their baby. But not everyone finds it easy to do this without feeling embarrassed or self-conscious. That's one reason why the games that parents traditionally play with their babies are so important. They provide a natural way for you to interact with your baby. Many of them involve simple repetitive rhymes and songs that even a baby quickly learns to recognize and that will help to stimulate his own language development. Here are some favorite games to play with your young child.

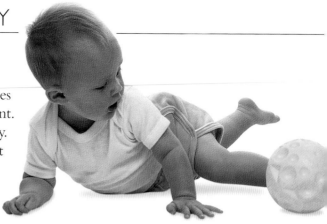

PLAYING CATCH

All children seem to love a game of simple catch. Sit down on the floor, with your baby directly opposite you, and gently roll a soft ball or wheeled toy toward him. He may pick the toy up and want to return it to you. Alternatively, he may simply want to hold the toy and examine or even chew it. He may even puzzle you by holding out the toy for you to take and then pulling it back again. This is quite common— although he's learned to grasp something, he may not yet have learnt to let it go. Don't try to pull the toy away from him. Just tell him what a nice toy it is and keep on chatting to him.

ACTIVITY GAMES

Games that involve riding and bouncing on a parents knee, such as "Yankee Doodle went to town," can be as boisterous or as gentle as the baby's own age and temperament dictate. Your baby will very quickly learn to indicate when he wants to do it again—and when he has had enough.

HIDING AND FINDING GAMES

Search and find games can be fascinating right from babyhood to primary school age. A baby's first "treasure hunt" is to see you hide one of his toys under a blanket or towel right in front of him, and then, when you say "Where did the toy go?" make the discovery that the hidden toy is actually still there, under the blanket. You can step up the excitement by using three towels— which one is the toy under? To find it the baby has to follow rudimentary rules—the toy is under a towel, not somewhere else quite different—and to remember under which towel his toy has gone.

"Peek-a-boo" is an immensely popular variation on this. The surprise of seeing your face dip out of sight and then come back into view can send a little one squealing with pleasure. And even if your baby loved it when he was only six months old, he will still enjoy variations on this search and find game later on. As he grows older he'll imitate you and

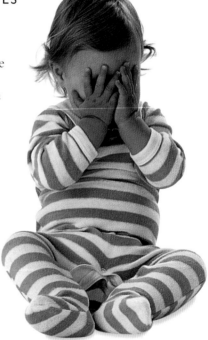

may "hide" from you behind his hands or under a towel. He'll pass through a stage where he thinks you can't see him simply because he can't see you. This is normal and can be fun when you turn it into a game.

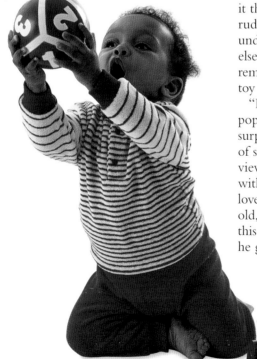

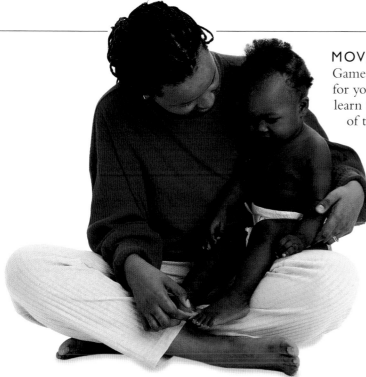

MOVEMENT AND TOUCHING GAMES

Games that involve you lovingly handling his body are fun for your baby, and you will be surprised at how soon he will learn to understand and respond when you start to play one of them. When you sing "The wheels on the bus," you can involve his whole body, his legs becoming the wheels, his arms the opening and closing doors and the wipers. He will enjoy having his toes wiggled in "This little piggy," and having you lightly run your fingers from his toes to his head for "all the way home."

SINGING AND LANGUAGE GAMES

Nursery rhymes and songs are part of your child's heritage. A few of the many excellent tapes of music and songs for small children are invaluable on car journeys. Best of all though, is to sing to your baby yourself. All babies seem to love being sung to. Singing lullabies to your baby such as "Twinkle, twinkle little star," and "Rock-a-bye Baby," can help soothe him. He will enjoy the rhythm and rhymes of these and other lullabies. In finger play songs such as "Incy Wincy Spider," the action of your hands can reinforce the meaning of the songs and help your baby to remember them.

Songs are one of the best ways to encourage your baby's language development and help him to understand and identify the world around him. "This little piggy" for example, explores the concepts of going and coming and opposites ("went to market," "stayed at home," "had roast beef," "had none"). "Old McDonald had a farm," will teach him about animals and animal noises.

In his third and fourth years, your child will start to appreciate rhyming and nonsense rhymes. You can reduce him to helpless laughter with your own nonsense variation on a song he knows well ("Hickory dickory dee, The mouse ran up the tree...") and you will find he will very soon start imitating you and making up his own versions.

READING

Your baby will like to have you read to him long before he has any idea of what reading is all about. He'll enjoy the physical closeness as he sits on your knee and is cuddled. He'll like the sound of your voice as you talk to him about the pictures in the book. He'll like the bright colors of the pictures themselves. To begin with, reading is just another opportunity for you to spend time with your baby and talk to him. But eventually he will even understand what it is you are talking about.

BECOMING A PERSON

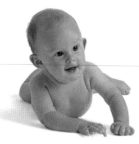

You will quickly become familiar with your baby's own particular temperament. She may be placid and "easy," she may cry a lot and be hard to comfort, or she may have a rather suspicious attitude toward anything new. Those characteristics will tend to persist as she gets older, but her personality is also shaped by what happens to her, and the way others behave toward her—particularly you and your partner. You can help her to be secure, confident, and outgoing by showing her, right from the beginning, how special she is to you. Treating your child as an individual with her own wishes and opinions will give her confidence in herself. There will be times during toddlerhood when her enthusiasm outstrips her still limited abilities, and you will need all your tact to help her succeed without letting her think that you're taking over. But if you are able to think yourself into your baby's shoes and understand her frustrations, the pre-school years should be a time of tremendous enjoyment and discovery for both of you.

GETTING ALONG TOGETHER

Learning to get along well together in the pre-school years is a process of adjustment for both of you. Your child has to learn the boundaries of acceptable behavior, while you may have to adapt your own natural style as a parent, which may not always make you tolerant, consistent, and fair. Your child needs you to show her, not just tell her, how to behave well. Kindness, politeness, thoughtfulness—all this she will only learn by copying you when you show the same behavior to her.

Learning for himself
Give your child help when he needs it, but don't take over—it's his toy, and he needs to feel he can succeed.

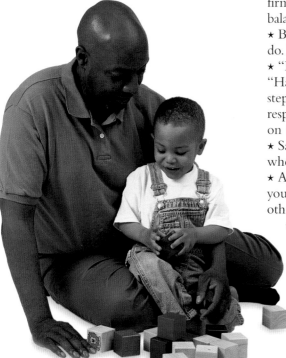

How to handle your child
Your child will respond best to you and do as you say more willingly if you can be both affectionate and firm. But it isn't easy to get the balance right.
★ Be consistent in what you say and do. Do not spank your child.
★ "Do's" work better than "Don'ts". "Hang your coat up so no one will step on it," elicits a more positive response than "Don't drop your coat on the floor."
★ Say please—and thank you—when you ask her to do something.
★ Agree with your partner what you will allow, and always back each other up.
★ Try to persuade rather than coerce. If she's in the middle of some absorbing activity, try "Let's finish this and then it'll be time to go to bed," rather than "Clear away those toys now it's bedtime."
★ Don't be too restrictive. Try listening to the way you talk to your child. Do you find you're nearly always issuing orders—"Stop that, Do as you're told, Don't touch?"
★ If you were unreasonable over something, say so, and apologize.
★ Don't assert your authority unnecessarily—avoid a clash of wills.
★ Always explain *why* she mustn't do something as well as *what* it is she mustn't do, even if she's too young to understand fully.

Rules to keep your child safe
Until your child has reached at least two-and-a-half, you can't expect her to understand reasons for not doing things, nor to remember what she mustn't do. It's your responsibility to make sure her curiosity can't lead her into much danger, and that the important rules are enforced.

For example, "You must never go out of the yard on your own" is an abstract rule that your toddler cannot comprehend, much less remember when she's busy playing or absorbed in her toys. You can only keep an eye on her and *make sure*—with a secure catch on the yard gate—that she doesn't stray out.

Childproof your home to minimize any dangers and so that you don't have to keep reprimanding her—otherwise her curiosity will lead the two of you into conflict (see pages 234-6). Move the television out of her reach, don't let electrical cords hang loose, use a fireguard, put child-resistant locks on drawers, cupboards, and fridges, and put socket covers over electrical sockets. Sometimes keeping her out of the way is the only answer: a child gate across the kitchen door may be the best way to keep her safe when you're cooking.

Loving and spoiling

You may worry that the normal affection you give your child will spoil her. It won't. She needs your love, combined with plenty of attention. But you *can* spoil her by being over-lenient in the face of bad behavior. Letting her get her own

way through tears and tantrums will not help her in her relations with friends and adults.

If you go out to work, you may find yourself "making up" to your child for not being there by lavishing toys on her. Toys can't take your place, and you may be giving her unrealistic expectations. Instead, when you *can* be around give her your time, your love, and plenty of affection.

Showing your love
Your child will prefer your love and attention to any toys. Don't worry about spoiling him with love, you can't.

DEVELOPING A SENSE OF IDENTITY

At around the age of 18 months or so, your child begins to realize that he is a separate person. He will start to refer to himself by name, and he'll enjoy looking at photos of himself too. From now on, he'll want to take charge of his own life more and more, and assert his own wishes and personality. You can help to foster this burgeoning sense of identity and determination to do things for himself.

Encouraging independence

★ Make things easy. From two on, organize his possessions so that he can do as much as possible for himself. Buy clothes that are easy to manage, so he can dress and undress himself as far as possible; put a step by the sink so he can wash his hands without your help; and fix a low hook so he can hang up his own coat.
★ Encourage him to help you. "Helping" is a game at the moment, not a chore. Simple jobs, such as unpacking the shopping, setting the table, or sweeping the kitchen floor, make your child feel he's achieved something, and show him that helping is part of family life.
★ Let him make decisions. The opportunity to make simple decisions gives your child the feeling that he has some control over his own life. So let him choose which T-shirt he wants to wear, or how his room is arranged, or where he'd like to go for a walk.

Helping your child to feel special

Your child, just like every child, needs to feel that he's special—that you love him and that he is worth loving. It's this message that helps to make him emotionally strong and able to cope away from the security of home. There are plenty of little ways you can show how special he is to you:
★ Don't forget to say you love him, or be too busy to give a hug or a cuddle when he wants one.
★ Respect his feelings and respond to his needs. When he's miserable, he needs to cry and be comforted. Saying "Don't be a crybaby" is denying him the right to feel sad.
★ Praise him and be enthusiastic about each fresh achievement.
★ Listen and show interest when he talks to you.

Becoming a person
Try to appreciate your toddler for the lively, fascinating, and independent individual he is fast becoming.

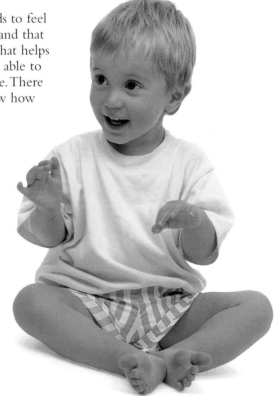

GOOD AND BAD BEHAVIOR

When they are well and happy, most children usually behave acceptably. But every child has off days, and every child wants to test her limits—and yours—by seeing how far she can go. Bad behavior is often an effective way of gaining your attention, too. The time of greatest conflict will probably come at some stage during her third year: tears and tantrums often go hand in hand with being two.

Dealing with bad behavior

Act quickly and remove the source of the trouble and pick your child up and remove her with a firm "NO." At the same time distract her attention with some other activity or toy.

Some types of bad behavior, fussing and whining, for example, are best ignored. If your child never manages to elicit a response from you, and is *never* allowed to win any arguments by such behavior, she will soon stop. Even tantrums are best ignored. Just be calm and carry on as normal. If necessary, put her outside the room until she calms down.

Rewards for good behavior

It's very easy to give your child more attention when she behaves badly and least when she behaves well and you feel you can relax. But rewarding your child with praise and affection, or a story on your lap when she behaves well is much more effective. You will encourage the behavior you want, and teach her a very useful lesson—that being nice to people works much better than being nasty in life.

Consequences for bad behavior

Whatever consequence you decide upon, it has to be immediate if it is to have any effect on your toddler. Threats of future action, perhaps the withdrawal of treats and privileges, are useless and unfair for young children. Your child will not be able to understand why she is having this delayed consequence.

An immediate consequence that your child *will* understand is to be isolated for a short time to cool off. A quarter of an hour spent somewhere safe but alone—the hall is often suitable—will be long enough for her to forget whatever it was that she wanted to do, and give you time to cool down.

Should I spank my child?

Do not spank or hit your child. It's not a good way to deal with bad behavior. What is more, you are teaching her that physical force is an acceptable way to make people do what you want. You must learn other ways to discipline your child.

How to avoid getting to the end of your rope

However clever you become at managing your child, there will be days when her behavior seems completely unbearable and you are close to losing control.

The solution is simple: take your child out. Whatever the weather, a trip to the park, the shops, or a friend will distract both of you from your respective moods and help you recover your sanity and sense of humor.

Dealing with agressive children

All small children fight occasionally, especially when they are bored or tired. When fights get out of hand, step in quickly:
★ separate the fighting children
★ divert them by introducing some other game or change of scene
★ don't take sides—it's nearly always impossible to work out the rights and wrongs of any situation.
If your child bites another child:
★ give all your attention and concern to the bitten child
★ remove the biter right away and put her somewhere else, safe, but alone, for a quarter of an hour.

Your child is bound to snatch and grab when she first starts playing with other children, but with help from you she will soon learn to share. It helps to get your child used to playing with other children from an early age, so ask about local toddler groups. A few children will continue to be very rough and agressive, and their behavior will eventually make them very unpopular. For your child's sake, help her to be gentle with others:
★ give her a good model to follow by always trying to be gentle, patient, and loving toward her.
★ make it clear through the way you act that it's your child's *behavior* you dislike, not her.
★ always step in and stop your child immediately if she starts to hit another child. Be firm, but don't shout or be agressive yourself.
★ Never let her get her own way by behaving agressively or unpleasantly.

If your child's behavior continues to worry you, and you can't seem to find a way to deal with it, seek advice from your doctor.

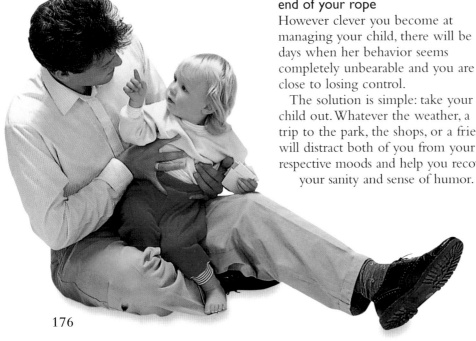

CHILDHOOD HABITS

Many small children develop habits such as thumb-sucking, head-banging, or breath-holding, which they resort to usually when they are angry, frustrated, bored, or simply in need of comfort. These habits are common and harmless, but they often worry parents. Although the child usually grows out of them by the time they are four, sometimes they can be hard to break.

Thumb-sucking and soothers

About half of three year olds suck their thumbs, and a few are still doing so when they are six or seven. Persistent thumb-suckers may gradually push their front teeth forward. Continually sucking a cuddly toy or blanket may have the same effect. However, unless the habit continues after the age of 6, when the second set of teeth come in, the distortion won't be permanent.

Head-banging, rolling, and rocking

Sometime in their first year many children develop a habit of rocking rhythmically on all fours in their crib, rolling their heads from side to side, or banging their heads on the head-board. Usually they'll do this as they are going off to sleep or as they wake up and often the rocking is violent enough to move the crib across the floor. Although this is alarming to watch, and to listen to, you really do not need to worry about it. Infants and young toddlers who do this seldom hurt themselves, though they may damage the furniture. These rhythmic behaviors nearly always disappear by the age of 3 or 4.

Some toddlers develop an equally worrying habit of banging their head on a hard surface during the day, usually to express frustration or boredom. Again, the child won't hurt himself, apart from the odd bruise. It's usually best to take no notice, though you may want to offer the child a pillow to soften the impact. If you ignore the habit, it will eventually disappear.

Head-banging or rocking that starts in older children, or persists after the age of four, needs to be taken more seriously. Discuss with your doctor; it may mean that your child has some emotional problem.

Breath holding attacks

A few young children deal with pain or frustration by holding their breath. They may do this for up to half a minute, and sometimes they will even pass out. Immediately this happens, the child will automatically start to breathe again, and no harm is done, but the child quickly discovers this is a splendid way to gain attention. Ignore the attacks as much as possible, and they will probably have stopped by the time your child is four.

Hold on to his security blanket

Even when your child seems to have outgrown his security blanket, don't throw it out. Even a year or two later, it can be surprising how happy your child will be to have his blanket back, especially if he is very stressed or ill.

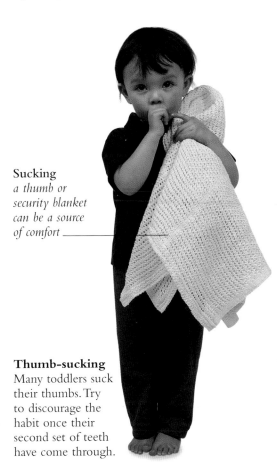

Sucking
a thumb or security blanket can be a source of comfort

Thumb-sucking
Many toddlers suck their thumbs. Try to discourage the habit once their second set of teeth have come through.

"BAD DREAMS" AND NIGHT TERRORS

Even a child as young as one may have nightmares about something that has frightened him during the day, even though he doesn't yet understand what a dream is and certainly couldn't tell you about it. If a very young child wakes from a nightmare, simply cuddle and comfort him till he calms down.

By the time he is two years old, he may try to tell you about it and you can reassure him that it was "only a dream", though he won't yet really understand this concept. By three or four he will have a much better idea of what is "real" and "not real". But he will still need you to soothe his fears and make it clear that you won't let anything bad happen to him. It may reassure him to have a nightlight in his room, and for the door to be left open.

A few children, however, have night terrors, which are quite different from nightmares. Nightmares usually occur in the second half of the night when the child is sleeping lightly and dreams are at their most plentiful. A night terror will start much earlier, usually between one and four hours after the child has gone to sleep, and is sleeping very deeply. You will hear your child screaming or moaning as if in terror, but when you rush into her she won't seem to recognize you, may push you away, and scream even more if you try to hold her. This is because she is not properly awake, and if left alone will quite quickly go back to sleep. So don't try to wake her or even hold her. Simply wait beside her so that you are there if she does wake. In the morning she will have no memory of what happened and be none the worse for it.

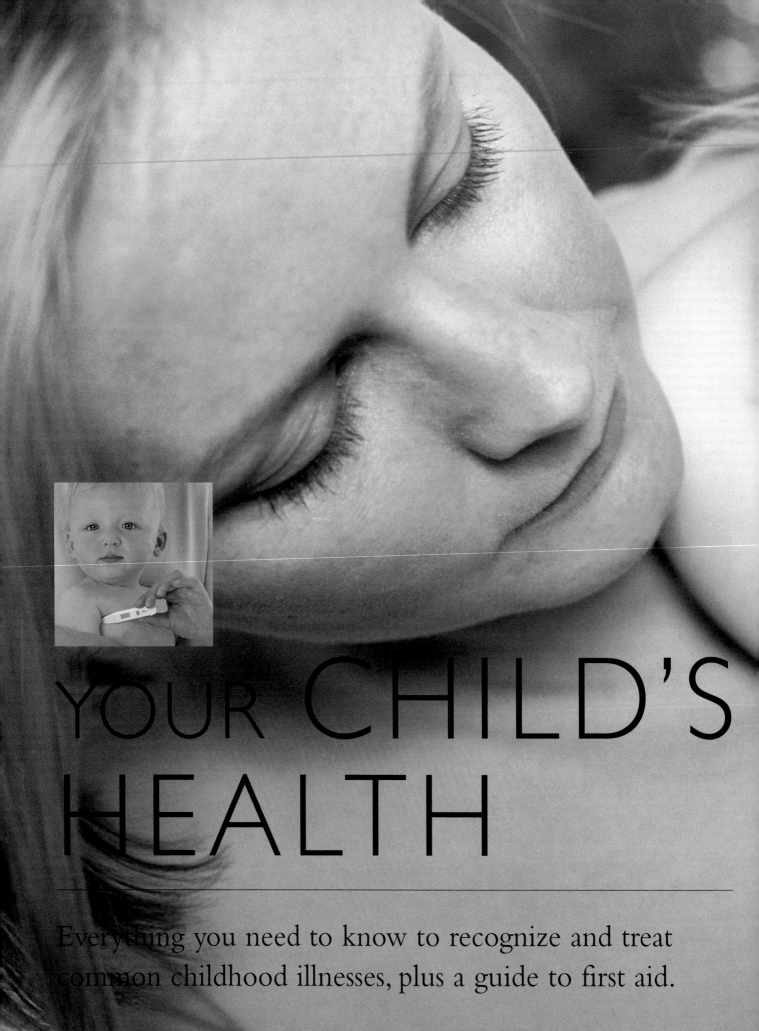

YOUR CHILD'S HEALTH

Everything you need to know to recognize and treat common childhood illnesses, plus a guide to first aid.

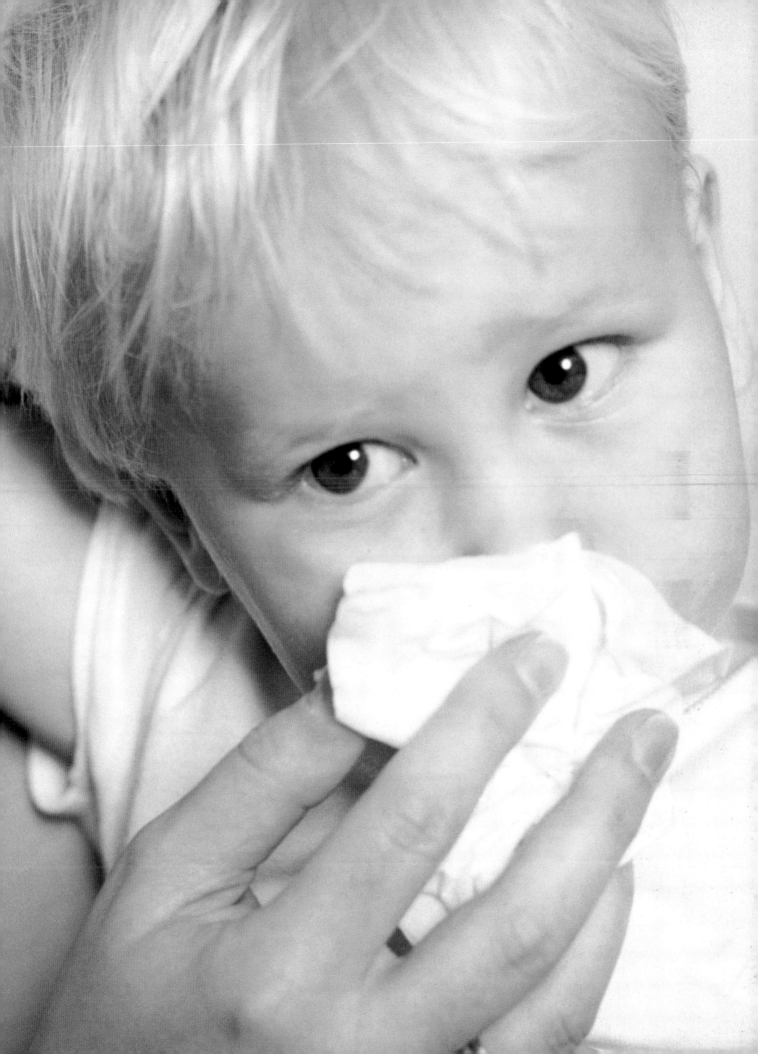

THE FIRST THREE MONTHS

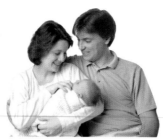

It is difficult to know when a baby is ill. If he is contented, and feeding normally, he is probably perfectly healthy. But babies can become ill quite quickly and any infection may be dangerous, so for the first three months you should be overcautious and call your doctor straight away if you think your baby is ill. If you notice any signs of illness, look at the symptoms listed here. These are the most common health problems for babies under three months old. This symptoms guide directs you to the relevant section on pages 182–5, but is not intended as a definite medical diagnosis – only a doctor can give that. If you can't find your baby's symptoms here, look at the pages 186–7, which covers illnesses for children of all ages. Babies are born with a natural immunity to many infections, since antibodies (which destroy germs) are passed to them from their mother's blood. Breast-fed babies also receive antibodies from their mother's milk. This immunity lasts for about six months and will give them some protection against disease.

EMERGENCY SIGNS

Call for help immediately or go to the Hospital Emergency Department if your baby:
★ brings up green vomit
★ has a temperature over 39°C (102.2°F) for more than half an hour
★ vomits AND cries uncontrollably as if in great pain
★ is breathing very noisily or rapidly

Fontanelle

★ has a taut, bulging fontanelle when he isn't crying
★ purplish rash on skin that does not fade if a glass is pressed against it.
★ passes stools containing blood and mucus, which resemble redcurrant jelly.

Loss of appetite
If your baby does not want to feed, but seems generally well and contented, there is no need to worry. If he refuses two feeds in succession, or does not demand a feed for six hours, **call your doctor now.**

CALL THE DOCTOR

Don't wait to call your doctor if your baby seems unwell or:
★ cries more than usual, or his crying sounds different from usual over a period of about an hour
★ seems abnormally quiet, drowsy, or listless
★ refuses two successive feeds, or does not demand a feed for six hours
★ seems particularly irritable or restless.

Crying
If you fail to calm your baby after an hour or so, or if his crying sounds unusual, **don't wait to call your doctor.** If your baby cries inconsolably for two or three hours at about the same time each day, but shows no other signs of illness, he might have colic (see page 118). This may continue for several weeks, but there is no treatment for it.

Slow weight gain
If your baby does not seem to be gaining weight at the normal rate (see charts on pages 254-7), consult your doctor. Occasionally an underlying illness can make a baby grow more slowly than normal.

PREMATURE BABIES

Babies who were very small at birth, or who were born a month or more before their due date, are very vulnerable to infections during their first weeks. Until your baby is older and has put on weight, keep him away from anyone who has a cough or cold, and don't take him into public places where he might pick up an infection.

Cold hands and feet, *see Chilling (page 184)*

Areas of dry, flaking skin *mean that your baby's skin needs moisturizing, so rub a little baby oil or baby moisturizer gently into the dry areas*

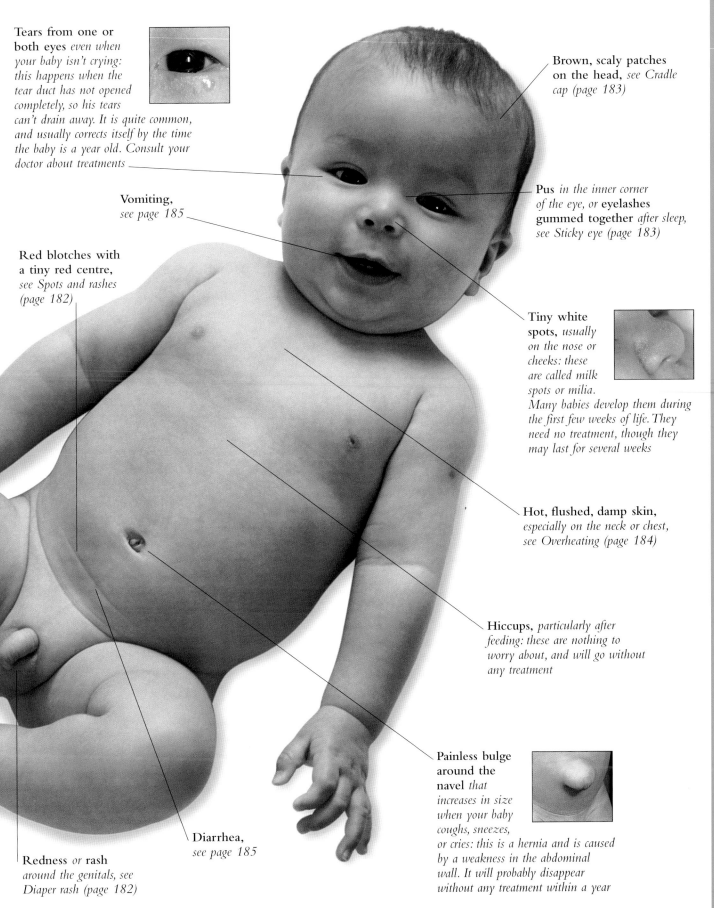

Tears from one or both eyes *even when your baby isn't crying: this happens when the tear duct has not opened completely, so his tears can't drain away. It is quite common, and usually corrects itself by the time the baby is a year old. Consult your doctor about treatments*

Vomiting, *see page 185*

Red blotches with a tiny red centre, *see Spots and rashes (page 182)*

Brown, scaly patches on the head, *see Cradle cap (page 183)*

Pus *in the inner corner of the eye, or* **eyelashes gummed together** *after sleep, see Sticky eye (page 183)*

Tiny white spots, *usually on the nose or cheeks: these are called milk spots or milia. Many babies develop them during the first few weeks of life. They need no treatment, though they may last for several weeks*

Hot, flushed, damp skin, *especially on the neck or chest, see Overheating (page 184)*

Hiccups, *particularly after feeding: these are nothing to worry about, and will go without any treatment*

Painless bulge around the navel *that increases in size when your baby coughs, sneezes, or cries: this is a hernia and is caused by a weakness in the abdominal wall. It will probably disappear without any treatment within a year*

Diarrhea, *see page 185*

Redness *or* **rash** *around the genitals, see Diaper rash (page 182)*

SPOTS AND RASHES

What are they?
Many newborn babies go through what might be called a spotty stage, so don't worry if your baby develops a few spots—they don't mean that he is sick; it's just that his skin is delicate. One of the most common rashes is newborn urticaria; it usually appears during the first week of life.

What can I do?
If your baby has newborn urticaria (see Symptoms box), the spots will disappear on their own within about two or three days, so don't put any lotions or creams on them. Don't alter your baby's feedings—the spots are not due to formula disagreeing with him.

SYMPTOMS

★ Red blotches, each with a tiny red center, which come and go on different parts of the baby's body, and last only a few hours.

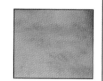

CALL THE DOCTOR

Call your doctor now if the rash is flat and dark red or purplish (a petechial rash—a sign of bleeding under the skin). Consult your doctor as soon as possible if:
★ a spot has developed a pus-filled center
★ you think a spot has become infected.

DIAPER RASH

What is it?
Diaper rash is an inflammation of the skin on a baby's bottom. It may occur if your baby has been left in a dirty diaper for too long, because as urine and feces are broken down, ammonia is released, which burns and irritates the skin. It can also be due to an allergy to laundry detergent or fabric conditioner. A similar-looking rash may be caused by thrush, a yeast infection, which normally starts in the mouth (see page 213), but can affect the skin around the anus.

SYMPTOMS

★ Red, spotty, sore-looking skin in the diaper area
★ smell of ammonia from your baby's diaper.

What can I do?

1 Change your baby's diaper frequently, and clean and dry her bottom thoroughly at each change (see pages 150–1). Inside cloth diapers, use an extra-absorbent type of liner.

2 Whenever possible, let your baby lie on a diaper with her bottom exposed to the air. Don't use plastic pants over cloth diapers until the rash subsides, since these prevent air from circulating to her bottom.

3 Look for white patches inside your baby's mouth. If you see any, she may have thrush (see page 213).

Spread the cream *evenly all over your baby's diaper area*

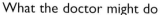

4 Don't use harsh detergents or fabric conditioner to wash her diapers, as they can trigger an allergy. Rinse her diapers thoroughly.

5 Use a diaper rash cream and apply it when you change her diaper.

CALL THE DOCTOR

Consult your doctor as soon as possible if:
★ the rash lasts several days or becomes worse
★ you think your baby has thrush.

What the doctor might do
The doctor may prescribe an antibiotic cream if the rash has become infected, or an antifungal cream if it looks like a rash caused by yeast.

CRADLE CAP

What is it?
Yellowish to brown, crusty patches on a baby's head are known as cradle cap. Sometimes it may spread to the baby's face, body, or diaper area, producing a red scaly rash. Although it looks as if it might be irritating, cradle cap doesn't seem to distress the baby.

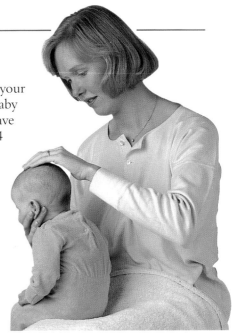

What can I do?
1 Rub the scales on your baby's head with baby oil to soften them. Leave the oil on for 12 to 24 hours, then comb his hair gently to loosen the scales. Finally, wash his hair—most of the scales should simply wash away.

SYMPTOMS
★ Yellowish to brown, scaly patches on the scalp.

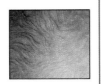

CALL THE DOCTOR
Consult your doctor as soon as possible if the rash spreads and:
★ seems to irritate the baby
★ looks infected or begins to ooze
★ does not clear up after five days.

2 If the rash spreads, keep the affected areas clean and dry.

What the doctor might do
If the condition proves obstinate, or if the rash looks infected or starts to ooze, your doctor may prescribe a cream to be rubbed gently on the area.

STICKY EYE

What is it?
This common mild eye irritation is caused by blood or fluid getting into the eye during birth. If your baby has any of these symptoms after she is two days old, she may have conjunctivitis (see page 209) or a blocked tear duct.

What can I do?
Clean your baby's eyes twice a day with a cotton ball dipped in warm boiled water. Wipe outward from the inner corner of her eye, and use a fresh cotton ball for cleaning each eye.

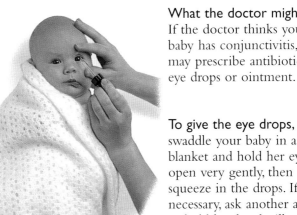

SYMPTOMS
★ Eyelashes gummed together after sleep
★ pus in the inner corner of the eye.

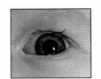

What the doctor might do
If the doctor thinks your baby has conjunctivitis, he may prescribe antibiotic eye drops or ointment.

CALL THE DOCTOR
Call your doctor now if your baby has a bad discharge of yellow pus or is very irritable.
Consult your doctor as soon as possible if:
★ your baby develops symptoms of sticky eye after the first two days of life
★ sticky eye does not clear up after three days.

To give the eye drops, swaddle your baby in a blanket and hold her eyes open very gently, then squeeze in the drops. If necessary, ask another adult to hold her head still.

CHILLING

Why are babies at risk?
For the first few weeks of his life, your baby will be unable to regulate his body temperature very efficiently. If he becomes too cold, his body temperature will drop and he may become dangerously chilled quite quickly. Babies who were born prematurely are particularly vulnerable to this.

What can I do?

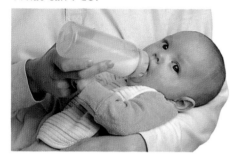

1 Warm your baby up by taking him into a heated room and feeding him. Once he has become chilled, it doesn't help just to pile on extra clothes or blankets.

2 Take your baby's temperature (see page 193) If it is below 35°C (95°F), he is dangerously chilled, so **call your doctor now.**

SYMPTOMS
First signs
★ Crying and restless behavior
★ cold hands and feet.
Signs of serious chilling
★ Quiet, listless behavior as the baby gets colder
★ cool skin on the chest and stomach
★ pink, flushed face, hands, and feet.

How can I prevent chilling?
Keep the room your baby sleeps in at about 20°C (68°F). When you undress and bathe him, the room should be warmer still. Be sensible about taking him out in cold weather— wrap him up well and don't stay out for too long. Be alert for any signs of chilling.

GET HELP
Call your doctor now if your baby:
★ shows signs of serious chilling
★ has a temperature below 35°C (95°F).

Put a hat *under the hood to keep his head warm*

In cold weather, dress your baby in an all-in-one outdoor suit, or wrap a shawl over his other clothes and use mittens and bootees.

OVERHEATING

Why are babies at risk?
Overheating is as dangerous for young babies as chilling, especially if they are feverish or unwell. Overwrapping of babies at night is thought to be one of the factors that contributes to crib death (see page 123).

What can I do?
1 Take your baby to a cooler place and remove a layer of clothing.

2 Take your baby's temperature and, if it is raised, administer an ASA-free medication containing acetaminophen (see page 194).

SYMPTOMS
★ Restless behavior
★ hot, sweaty skin
★ raised temperature.

How can I prevent overheating?
Dress your baby according to the weather—on very hot days, she can sleep in just a diaper and a shirt, but always remember the danger of chilling (see above). Never leave her to sleep in the sun, her skin will burn easily. Provide shade of some sort, and check her frequently as the sun moves round.

GET HELP
Call your doctor if your baby has a persistent temperature over 38°C (100.4°F).

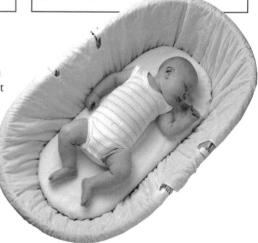

184

VOMITING

Why do babies vomit?
All babies spit up a small amount of milk during or just after a feeding. This is perfectly normal, and does not mean that your baby is ill, but until you are used to it, you may think that she is vomiting. If your baby vomits, she will bring up most of her feed. This is unlikely to happen in a breast-fed baby.

Frequent vomiting, especially if she also has diarrhea, may be caused by gastroenteritis (see page 222). This is very serious in a young baby because it can make her dehydrated very quickly.

FORCEFUL VOMITING
Sometimes a baby vomits with great force, so that the vomit shoots across the room. If your baby does this at two successive feedings, **consult your doctor as soon as possible.**

The most likely reason is that she has brought back part of her feeding with a large burp of gas. However, if it happens after every feeding, especially if she is hungry all the time, she may have a condition call pyloric stenosis, in which the outlet from the stomach becomes blocked. This condition runs in families, and usually develops when the baby is two to eight weeks old. If your baby has this she will need a simple operation.

What can I do?

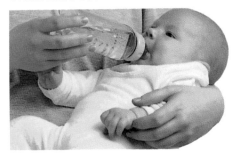

Bottle-fed (formula-fed) baby:
Stop formula feeding. Replace with commercial oral rehydration solution (ORS—ask your pharmacist to recommend a brand). Feed your baby small amounts frequently, either by bottle, medicine dropper, or small spoon—about 15ml (1tbsp) every 15 minutes. When vomiting stops, give 30 to 90ml (1 to 3oz) of ORS every hour. When vomiting has stopped and diarrhea is less frequent, replace the ORS with usual formula.

Do not give your baby any fluids other than those that are recommended above.

Get medical advice if your baby's condition has not improved within 24 hours.

Breast-fed baby:
Continue to breast-feed, and also offer your baby small amounts of an oral rehydration solution (ORS—ask your pharmacist to recommend a brand) between feedings. If your baby refuses the bottle, use a medicine dropper or a small spoon.

EMERGENCY SIGNS
Call for emergency help immediately if your baby:
★ vomits all feedings in a four- to six-hour period, despite treatment
★ has a dry mouth
★ has sunken eyes or a sunken fontanelle
★ has a dry diaper for more than six hours
★ is abnormally drowsy.

GET HELP
Call your doctor now if:
★ your baby vomits and shows any other signs of illness
★ your baby vomits the whole of two successive feedings.

What might the doctor do?
The doctor may prescribe a powder to be mixed with water for your baby to drink. If your baby has lost a lot of body fluid, the doctor might send her to hospital, where she may be given fluid intravenously.

How can I prevent an upset stomach?
Breast-fed babies rarely have upset stomachs. If you are bottle-feeding, sterilize all the equipment and discard any unfinished feedings. When making up bottles, cool them quickly under cold water and store in the fridge. Never keep a feed warm for a long period.

DIARRHEA

What is it?
Until babies start eating solid food, they will usually pass fairly runny bowel movements a few times a day. If your baby passes very watery, greenish bowel movements more often than usual, he has diarrhea. Diarrhea is serious in a young baby, since there is a danger that he may become dehydrated quite quickly.

What can I do?
It is important to prevent your baby from becoming dehydrated, so make sure that he has plenty to drink. Follow the advice above under Vomiting: What can I do?. Make sure your baby is wetting his diaper and staying alert.

GET HELP
If your baby is less than six months old and you suspect that he has diarrhea, call the doctor now.

DIAGNOSIS GUIDE

I f your child is unwell, try to identify her symptoms in the guide below. If she has more than one symptom, look up the most severe one. This gives you a possible diagnosis and refers you to a section covering the complaint. As well as giving a more detailed list of symptoms, the section contains a brief explanation of the nature of the illness, with information about how you can help your child, and advice on whether you need to call a doctor. Bear in mind that the guide is not intended to give an accurate diagnosis, only a doctor can do that, and that your child may not develop all the symptoms listed for an illness. If your baby is under three months old, look also at the guide on pages 180–81, which covers special health risks for young babies.

Fever
A raised temperature (fever) may mean that your child has an infection, so you should check for other signs of illness. However, healthy children may get a slight fever during energetic play or in very hot weather, so check your child's temperature again after she has rested for about half an hour. If it is still over 38°C (100.4°F), she may have an infection.

Changed behavior
If your child is less lively than usual, more irritable, whiny, or simply unhappy, she may be ill.

Unusual paleness
If your child looks much paler than usual, she may be ill.

Hot, flushed face
This may be a sign of a fever.

Loss of appetite
Although a child's appetite varies from meal to meal, a sudden loss of appetite may be a sign of illness. If your baby is under six months old and has refused two successive feeds, or has not demanded a feed for more than eight hours, **call your doctor now**. If your child goes off her food for more than 24 hours, look for other signs of illness (see page 189).

Eyes looking in different directions, *see Squint (page 210)*

Red, sore, or sticky eyes or eyelids, *see Eye problems (pages 209–10); if combined with a* **rash and fever**, *see Measles (page 204)*

Itchy eyes, *especially if accompanied by* **runny nose or sneezing**, *see Colds and flu (pages 200–1). Could also be hay fever, particularly if it occurs in summer—consult your doctor*

Aversion to bright light, *especially if accompanied by* **fever, headache, and stiff neck**, *see Meningitis and encephalitis (page 208)*

Runny or blocked nose, sneezing, *see Colds and flu (pages 200–1)*

Sore mouth, *see page 213*

Momentary lapses of attention, *see Absence attacks (page 233)*

Loss of consciousness, combined with stiffness and twitching movements, *see Major seizure (page 233)*

Itchy head or tiny white grains in the hair, *see Lice and nits (page 232)*

Earache, partial deafness, discharge from ears, itchy ears, *see Ear problems (pages 211–2)*

Puffy face, swollen glands, *at the angle of the jaw-bone and on the sides of the neck, see Mumps (page 206);* **swollen glands** *accompanied by* **sore throat**, *see Tonsillitis (page 214) and German measles (page 203)*

Stiff neck, *if accompanied by* **fever and headache**, *see Meningitis and encephalitis (page 208)*

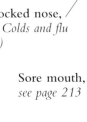

Red lump, perhaps with pus-filled center, *anywhere on the body, see Spots and boils (page 226)*

Red, raw skin, *see Chapped skin (page 229)*

Sore throat, *see Throat infections (page 214); if accompanied by* fever and general illness, *see Colds and flu (pages 200–1); if also accompanied by* a rash, *see German measles (page 203); if accompanied by* puffy face, *see Mumps (page 206)*

Spots or rash *anywhere on the body, if accompanied by* sore throat *or* fever, *see Infectious illnesses (pages 203–8); if without other symptoms, see Skin problems (pages 226–32) and Insect stings (page 252)*

Stomach pain, *see page 220; if accompanied by nausea, vomiting, or diarrhea, see Gastroenteritis (page 222)*

Abnormal-looking feces, *see page 223*

Diarrhea, *see page 223*

Constipation, *see page 221*

Intense itching around the anus, *see Pinworms (page 232)*

Pain when urinating, odd-colored urine, frequent urination, *see Urinary system infections (page 224)*

Vomiting with great force *in babies, see Forceful vomiting (page 185)*

Vomiting or nausea, *see page 222*

Sores around the mouth, *see Cold sores (page 230) and Impetigo (page 231)*

Faint red rash over the face or in skin creases, *see Heat rash (page 227)*

Cough, *see Coughs and chest infections (pages 215–9) and Whooping cough (page 207); if accompanied by a rash, see Measles (page 204)*

Breathing difficulty, wheezing, rapid breathing, *see Coughs and chest infections (pages 215–9)*

Areas of very itchy, dry, red, scaly skin *anywhere on the body, see Eczema (page 228)*

Red, tender skin *anywhere on the body, see Sunburn (page 229) or Burns and scalds (page 245)*

Dry, painless lump *anywhere on the body, see Warts (page 230)*

Soreness, itching or redness around the vagina, vaginal discharge, *see Genital problems in girls (page 225)*

Intense itching around the vagina, *see Pinworms (page 232)*

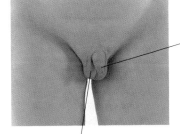

Sore tip of penis, *see Genital problems in boys (page 225)*

Painless bulge in the groin or scrotum, *see Genital problems in boys (page 225)*

White or brown lump on sole of foot, *see Warts (page 230)*

FIRST SIGNS OF ILLNESS

Even if your child has no definite symptoms, you can often tell he is sick by his whiny, clingy behavior. Children may become pale, lose their appetite, and drive their parents crazy with temper tantrums. With a teething baby, don't dismiss the change in behavior as new teeth on the way. No studies have confirmed the connection between illness and teething. Try to isolate the origin of all symptoms by using the guide here. Follow the directions for diagnosing and stay calm. Sick children can test even the most patient parents. If your child is under a year old, watch especially carefully, as babies can become very ill very quickly.

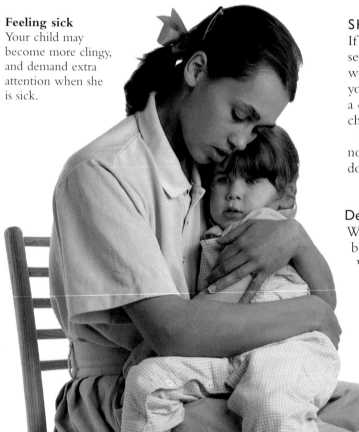

Feeling sick
Your child may become more clingy, and demand extra attention when she is sick.

SHOULD I CALL THE DOCTOR?

If you think you know what is wrong, read the relevant section about complaints on pages 203–233 to determine whether you need to call the doctor. As a general rule, the younger the child, the more quickly he should be seen by a doctor. When you phone your doctor, describe your child's symptoms and remind him of his age.

Don't ever hesitate to call your doctor, even if you are not absolutely certain that something is wrong. Your doctor may want to see your child.

Degree of urgency

Whenever you are instructed to call the doctor, you will be told how quickly your child needs medical help.
★ **Call for emergency help immediately:** this is a life-threatening emergency. Call 911 or an ambulance, or go to the nearest hospital emergency room.
★ **Call your doctor now:** your child needs medical help now, so contact your doctor immediately, even if it is the middle of the night. If you can't reach him, call 911 for immediate emergency help.
★ **Consult your doctor as soon as possible:** your child needs to be seen by a doctor within the next 24 hours.
★ **Consult your doctor:** your child should be seen by a doctor within the next few days.

SYMPTOMS

The most common early symptoms of illness in children are:
★ raised temperature—38°C (100.4°F) or more
★ crying and irritability
★ vomiting or diarrhea
★ refusal to eat or drink
★ sore or red throat
★ swollen glands in the neck or behind the jaw
★ rash.

EMERGENCY SIGNS

Call for emergency help immediately if your child:
★ is breathing very noisily, rapidly, or with difficulty
★ has a convulsion
★ loses consciousness after a fall
★ is in severe, persistent pain
★ has a fever and is unusually irritable or drowsy
★ has a flat dark red or purplish rash
(a petechial rash—a sign of bleeding under the skin).

CHECKING FOR SYMPTOMS

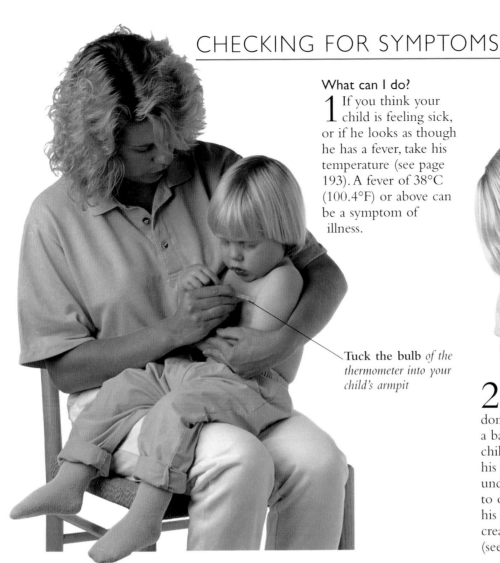

What can I do?

1 If you think your child is feeling sick, or if he looks as though he has a fever, take his temperature (see page 193). A fever of 38°C (100.4°F) or above can be a symptom of illness.

Tuck the bulb *of the thermometer into your child's armpit*

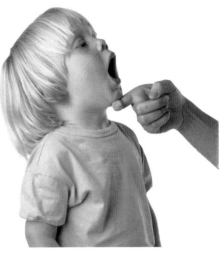

2 Check your child's throat to see if it's inflamed or infected, but don't try to examine the throat of a baby under a year old. Ask your child to face a bright light and open his mouth. If he is old enough to understand, tell him to say "Aah" to open the back of his throat. If his throat looks red or you can see creamy spots, he has a sore throat (see Throat infections, page 214).

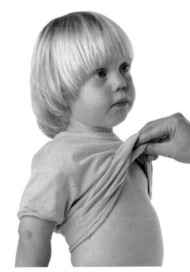

3 Feel gently along your child's jaw-bone and down either side of the back of his neck. If you can feel tiny lumps under the skin, or if any of these areas seem swollen or tender, your child has swollen glands, which are common signs of illness.

4 Check your child for a rash, particularly on his chest and behind his ears—the most common areas for one to start. If he has a rash and a fever, he may have one of the common childhood infectious illnesses (see pages 203–08).

"Is my child in pain?"

Q&A

If your baby is in pain, his crying may sound different from normal. When a baby or a small child cries or complains of pain, it can be difficult to discover where the pain is, let alone how bad the pain is.

Serious pain will affect your child's behavior, so watch him to find out how severe his pain is. Does it make him cry or stop him from sleeping, eating, or playing? Does his face look drawn or has his color changed? Would you know he was in pain if he didn't tell you? If not, his pain isn't severe.

Call your physician and describe your child's symptoms before offering pain medication.

THE DOCTOR'S EXAMINATION

The doctor will ask you about any symptoms you have noticed in your child and how long he has had them, and will then examine your child. If your child is old enough to understand, explain what will happen when he visits the doctor. If the doctor suspects any particular illness, he may do other investigations as well as or instead of those shown below.

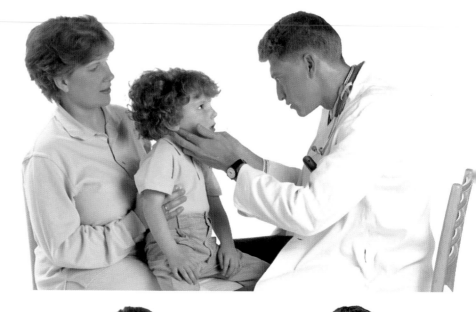

1 The doctor may feel the glands that lie along your child's jaw-bone, down the back of his neck, and in his armpits and groin. These may become swollen during an infectious illness.

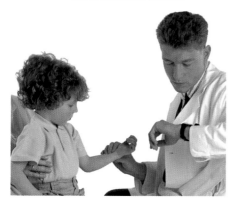

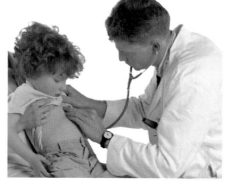

2 He may feel your child's pulse to check if his heart is beating faster than usual. This is often a sign of a raised temperature. The doctor may also take your child's temperature.

3 By listening to your child's chest and back through a stethoscope, and asking your child to breathe deeply, the doctor will check the health of his heart and lungs.

4 If your child has a sore or inflamed throat, the doctor will examine his throat using a small light, pressing his tongue down with a spatula.

5 The doctor may ask your child to lie on the examining couch so that he can gently feel his abdomen. He will check for swelling or tenderness in any of the internal organs.

QUESTIONS TO ASK THE DOCTOR

Don't hesitate to ask the doctor about anything that is worrying you. In particular, find out:
★ how long your child may be ill, and what symptoms to expect
★ whether he is infectious, and whether you should isolate him, particularly from small babies and pregnant women
★ how you can make your child more comfortable while he is ill.

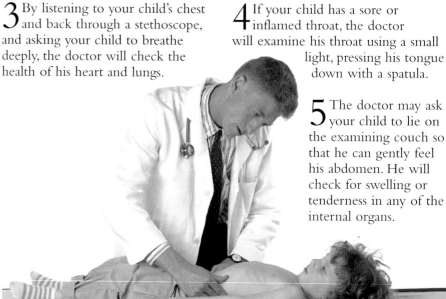

GOING TO THE HOSPITAL

Going into the hospital is stressful for anyone. For a child who is too young to understand why he is there, it can be terrifying, especially if he is separated from his parents. While it helps to explain to your child what is happening, you can't do much to prepare a child under two—all he really needs at this age is your

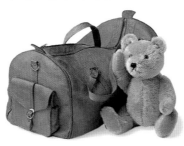

presence. If your child is over two, playing with a favorite toy may help: explain that teddy bear goes to the hospital to be made better, not as a punishment, and soon the teddy bear comes home again. Keep explanations simple but truthful; your child will feel let-down and mistrustful if you promise something won't hurt, and then it does.

VISITING YOUR CHILD

Hospital staff know how important it is for a parent to be with a child to comfort and reassure him, and should make it easy for you to visit him at any time. Some even provide accommodation so that you can live in with your child—find out about this before his admission. He won't find the hospital so frightening if you continue to care for him as you would at home, so ask the nurses whether you can still bathe and feed him.

If you can't stay in the hospital with your child, visit him as often as you can, and bring brothers and sisters to see him. Even if he cries when you leave, don't feel that he might settle better without your visits. It would only make him even more anxious, unhappy, and abandoned. Make a special effort to be with him for the first day or two, and when he has any unpleasant procedures such as injections, or having his stitches removed.

WHAT TO PACK

Your child will need the following things while she is in the hospital. Pack diaper changing equipment as well, if necessary. Label everything, particularly her toys.

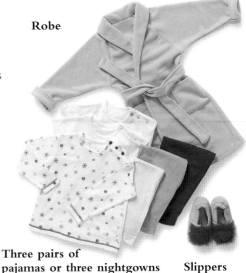

Robe

Three pairs of pajamas or three nightgowns

Slippers

Bib and feeding equipment

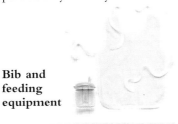

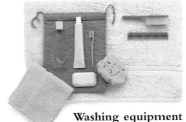

Washing equipment

Pack soap, a washcloth, a sponge, her toothbrush and toothpaste, her brush, comb, and a towel.

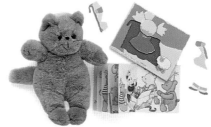

Favorite toys

HAVING AN OPERATION

If your child is old enough to understand, it will help to explain what will happen on the day of his operation. Ask the doctor how the anesthetic will be given (it may be injected or inhaled through a mask), and find out whether you will be allowed to stay with your child while he is given the anesthetic.

Try to be with him when he wakes up after the operation since he may be frightened.

1 Warn your child that he may not be allowed to eat or drink anything on the day of his operation.

2 Tell your child that he will be dressed up for the operation in a hospital gown, and will wear a bracelet with his name on it.

3 While he is still in the ward, your child will be given a "pre-med" to make him sleepy.

4 Your child will be wheeled to the anesthetic room, where he will be given an anesthetic. He will fall asleep quickly.

5 Warn your child that he may vomit when he wakes up.

6 If your child has stitches, discourage him from scratching them. It will hurt only momentarily when they are removed.

THE CHILD WITH A FEVER

In children, normal body temperature is between 36° and 37.5°C (96.8° and 99.5°F). A temperature above 38°C (100.4°F) may be a sign of illness. A child's temperature can shoot up alarmingly quickly when she is ill, but a slightly raised temperature is not a reliable guide to her health. Babies and children can be ill with a normal, or below normal, temperature,

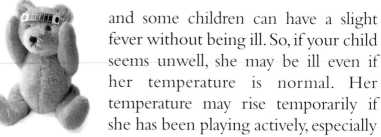

and some children can have a slight fever without being ill. So, if your child seems unwell, she may be ill even if her temperature is normal. Her temperature may rise temporarily if she has been playing actively, especially in hot weather. If it is still above 38°C (100.4°F) after she has rested for about half an hour, she may be ill, so check for other signs of illness.

READING A THERMOMETER

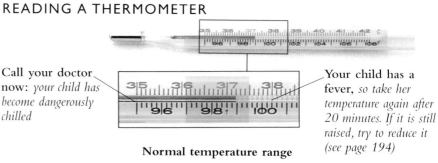

Call your doctor now: *your child has become dangerously chilled*

Your child has a fever, *so take her temperature again after 20 minutes. If it is still raised, try to reduce it (see page 194)*

Normal temperature range

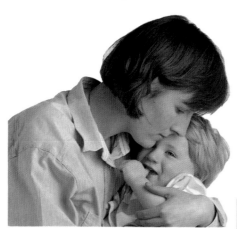

Feel your child's forehead with your cheek if you think he has a fever – don't use your hand because, if it is cold, your child's skin will feel warm by comparison. If his forehead feels hot, take his temperature.

SIGNS OF A FEVER

Your child may have a fever if:
★ she complains of feeling unwell
★ she looks pale and feels cold and shivery
★ she looks flushed and her forehead feels hot.

CALL THE DOCTOR

Call the doctor now if your child:
★ has a fever over 39.4°C (103°F)—over 38.3°C (101°F) if she is under a year old—and you can't bring it down
★ has a fever for 24 hours.

CHOOSING A THERMOMETER

Your choice of home thermometer depends on your child's age, your budget and what you are comfortable using. A rectal thermometer is the most accurate in children under 2, but many parents feel uneasy using it. Ask your doctor for advice. From birth to 2 years, the easiest method is to check the armpit, using a mercury thermometer. From 2 to 5 years, as well as using the armpit method, you can use an ear thermometer. An ear thermometer is more accurate than the armpit method. You can use these methods in children over 5, or use a digital thermometer in the mouth. Indicator strips are not very reliable, but can be used if your child is uncooperative.

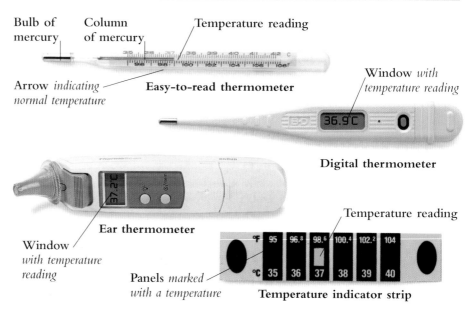

Bulb of mercury **Column of mercury** Temperature reading

Arrow *indicating normal temperature* **Easy-to-read thermometer**

Window *with temperature reading*

36.9°C

Digital thermometer

Ear thermometer

Window *with temperature reading*

Panels *marked with a temperature*

Temperature reading

Temperature indicator strip

TAKING YOUR CHILD'S TEMPERATURE

When your child is unwell, take her temperature at least twice a day, morning and evening. One method is to place the thermometer under her arm, which gives a reading 0.6°C (1°F) lower than her true temperature. Never put a mercury thermometer into a young child's mouth, since it can break easily. The digital thermometer is not breakable so it is safe to put it into a young child's mouth, but if she can't hold it correctly under her tongue, place it in her armpit, as for a mercury thermometer. The ear thermometer is also suitable for young children. The temperature indicator strip is much the easiest way of taking a young child's temperature, but the reading is less accurate than that of a thermometer.

USING A MERCURY THERMOMETER

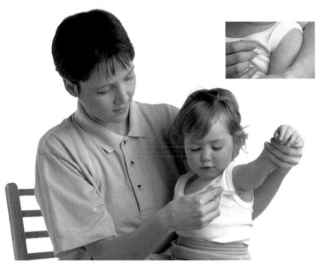

1 Hold the thermometer firmly and shake it sharply several times, with a downward flick of your wrist, to shake the mercury back into the bulb. Then sit your child on your knee and lift her arm. Tuck the bulb end of the thermometer into her armpit.

2 Bring your child's arm down and fold it over her chest. Hold the thermometer firmly in place for the recommended time—usually three minutes. Then remove the thermometer from under your child's arm.

The **number** *aligning with the top of the mercury column is your child's temperature*

3 Turn the thermometer around until you can see the column of mercury next to the scale. After use, wash it in cool water and store it out of your child's reach.

USING AN EAR THERMOMETER

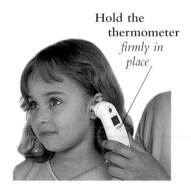

Hold the thermometer *firmly in place*

Make sure a clean lens filter is in place. Pull the ear back and insert the thermometer until the ear canal is sealed off. Press the button on top of the thermometer for one second, then remove the thermometer and read your child's temperature.

USING A DIGITAL THERMOMETER

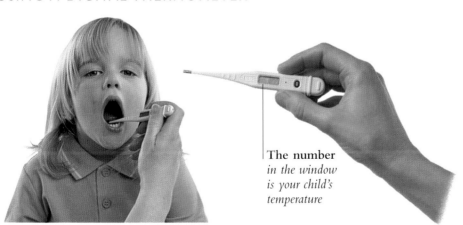

The **number** *in the window is your child's temperature*

1 Switch the thermometer on and ask your child to open her mouth. Place the thermometer under her tongue and ask her to close her mouth. Wait for about three minutes.

2 Remove the thermometer and read your child's temperature. Anything over 38°C (100.4°F) is a fever. Switch the thermometer off, then wash it in cool water and dry it.

USING AN INDICATOR STRIP

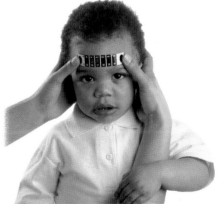

Hold the indicator strip on your child's forehead for about 15 seconds. The highest panel that glows indicates your child's temperature. Any reading over 37.5°C (99.5°F) is a fever.

BRINGING DOWN A FEVER

KEEPING HIM COMFORTABLE

If your child has a fever, remove extra blankets and clothing and make sure that he has plenty of fluids.

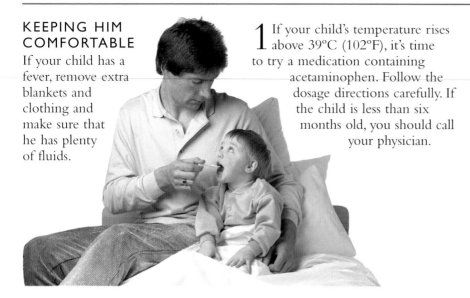

1 If your child's temperature rises above 39°C (102°F), it's time to try a medication containing acetaminophen. Follow the dosage directions carefully. If the child is less than six months old, you should call your physician.

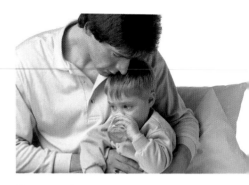

2 Your child may sweat profusely as his temperature falls, so give him plenty to drink to replace the lost fluid. Cover him with a warm cotton sheet to discourage shivering, which produces heat.

ADDITIONAL MEASURES

You can make your child more comfortable by changing the sheets and putting on fresh pajamas when her temperature is normal again.

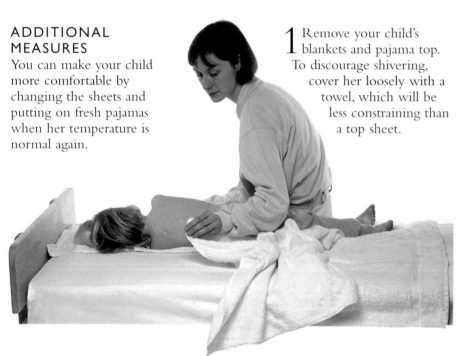

1 Remove your child's blankets and pajama top. To discourage shivering, cover her loosely with a towel, which will be less constraining than a top sheet.

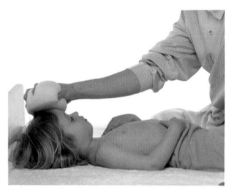

2 Gently wipe your child's face, neck, and arms with lukewarm water. Do not put her in water. Let her skin dry naturally. Continue for about half an hour. If her temperature is still above 39°C (102°F), **call your doctor now.**

FEVERISH CONVULSIONS

A rapid rise in temperature can cause convulsions in some children. They'll lose consciousness and go rigid for a few seconds, then twitch uncontrollably.

What can I do?

Put your child on the floor and stay with her, but do not try to restrain her. Put her in the recovery position (see page 233). Call your doctor when the convulsions stop.

How can I prevent feverish convulsions?

If a tendency to have feverish convulsions runs in your family, keep your child's temperature as low as you can when she is ill. Follow the cooling methods shown above, and try not to let her temperature rise above 39°C (102°F). Your doctor may instruct you to give her children's medicine with acetaminophen at the first signs of illness, to prevent a fever.

DELIRIOUS CHILDREN

Some children become delirious when they have a high fever. A delirious child will be very agitated, and may hallucinate and seem very frightened. This state is alarming for a parent to witness, but it isn't dangerous for your child. Stay with her to comfort and calm her. When her temperature drops, she should be begin to be calmer and seem much better.

ALL ABOUT MEDICINES

Most minor illnesses get better on their own. Your doctor may not prescribe medication, but if he does, he will tell you how often, and for how long, your child should take it. Follow the directions carefully. Always shake the bottle before pouring out liquid medicine, and measure doses exactly. You can buy child-sized medicine spoons, droppers, and tubes for giving medication to babies at most drugstores. Never mix medicine into your baby's food or bottle or a child's drink, since he may not finish it, or somebody else may unwittingly drink it. If your baby or child struggles when you give him medicine or put drops into his nose, ears, or eyes, ask another adult to help. Wrap a baby firmly in a receiving blanket. If the doctor prescribes antibiotics, your child must take the full course, even if he seems better before the course is finished; otherwise the infection may recur. However, antibiotics aren't effective against all illnesses: infectious diseases are caused by either viruses or bacteria, and antibiotics destroy bacteria, but don't affect viruses. This means that there is no real cure for viral illnesses such as colds. They simply have to run their course.

GIVING MEDICINE TO BABIES

Put a bib on him in case of a spill, and keep some tissues handy. Wash your hands and all the equipment carefully before giving medicine. If your baby cannot sit up yet, hold him as if you were going to feed him. If he can sit up, hold him on your lap and tuck one of his arms behind your back. Keep your hand on his other arm to prevent him from struggling.

Using two spoons
Measure the exact dose and pour half into a clean teaspoon, so it won't spill easily.

MEDICINE SPOON

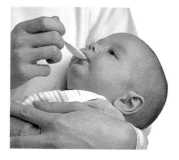

Measure your baby's dose and pour half into another spoon (see above). Keep both spoons nearby, then pick up your baby. Hold him so that he can't wriggle, then pick up one spoon and rest it on his lower lip. Let him suck the medicine off, then repeat with the rest of the dose.

MEDICINE DROPPER

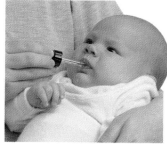

Measure the dose in a measuring spoon. Squeeze the end of the dropper and suck some of it up into the tube. Put the dropper into your baby's mouth and squirt in the medicine. Repeat until your baby has taken an accurate dose. Don't use a glass dropper if your baby has teeth.

MEDICINE TUBE

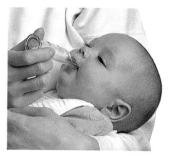

Measure the correct dose and pour it into the medicine tube, then pick up your baby and rest the mouthpiece of the tube on his lower lip. Tilt the tube slightly so that the medicine runs into your baby's mouth, but don't tilt it too much, or the medicine will run out too quickly.

FINGERTIP

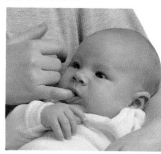

When all else fails, try letting her suck medicine off your finger. Measure the dose in a medicine spoon, then pick up your baby, keeping the spoon nearby. Dip your finger into it and let her suck the medicine off. It may take time, but continue until she has taken the whole dose.

GIVING MEDICINES TO CHILDREN

Most medicines for children are made to taste fairly pleasant, but if your child dislikes the taste, the following tips may help.

★ Have your child's favorite drink ready to take away the taste of the medicine, and try bribery—a small treat or reward may help.

★ Tell your child to hold her nose so that she can't taste the medicine, but never do this forcibly for her.

★ If your child is old enough to understand, explain why she has to take the medicine—if she knows that it will make her feel better, she may be more inclined to take it.

★ If you really find it impossible to get the medicine into your child, ask your doctor if he can prescribe it with a different flavor or in another form.

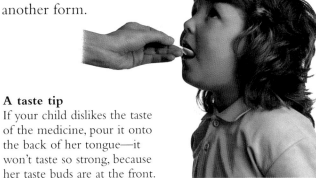

A taste tip
If your child dislikes the taste of the medicine, pour it onto the back of her tongue—it won't taste so strong, because her taste buds are at the front.

MEDICINE AND SAFETY

Make sure that your child can't help herself to any medicines in your home.

★ Keep all medications out of her reach, preferably in a locked cabinet.

★ Buy medicines with childproof lids or packaging.

★ Don't pretend to your child that her medicine is a soft drink.

Medicine and tooth decay

Try to clean your child's teeth after giving her medicine. This is because many medicines for children contain sugar and may cause tooth decay. If your child has to take medicine over a long period, ask your doctor or pharmacist whether a sugar-free alternative is available.

WARNING

Never give ASA (Acetylsalacylic acid) to your child when she is ill; give her acetaminophen instead. A few children who have been given ASA for a mild illness such as the flu have developed a rare, but very serious illness called Reye's syndrome. If your child suddenly vomits and develops a high fever while she is recovering from an illness, **call for emergency help immediately.**

GIVING NOSE DROPS

CHILDREN

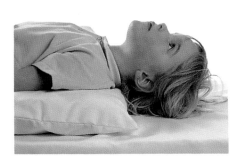

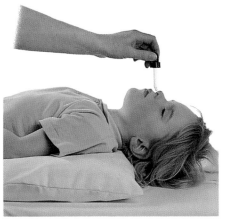

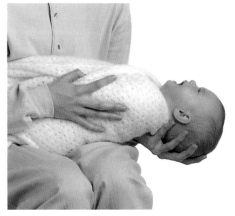

1 Place a small pillow or cushion on a bed and help your child to lie on her back with the pillow beneath her shoulders and her head dropped back. If your child is likely to wriggle as you give her the drops, ask another adult to help you by holding her head.

2 Put the tip of the dropper just above your child's nostril and squeeze out the prescribed number of drops. Don't let the dropper touch her nose—if it does, wash it before using it again. Keep your child lying down for about a minute.

BABIES

Wrap your baby in a blanket, then lay her on her back across your knee, so that her head falls back over your left thigh. Put your left hand beneath her head to support it, then give the drops as instructed for a child.

GIVING EAR DROPS

CHILDREN

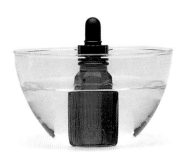

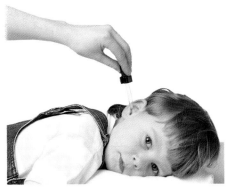

1 Most children find ear drops too cold as they are squeezed into their ears, so ask your doctor whether you can warm them up (some medicines deteriorate if they are warmed). To warm the drops, place the bottle in a bowl of warm, not hot, water for a few minutes. Before giving to your child, check the temperature on the inside of your wrist.

2 Ask your child to lie on his side with the affected ear uppermost. You may have to hold your child's head gently, to prevent him from making any sudden movements. Place the dropper close to his ear and gently squeeze the prescribed number of drops into the ear canal. Keep your child lying down for approximately a minute to stop the drops running out.

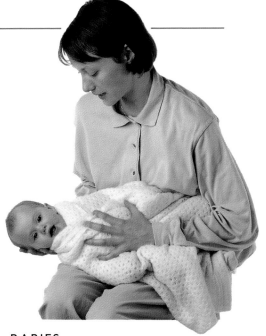

BABIES
Wrap your baby and lay her on her side across your lap. Support her head with one hand, then give the ear drops as instructed for a child.

EYE DROPS

CHILDREN

Hold your child's head *steady and pull her lower eyelid down gently with your thumb*

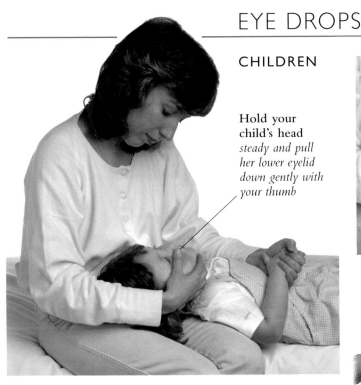

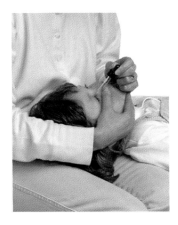

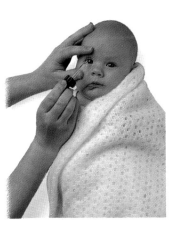

1 Bathe your child's affected eye (closed) with cotton wool dipped in warm boiled water, then ask your child to lie on her back across your knee or with her head in your lap. Put one arm round your child's head with your palm against her cheek, then tilt her head so that the affected eye is slightly lower than the other. Draw her lower eyelid gently down with your thumb.

2 Hold the dropper over the gap between the lower lid and the eye, angling it so that it is out of your child's sight. If necessary, ask someone to hold her head steady. Squeeze out the prescribed number of drops, being careful not to touch the eye or the lid. Even if she cries, enough of the medicine is likely to stay in her eye.

BABIES
Choose a time when your baby is relaxed, then wrap her and lay her on a firm surface or across your knee. Give your drops as for a child.

EYE OINTMENT
If your child is prescribed eye ointment, squeeze a tiny amount into the outer corner of her eye.

CARING FOR A SICK CHILD

While your child is feeling ill, she may demand a great deal of attention, and may be irritable and easily bored. Most children become more babyish when they are ill, and need a lot of extra hugs and reassurance. Keep your baby with you during the day, so that you can check on her frequently. Let your child lie down in the family room, so that she is near you. At night, sleep in the same room as your child if she is very unwell, so that

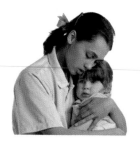

you are nearby if she needs you. Many children vomit when they are ill, so keep a small bowl nearby. Vomiting is only rarely a serious symptom and, while it is often a sign of illness, it can also be brought on by emotional upset or excitement. Frequent or persistent vomiting can be a sign of a serious condition, and may lead to dehydration; see page 222 for when to call your doctor and how to prevent dehydration.

EATING AND DRINKING

Your child will probably have a smaller appetite than usual while she is ill. Don't worry if she doesn't want to eat much for a few days—it won't do her any harm. Allow her to choose her favorite food, and offer small helpings. Let her eat as much or as little as she wants: when she is feeling better, her appetite will return. Babies may demand to be fed more frequently than usual, but take very little milk each time. Be patient if your baby behaves like this—she needs the comfort of feeling close to you as she sucks. Drink is much more important than food while your child is ill. Make sure that she has plenty to drink—about 1½ liters (3 pints) a day, especially if she has a raised temperature, or has been vomiting or had diarrhea— to make sure that she doesn't get dehydrated.

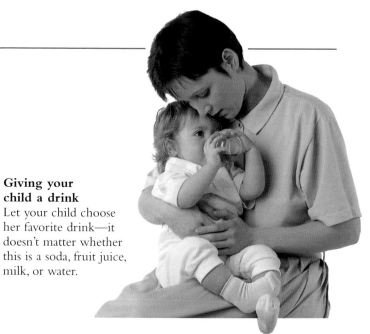

Giving your child a drink
Let your child choose her favorite drink—it doesn't matter whether this is a soda, fruit juice, milk, or water.

ENCOURAGING YOUR CHILD TO DRINK
If it is difficult to persuade your child to drink enough, make her drinks seem more appetizing by trying some of the ideas suggested below.

Small container
Offer frequent small drinks from a doll's cup or an egg cup, rather than giving large amounts.

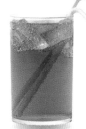

Straws
Make drinks look appetizing and more fun by letting your child use a straw.

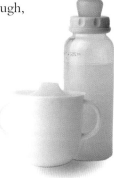

Training cup
Offer drinks in a training cup or bottle if your child has just grown out of either of these.

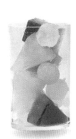

Ice cubes
For a child over a year, freeze diluted fruit juice into cubes, then let her suck the cubes.

Ice Popsicle
Your child may prefer an ice pop—the "drink on a stick." Try to avoid ones with artificial coloring.

SICKNESS AND VOMITING

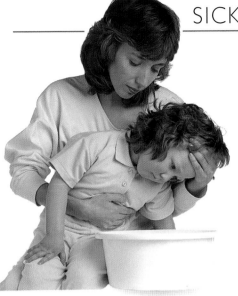

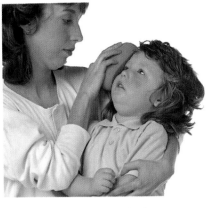

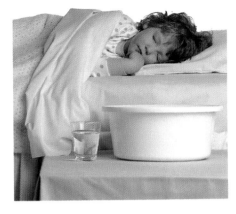

1 Hold your child while she is vomiting to comfort her. Support her head with one hand on her forehead, and put your other hand over her stomach, just below her rib cage.

2 After she has finished vomiting, do your best to reassure your child. Then sponge her face and wipe around her mouth. Give her a few sips of water, let her rinse her mouth out, or help her to clean her teeth, to take away any unpleasant taste that she may have.

3 Let your child rest quietly after vomiting; she may want to lie down and perhaps sleep for a while. Wash out the container and put it within easy reach, in case she vomits again. If your child vomits frequently, she may have gastroenteritis (see page 222).

COMFORT AND ENTERTAINMENT

STAYING IN BED

There is no need to insist that your sick child stays in bed, though if he is feeling very ill, he will probably prefer to stay there. If he wants to get up, make sure that he is dressed warmly and that the room he is playing in isn't too drafty. However, your child may want to lie down and go to sleep during the day, even if it isn't his usual naptime. If he doesn't want to be left alone, let him snuggle up with a pillow and a blanket and his favorite soft toy on the sofa in the sitting room, or make up a bed for him wherever you are (a folding guestbed is ideal). In this way your child still feels like he is a part of the family and does not get too bored or lonely.

Playing in bed
If your child feels like staying in bed, but wants to sit up, prop him up with pillows. Make a tray-table by resting a large tray or board on piles of books.

ENTERTAINING YOUR CHILD

Try to keep your child occupied, so that he doesn't get too bored, but remember that he will probably act younger than his age while he is feeling unwell. He won't be able to concentrate for very long, and he won't want to do anything too demanding. Bring out an old favorite toy that he hasn't played with for a while. If you give him small presents to keep him entertained and cheer him up, don't be tempted to buy toys that are advanced for his age. Babies will enjoy a new mobile or a rattle that makes a new sound. Quiet activities such as interlocking building bricks, felt pictures, simple jigsaw puzzles, crayons or felt-tip pens, a kaleidoscope, or modeling clay are ideal for sick toddlers and children. Protect the bedding with a towel if your child wants to play with something messy while he is in bed.

COLDS AND FLU

All children get colds and flu. As soon as your child comes into contact with other children, he may get one cold after another—some children under six have up to seven a year. As a child grows older, he develops resistance to many of these viruses.

Wiping your child's nose
If your child has a runny nose, dab it gently with a tissue to prevent it becoming sore from frequent wiping. Throw the tissue away immediately, to avoid spreading infection.

CALL THE DOCTOR

If your child has been feeling absolutely miserable, and especially if he is not yet one year old, consult your doctor as soon as possible if he has:
★ a temperature over 39°C (102.2°F)
★ wheezy, fast, or labored breathing
★ earache
★ a throat so sore that swallowing is painful
★ a severe cough
★ no improvement after three days.

COLDS

What are they?
Perhaps the most common of all illnesses, a cold is a viral infection that irritates the nose and throat, so children don't catch a cold simply by being cold, by going out without wearing a coat, or by getting their feet wet. While it is not a severe illness, a cold should be taken more seriously in babies and children than in adults, because of the risk of a chest or ear infection developing. If your child develops a rash in addition to the symptoms of a normal cold, contact your doctor to determine what the rash could be.

SYMPTOMS

★ Runny or blocked nose and sneezing
★ slightly raised temperature
★ sore throat
★ cough.

WHAT MIGHT THE DOCTOR DO?
If your baby has trouble sucking because her nose is blocked, your doctor may prescribe nose drops to be given just before a feeding.

NOSE DROPS
Use these only if your doctor has prescribed them, and never use them for more than three days. When overused they can increase mucus production, which will make your child's nose even more blocked.

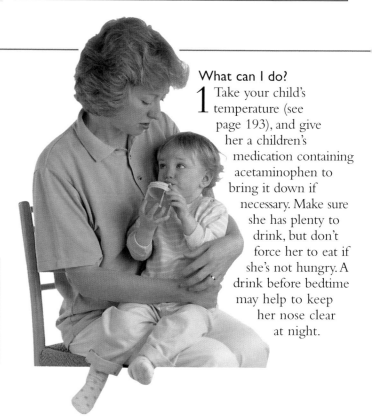

What can I do?
1 Take your child's temperature (see page 193), and give her a children's medication containing acetaminophen to bring it down if necessary. Make sure she has plenty to drink, but don't force her to eat if she's not hungry. A drink before bedtime may help to keep her nose clear at night.

SINUSITIS
The sinuses are air-filled cavities in the bones of the face. The lining of the nose extends into them, so they can easily become infected after a cold. This infection, sinusitis, often seems like a cold that won't go away, with nasal congestion, cough, and bad breath. These sinuses don't develop until age three or four, so for younger children, sinusitis isn't a problem.

FLU

What is it?

The flu (also known as influenza) is a very infectious illness caused by hundreds of different viruses. It tends to occur in epidemics every two or three years, when a new strain of the virus appears to which people have not yet developed immunity. If your child has caught the flu, he will develop symptoms a day or two later, and will probably be sick for about three or four days. He may be sick enough to want to stay in bed and could remain weak for several days after his temperature goes down. A few children develop a chest infection such as bronchitis or pneumonia (see page 218) after having the flu.

SYMPTOMS

★ Raised temperature
★ headache
★ aching all over the body
★ shivery feeling
★ runny nose
★ cough
★ sore throat.

What can I do?

Take your child's temperature (see page 193) and give him medicine with acetaminophen to reduce his fever if necessary. Make sure he has plenty to drink. Offer your baby cooled water.

"Should I have my child vaccinated against the flu?"

A vaccination may be a good idea, even for healthy children, so discuss it with your doctor. It will protect him from the illness for about a year. The flu vaccine is especially important for children with ongoing health problems, such as heart, kidney, or lung disease. Since new strains of the virus develop every two or three years, the vaccine (which can only be made from existing forms of the virus) does not give lifelong protection from the illness.

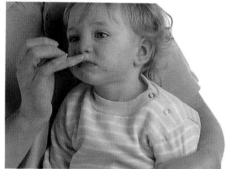

2 Spread a barrier cream, such as petroleum jelly, under your child's nose and around her nostrils if the area has become red and sore from a constantly runny nose or frequent wiping.

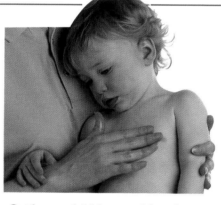

3 If your child has a cold, sit her on your lap—it will ease her cough and help her to settle before bed.

4 If your baby has a cold, she will be able to breathe more easily if you raise the head of the crib mattress slightly. Put a small pillow or a folded towel underneath it, then lay your baby in her crib so that her head and chest are slightly raised.

5 Make sure that the air in your child's room isn't too dry, since breathing very dry air can be uncomfortable. Use a humidifier if you have one, to add moisture to the air.

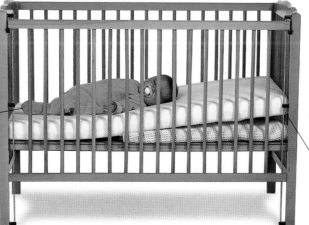

Put *your baby to sleep on her back.*

Make sure *that there are no gaps between the mattress and the head of the crib*

HAVING YOUR CHILD IMMUNIZED

At the two-month well-baby checkup, your baby will probably receive her first in a series of vaccination shots designed to protect her from severe infectious diseases. A vaccine is nothing more than a small harmless dose of the germ that causes the disease. It's too weak to endanger your baby but it will make her body produce special proteins called antibodies that will then protect her from the disease. Some babies become fussy or run slight fevers after certain immunizations such as the DPT (diphtheria, pertussis, and tetanus) shot.

Why should my baby be immunized?

Childhood immunization means protection against many serious diseases: polio, measles, mumps, rubella (German measles), whooping cough (pertussis), diphtheria, tetanus, Haemophilus influenzae type B (Hib), and Hepatitis B infections. Vaccines are also available for chickenpox (varicella), Strep pneumoniae (which is a cause of ear infections and meningitis) and Meningococcus (a cause of meningitis).

All these major diseases of childhood are preventable through immunization. By having your child immunized, not only do you protect her but you also help to eradicate the disease itself.

The table shown on this page is an example of a typical immunization schedule. Consult your doctor for more information on when immunizations are given.

What are the after-effects?

Immunization may induce a slight fever, so watch your child's temperature for 24 hours. You may want to give her the recommended dose of children's medication containing acetaminophen beforehand to prevent a temperature increase.

Your baby may develop a small, hard lump at the injection site. This will disappear in a few weeks. The measles vaccine may give her a rash and a fever six to 10 days later, and the mumps vaccine might make her face swell slightly three weeks later. If her crying sounds unusual, her temperature rises above 40°C (104°F), or she develops any other symptoms, **call your doctor immediately.**

IMMUNIZATION PROGRAM

Age	Vaccine	How given
2, 4, 6 month	Diphtheria pertussis tetanus poliomyelitis Hib	Combined injection
12 to 15 months	Measles mumps rubella	Combined injection
18 months	Diphtheria pertussis tetanus poliomyelitis Hib	Combined injection
4 to 6 years	Diphtheria pertussis tetanus poliomyelitis	Combined injection
	Measles	Separate injection
14 to 16 years	Diphtheria tetanus poliomyelitis	Combined injection
Every 10 years	Diphtheria tetanus	Combined injection
Also available	Chicken pox pneumococcal meningococcal	Separate injection

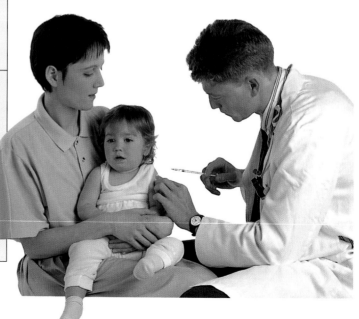

INFECTIOUS ILLNESSES

Because most children are immunized, many ailments in this section are uncommon. Most infectious diseases are caused by viruses, so medicines cannot cure them (see page 195), but recovery is ordinarily quick and uneventful. If your child catches a virus, she will become immune to that virus for the rest of her life. Some infectious diseases are caused by bacteria. These require prompt treatment with antibiotics. Many diseases are most infectious just before symptoms appear. It is helpful to inform the parents of your child's playmates.

WARNING

If your child has a raised temperature while she is ill with one of these diseases, **DO NOT** give her ASA to bring the fever down. Give her children's medication containing acetaminophen.

EMERGENCY SIGNS

Call for emergency help immediately if your child has an infectious disease and develops any of these signs:
* unusual and increasing drowsiness
* headache or stiff neck
* convulsions
* flat, dark red or purplish rash.

RUBELLA (GERMAN MEASLES)

What is it?
Rubella, also known as German measles, is a very mild illness, so your child may feel perfectly well and may not want to stay in bed. She will develop symptoms two to three weeks after she has been infected.

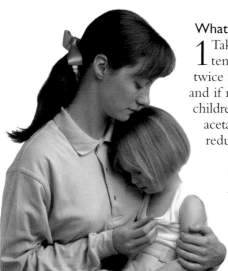

What can I do?
1 Take your child's temperature at least twice a day (see page 193), and if necessary give her children's medication with acetaminophen to reduce her fever.

2 Make sure that your child has plenty to drink, especially if she has a fever.

SYMPTOMS

Days 1 and 2
* Symptoms of a mild cold
* slightly sore throat
* swollen glands behind the ears, on the sides of the neck, and on the nape of the neck.

Day 2 or 3
* Blotchy rash of flat, pink spots appearing first on the face, then spreading down the body
* slightly raised temperature.

Day 4 or 5
* Fading rash and general improvement.

Day 6
* Your child is back to normal.

Day 9 or 10
* Your child is no longer infectious.

CALL THE DOCTOR

Call for emergency help immediately if your child develops any of the emergency signs above. Consult your doctor as soon as possible if you think your child has rubella, but check with him before taking your child to his office, to avoid the possibility of her coming into contact with a pregnant woman.

What the doctor might do
Your doctor will confirm that your child has rubella, but there is no treatment for it.

Rubella and pregnancy
While your child is infectious, don't let her come into contact with pregnant women. Although rubella is a mild disease, it can cause defects in a fetus if a pregnant woman catches it.

MEASLES

What is it?
Measles is a very infectious illness that causes a rash, fever, and a cough, and sometimes more serious complications. It used to be common, but widespread immunization has made it a rare disease.

What can I do?
1 Try to bring down her temperature (see p.196) and give plenty of fluids. She may feel very miserable and want to stay in bed.

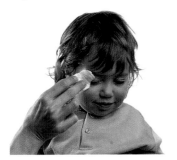

2 If her eyes are sore, bathe them with a cotton ball dipped in cool water. Keep her room dark if this makes her more comfortable.

What the doctor might do
Your doctor will confirm the diagnosis and may want to keep a check on your child until she has recovered. He will treat any complications if they develop.

CALL THE DOCTOR
Call for emergency help immediately if your child develops any of the signs listed on page 203. Consult your doctor as soon as possible if you think your child has measles. Call him again if:
★ your child is no better three days after the rash develops
★ your child's temperature rises suddenly
★ her condition worsens after she seemed to be improving
★ your child has an earache
★ your child's breathing is noisy or difficult.

ROSEOLA INFANTUM

What is it?
Roseola is a mild illness that is very common in early childhood. It is characterized by a high fever that lasts for about three days, followed by a rash of pink spots. Most children will have had it by the time they are two.

SYMPTOMS
Symptoms appear 5–15 days after infection
Days 1 to 4
★ High temperature
★ sometimes a mild cold or cough.

Days 4 to 8
★ Temperature suddenly returns to normal
★ rash of pink, slightly raised spots appears over head and trunk.
★ rash fades and child is back to normal.

What can I do?
1 Call your doctor if your child's temperature is 39°C (102.2°F) or above.

2 Try to bring down the fever to make your child more comfortable (see p.196). Acetaminophen may bring his temperature down briefly.

3 Make sure your child has plenty to drink.

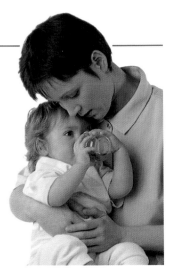

CALL THE DOCTOR
Call for emergency help immediately if your child develops any of the emergency signs on p. 203.

CHICKEN POX

What is it?

This very infectious illness produces a rash of very itchy spots. Your child may not feel very ill, but if she has a lot of spots, she may itch all over. Symptoms appear two to three weeks after your child has been infected.

The chicken pox virus causes shingles in adults, particularly in the elderly. It is possible to catch chicken pox from someone with shingles, but not vice versa.

SYMPTOMS

Days 1 to 4

★ Groups of small, red, very itchy spots with fluid-filled centers, appearing in batches first on the child's chest, abdomen, and back, and later elsewhere on the body
★ fluid within the spots becomes white and cloudy
★ slight temperature.

Days 5 to 9

★ The spots burst, leaving small craters
★ scabs form over the spots and drop off after a few days.

Day 6

★ Counting the first day that the spots appear as Day 1, your child is no longer infectious by Day 6.

Day 10 or sooner

★ Your child is back to normal.

CALL THE DOCTOR

Call for emergency help immediately if your child develops any of the emergency signs listed on page 203. Consult your doctor as soon as possible if you think your child has chicken pox, and call him again if your child has any of these symptoms:

★ severe itching
★ redness or swelling around any spots, or pus oozing from the spots—this means they have become infected
★ severe cough
★ confusion or difficulty walking.

What can I do?

1 Take your child's temperature (see page 193), and, if raised, give her the recommended dose of a children's medicine containing acetaminophen to bring it down, and plenty to drink.

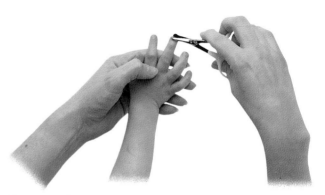

2 Try to discourage your child from scratching the spots, because they can become infected and cause scarring when they heal. Cut your child's fingernails short and keep them clean so that the spots are less likely to become infected if she does scratch them.

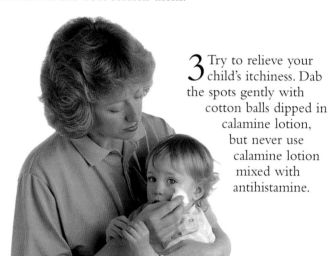

3 Try to relieve your child's itchiness. Dab the spots gently with cotton balls dipped in calamine lotion, but never use calamine lotion mixed with antihistamine.

4 Give your child regular warm baths, each with a handful of baking soda dissolved in the water to help reduce the itching.

5 If your child is very itchy, she will probably find loose cotton clothes the most comfortable.

What the doctor might do

Your doctor will confirm the diagnosis and may prescribe medicine to relieve your child's itching if it is very severe. If any of the spots have become infected, he may prescribe an antibiotic cream.

MUMPS

What is it?
Mumps is an infection that is rare, now that immunization is widespread. It causes swollen glands, specifically the glands in front of the ears, making your child's cheeks look puffy. Mumps can occasionally cause inflammation of the testicles, but this is very rare in a pre-pubescent boy.

What can I do?
1 Give plenty of drinks. Let your child drink through a straw if he wants.

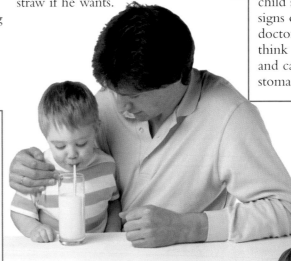

2 Check his temperature (see page 187) and give him children's medication with acetaminophen to reduce his temperature if it is raised.

3 Give him liquid or soft foods to eat, such as soup or ice cream.

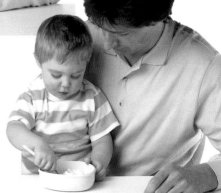

CALL THE DOCTOR
Call for emergency help if your child shows any of the emergency signs on page 203. Consult your doctor as soon as possible if you think your child has the mumps, and call him again if he develops stomach pain or a red testicle.

What the doctor might do
Your doctor can offer suggestions for making your child as comfortable as possible.

SYMPTOMS
Symptoms appear 14–24 days after infection.
* raised temperature
* one or two days later the child develops painful swellings on one or both sides of the face. This lasts 4–8 days.

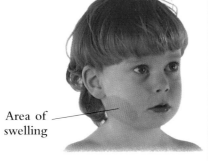

Area of swelling

ERYTHEMA INFECTIOSUM (FIFTH DISEASE)

What is it?
Erythema infectiosum is a mild, and mildly infectious, illness that usually occurs in small outbreaks in the spring and mostly affects children over the age of two years. The disease is characterized by a bright red rash that suddenly appears on both cheeks, hence its other name of "slapped cheek disease."

What can I do?
Give your child acetaminophen to reduce the fever. Make sure she drinks plenty of fluids. If your child has a blood disorder (for example, sickle-cell anemia or thalassemia), consult your doctor. Erythema infectiosum can sometimes cause severe illness in such children. If your child has Erythema infectiosum, keep her away from anyone who might be pregnant. Contact your doctor if your child has erythema infectiosum and you are pregnant.

SYMPTOMS
Symptoms appear 4–14 days after infection.

Day 1
* Bright red cheeks, with a contrasting pale area around the mouth
* mild fever.

Day 2–5
* Blotchy, lace-like rash spreading over trunk and limbs.

Day 7–10
* Rash fades. The rash may recur over the next few weeks or months, particularly if your child gets hot or is exposed to sunlight.

WHOOPING COUGH

What is it?

One of the most serious childhood diseases, whooping cough is a severe and persistent cough. It is highly infectious, so keep your child away from babies and children who have not been immunized. Even a child who has been immunized can get a mild form of the illness. A few children with whooping cough also develop a secondary infection, such as bronchitis or pneumonia (see pages 218–19).

What can I do?

1 Stay with your child during coughing fits, since he may be very distressed. Sit him on your lap and hold him leaning slightly forward. Keep a bowl or plastic container nearby so that he can spit out any phlegm he coughs up, and in case he vomits afterward. Clean the bowl thoroughly with boiling water, to make sure that the infection doesn't spread.

2 If your child often coughs and vomits after meals, offer him small meals at frequent intervals, if possible just after a coughing fit.

3 Keep your child entertained—he will have fewer coughing fits if his attention is distracted, but don't let him get too excited or overtired since this may bring on a coughing fit.

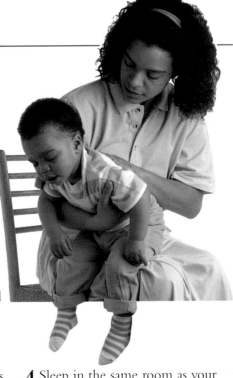

4 Sleep in the same room as your child, so that you can be with him if he has a coughing fit at night.

5 Don't let anyone smoke near your child, and don't give him any cough medicines, unless prescribed.

SYMPTOMS

Week 1
* Symptoms of a normal cough and cold
* slight temperature.

Week 2
Worsening cough, with frequent coughing fits lasting up to a minute, after which your child has to fight for breath
* if your child is over 18 months, he may learn to hold his coughs in with a "whooping" sound
* vomiting after a coughing fit.

Weeks 3 to 10
* Cough improves, but may worsen if your child gets a cold
* your child is unlikely to be infectious after the third week.

EMERGENCY SIGNS

Call for emergency help immediately if your child turns blue during a coughing fit.

CALL THE DOCTOR

Consult your doctor as soon as possible if you suspect that your child has whooping cough.

What the doctor might do

The doctor might prescribe a cough suppressant and an antibiotic. The antibiotic won't cure your child's cough, but it may reduce its severity and make your child less infectious. This is particularly important if you have a baby who is at risk of catching whooping cough from an older sibling who already has the disease. However, the antibiotic is only really effective if it is given right at the beginning of the infection.

CARING FOR A BABY

Whooping cough is dangerous in babies since they may not be able to draw breath properly after coughing. Your baby will need careful nursing and may be admitted to the hospital. She may find sucking difficult if she vomits frequently, so abandon your regular feeding schedule, and feed her as soon as she has calmed down after coughing or vomiting.

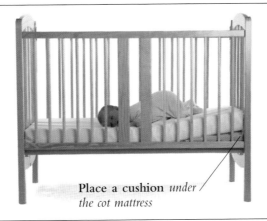

Place a cushion *under the cot mattress*

Coughing fits

When your baby has a coughing fit, lay her in her crib on her stomach with the foot of her crib mattress slightly raised, or face down across your lap. Stay with her until she has stopped coughing and is breathing normally again. Hold her to comfort her and put her down to sleep on her back as usual.

MENINGITIS

What is it?

Meningitis is an inflammation of the tissues covering the brain. It can be caused by infection with bacteria or by viruses. It can occur at any time in the year. In Canada, the Hib vaccination has wiped out one type of bacterial meningitis. Unfortunately there are others, of which the most common are strep pneumoniae and meningococcus. Fortunately, vaccines are now available for both of

The meninges

Three protective layers, known as the meninges, cover the brain and spinal cord. Meningitis occurs when the meninges become infected by viruses or bacteria.

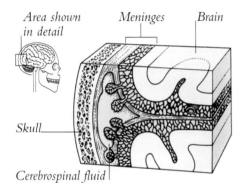

Area shown in detail   *Meninges*   *Brain*

Skull

Cerebrospinal fluid

these diseases. Although bacterial meningitis can occur at any age, it is most common in children under the age of 5.

The early symptoms of bacterial and viral meningitis are very similar, and unfortunately can easily be mistaken for those of flu. However, the symptoms of bacterial meningitis are usually more severe. What makes bacterial meningitis so dangerous and frightening for parents is that it can develop very rapidly, so that the child may become seriously ill within a few hours, with symptoms that include increasing drowsiness and sometimes loss of consciousness or convulsions.

Meningitis rash

Some children with meningitis develop a characteristic rash of tiny blood-spots under the skin, which can appear anywhere on the body, and don't disappear when pressed with a glass (see below). The spots are flat and look like pin-pricks at first, and then like fresh bruises.

What can I do?

Call your doctor immediately, or take your child to the nearest hospital emergency department if she seems abnormally drowsy or if she has any two of the symptoms listed in the emergency signs box below. Do not delay, because early treatment of bacterial meningitis is crucial.

What might the doctor do?

The doctor may send your child to the hospital to confirm the diagnosis.

If viral meningitis is diagnosed, no further treatment is necessary except for painkillers, and your child will recover within a week or two.

Bacterial meningitis will be treated with antibiotics and, if convulsions occur, with anticonvulsant drugs as well. If the disease is picked up early and treated promptly, most children recover completely from bacterial meningitis. Rarely, the disease may be fatal. Even with early diagnosis and treatments, meningitis can leave lasting health complications. The best "treatment" is prevention, when available, through vaccination.

EMERGENCY SIGNS

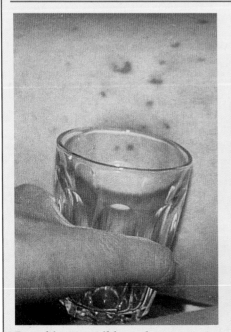

Petechiae (possible early purpura)

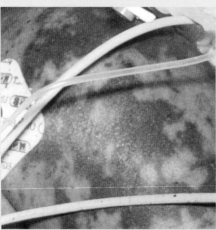

Purpura

Obtain emergency help immediately if your child has two or more of the following symptoms:
★ Abnormal drowsiness
★ fever with cold hands and feet
★ vomiting
★ stiff neck
★ refusing feeds
★ restlessness and irritability
★ tense or bulging fontanelle
★ purple-red rash that does not fade when pressed
Older children may also have:
★ severe headache
★ dislike of bright light and noise.

If your child has a dark, purplish rash, check to see whether it fades when pressed. To do this, press the side of a glass on to the rash. If the rash is still visible through the glass, it may be a petechial rash, which may be an early sign of a purpural rash. This requires immediate medical attention. Take your child to the nearest hospital emergency department.

EYE PROBLEMS

Although most eye disorders clear up quickly when treated, all eye problems should be taken seriously. Eye infections spread easily, so give your child her own washcloth and towel, and change them frequently. Dry her eyes with tissues, using a clean one for each eye. Keep her hands clean and try to stop her from rubbing her eyes.

BLEPHARITIS

What is it?
Blepharitis is an inflammation of the edges of the eyelids, which usually affects both eyes. Children with dandruff often have blepharitis.

SYMPTOMS
* ★ Red and scaly eyelids.

What can I do?
1 Dissolve a teaspoon of baking soda or salt in a glass of warm boiled water. Soak a ball of cotton in the solution and use this to bathe your child's eyelids. Wash your hands before and afterward, and use a fresh cotton ball for each eye. Do this twice a day, making a fresh solution each time.

2 If your child has dandruff, wash her hair with an antidandruff shampoo. Use an anticradle cap shampoo for a baby.

CALL THE DOCTOR
Consult your doctor as soon as possible if:
* ★ your child's eyes are sticky
* ★ there is no improvement after about a week of home treatment.

What might the doctor do?
The doctor might prescribe a cream to soothe your child's eyelids, or an antibiotic ointment.

CONJUNCTIVITIS

What is it?
Also known as "pink eye," because the white of the eye may turn pink, conjunctivitis is an inflammation of the lining of the eye and the eyelid. It can be caused by either a virus or bacteria. It is milder when caused by a virus. If your child's eyelids are gummed together with pus when she wakes up, she probably has bacterial, rather than viral, conjunctivitis. If your baby develops any of the symptoms in the box (right) in the first day or two of life, see Sticky eye, page 183.

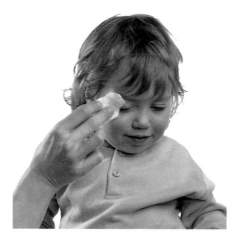

SYMPTOMS
* ★ Bloodshot eye
* ★ gritty, sore eye
* ★ discharge of pus
* ★ eyelids gummed together after sleep.

CALL THE DOCTOR
Consult your doctor as soon as possible if you think your child has conjunctivitis or if her eyes are bloodshot and sore.

What can I do?
1 Try to find out whether or not your child's symptoms are caused by something other than conjunctivitis. She might have an allergy such as hay fever, or she may have a speck of dust or an eyelash in her eye. If she has an allergy, her eyes may be itchy and watering as well as red and sore.

2 If you think she has conjunctivitis, dissolve a teaspoon of salt in a glass of warm boiled water, and dip a cotton ball in the solution. Bathe both eyelids, using fresh cotton balls for each one. Start with the infected one, and wipe from the outside corner to the inside. Wash your hands before and after this procedure.

What the doctor might do
The doctor may prescribe antibiotic drops or ointment for a bacterial infection, which will cure it quickly. Viral conjunctivitis needs no treatment, but may last a few days.

STYE

What is it?
A stye is a painful, pus-filled swelling on the upper or lower eyelid, caused by infection at the base of an eyelash. Some styes simply dry up, but most come to a head and burst within a week, relieving the pain. Styes are not serious and you can treat them at home.

SYMPTOMS

* ★ Red, painful swelling on the eyelid
* ★ pus-filled center appearing in the swelling.

CALL THE DOCTOR

Consult your doctor as soon as possible if:
* ★ the stye does not improve after a week
* ★ your child's whole eyelid is swollen
* ★ the skin all around your child's eye turns red
* ★ your child also has blepharitis.

What can I do?

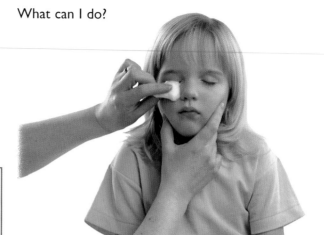

1 Dip a cotton ball in hot water, squeeze it, and press it gently onto your child's stye for two or three minutes, to help bring the stye to a head more quickly. Repeat this three times a day until the stye bursts.

2 When the stye bursts, the pain is relieved. Wash the pus away very gently using a fresh cotton ball dipped in warm boiled water for each wipe.

STRABISMUS (CROSS-EYE)

What is it?
Normally, both eyes look in the same direction at the same time, but in a child with strabismus, one eye focuses on an object, while the other does not follow it properly.

A newborn baby's eyes do not always work together correctly, so intermittent cross-eyes is common. This is nothing to worry about—your baby is simply learning to use his eyes. But if your baby's eyes don't move together after he is about three months old, he may have strabismus.

Strabismus may be constant, but in some children it comes and goes. However, children do not grow out of strabismus, so it is essential to have it treated. The younger the child, the more successful the treatment.

SYMPTOMS

* ★ Eyes looking in different directions

CALL THE DOCTOR

Consult your doctor if you think your child has strabismus.

How can I check for strabismus?
When your baby is about three months old, hold a toy 20cm (8in) from his face and move it slowly from side to side. Check that his eyes work together to follow the moving object.

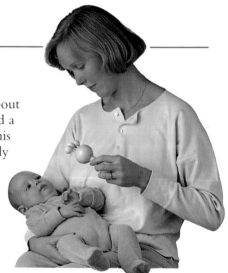

What the doctor might do
The doctor will check your child's vision and may give him a patch to wear over his stronger eye for several hours each day. This forces him to use his weak eye. A toddler may need to wear glasses. If your child is under two, this treatment will probably cure his strabismus in a few months. If your child has severe strabismus caused by muscle weakness, he may need to have surgery to correct the problem.

EAR PROBLEMS

Most ear problems in small children come from an infection of the outer or middle ear, or when the tube connecting the ear and throat becomes blocked. Infections should be taken seriously, but are dangerous only if not treated promptly: there is a risk that pus may build up behind the eardrum, and eventually burst it, or that infection might spread into a bone behind the ear (mastoiditis).

Anatomy of the ear

The ear consists of three parts. From the outer ear (the only visible part) a slightly curved canal leads to the eardrum. The middle ear lies behind the eardrum and is a cavity housing three small bones that transmit sound vibrations. The inner ear contains the delicate structures that allow you to hear and balance yourself.

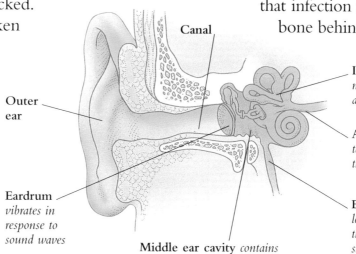

Canal

Outer ear

Eardrum *vibrates in response to sound waves*

Middle ear cavity *contains three tiny bones that transmit sound signals to the inner ear*

Inner ear *contains the mechanisms for hearing and balance*

Auditory nerve *takes sound signals to the brain*

Eustachian tube *leads to the back of the throat. It is much shorter in children than in adults, so infection can spread easily*

OUTER EAR INFECTION

What is it?

The skin lining the outer ear canal becomes inflamed when your child has an outer ear infection. This may happen if he swims in chlorinated water a lot, or because he has poked or scratched his ear and it has become infected. Children with eczema are especially prone to such infections if they get water in their ears.

SYMPTOMS

★ Pain in the ear that is worse when the child touches his ear or lies on it
★ redness in the ear canal
★ discharge from the ear
★ itchiness inside the ear.

CALL THE DOCTOR

Consult your doctor as soon as possible if you think your child has an outer ear infection.

What can I do?

1 Give your child the recommended dose of a children's medication containing acetaminophen.

2 Make sure that water doesn't get into the affected ear at bathtime, and just sponge his hair clean. Don't let your child go swimming until the infection clears up.

What the doctor might do

Your doctor will probably prescribe antibiotic or anti-inflammatory ear drops to treat the infection.

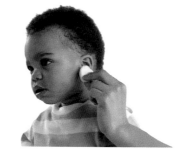

WAX IN THE EAR

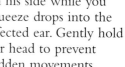

Wax can sometimes accumulate in the ear, giving a feeling of fullness or partial deafness. If your child has a lot of ear wax, very gently wipe away any visible wax with a cotton ball, but don't poke anything into the ear. If this doesn't help, consult your doctor.

To administer ear drops, ask your child to lie still on his side while you squeeze drops into the affected ear. Gently hold her head to prevent sudden movements.

MIDDLE EAR INFECTION

What is it?
If your child has a middle ear infection, the cavity behind his eardrum becomes inflamed, usually because an infection has spread from the throat. The tube that runs from the throat to the ear is very short and narrow in a child, allowing infection to spread extremely easily. Generally only one ear is infected. Once your child has had a middle ear infection, especially if this happens during his first two years, he is likely to have one whenever he has a cold or throat infection.

What can I do?
1 Try to relieve your child's earache. Fill a hot water bottle with warm, not hot, water and wrap it in a towel, then let him rest his ear against it. Don't give a hot water bottle to a baby who is too young to push it away if it is too hot: heat a soft cloth and hold it against his ear instead.

2 If your child's ear is very painful, give him the recommended dose of children's medication containing acetaminophen.

3 If you notice a discharge, don't clear it away or probe into his ear—just put a clean handkerchief over his ear. Encourage him to rest his head on the affected side, so that any discharge can drain away.

What the doctor might do
Your doctor might prescribe an antibiotic to clear the infection. Rarely, if this is not effective, your child may need the minor surgery described below.

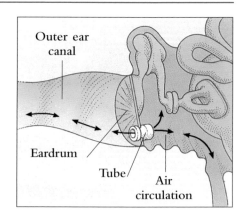

SYMPTOMS

★ Very painful ear, which may stop your child from sleeping
★ crying and rubbing or tugging at the ear, if your child can't talk yet or easily explain that his ear aches
★ crying, loss of appetite, and general signs of illness in young babies, especially following a cold
★ fever
★ partial deafness.

CALL THE DOCTOR

Consult your doctor as soon as possible if your child's ear is infected or has a discharge.

GLUE EAR (EFFUSION)

What is it?
Repeated middle ear infections can lead to glue ear, an accumulation of sticky fluid (effusion) in the middle ear.

SYMPTOMS

★ Partial deafness after repeated middle ear infections.

CALL THE DOCTOR

Consult your doctor as soon as possible if you think your child has glue ear.

What the doctor might do
Your doctor may prescribe an antibiotic to clear up the infection, but the majority of cases of glue ear clear up on their own in six to 12 weeks with no treatment. Occasionally, a simple operation may be necessary. Under anesthesia, a small hole is made in the eardrum and a tiny tube is inserted through this. The tube is not uncomfortable and will not affect your child's hearing, but he can't go swimming while it is in place. After several months it will fall out, the hole will heal, and his hearing will be back to normal.

The tube is implanted in the eardrum, to equalize air pressure on either side of the eardrum and to allow the ear to dry out.

MOUTH INFECTIONS

When a baby or young child has a mouth infection, two of life's simple pleasures —sucking and eating—become very painful.

Thrush is the most common mouth affliction in babies, while older children may be prone to cold sores (see page 230).

Helping the child with a sore mouth

If your child's mouth is sore, try to make eating and drinking as painless as you can. Allow warm meals to cool before giving them to your child, since hot food generally hurts more than cold, and offer her plenty of very cold drinks. If she is reluctant to eat or drink, try some of the suggestions given here.

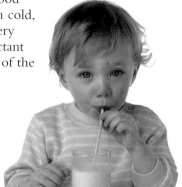

Let your child drink

through a straw or use a training cup, since this may be less painful than drinking straight from a glass.

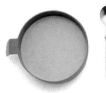

Soup
This is nourishing, easy to eat, and can be served cold. Mix or chop solid food into very small bites.

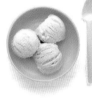

Cold drinks
Serve drinks very cold; avoid fruit juice, since it is very acidic.

Ice cream
Your child may find cold food such as ice cream easy to eat.

Water

Cheese
Your child may also like cheese. A drink of water will help rinse her mouth.

THRUSH

What is it?

Thrush is an infection caused by a yeast that lives in the mouth and intestines. The yeast is normally kept under control by bacteria, but sometimes it multiplies wildly, producing a sore, irritating rash. Occasionally, it spreads through the intestines and causes a rash around the anus. It is not a serious infection and, although it does not ordinarily respond to home remedies, it usually clears up quickly under a doctor's care.

SYMPTOMS

★ Reluctance to eat due to a sore mouth

★ creamy yellow, slightly raised patches on the inside of the cheeks, tongue, or the roof of the mouth, which do not come away easily if you try to wipe them off

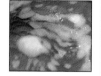

★ in babies, a rash around the anus that looks like diaper rash.

CALL THE DOCTOR

Consult your doctor if you think your baby or child has thrush.

What can I do?

1 Wipe the patches in your child's mouth very gently with a clean handkerchief. If they don't come off easily, she probably has thrush. Don't rub them hard, because if you scrape them off there will be sore, bleeding patches beneath.

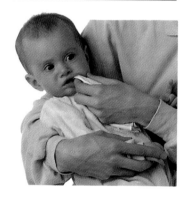

2 Give your child food that is easy to eat (see above). If you are bottle-feeding, buy a special soft nipple and clean it carefully, then sterilize it after each feeding.

3 If you are breast-feeding, continue to nurse normally, but take extra care with nipple hygiene to prevent your nipples from becoming infected. Wash them in water only, not soap, after each feeding, and don't wear breast pads. If they are sore or develop white spots, consult your doctor.

What the doctor might do

Your doctor may prescribe a medicine to be dropped into your baby's mouth just before a feeding. If you are breast-feeding, the doctor may check your nipples for signs of infection.

THROAT INFECTIONS

Sore throats are common in children of all ages, and often accompany a cold or the flu. Most are caused by viruses and clear up quickly. Call your doctor because it's important to rule out more severe ailments, which might require a prescription medication or signal a bacterial infection of the tonsils.

CALL THE DOCTOR

Consult your doctor as soon as possible if your child:
* ★ has a throat so sore that swallowing is painful
* ★ seems generally sick with a fever or rash
* ★ has infected tonsils
* ★ has not had a diphtheria-pertussis-tetanus (DPT) shot.

SORE THROAT

What is it?
A sore throat is an infection of the throat that makes the area painful and red. It may be part of a cold or the flu (see pages 200–201), or it may be caused by a bacteria called streptococcus ("strep"). Children are prone to earaches when they have a throat infection (see page 212).

SYMPTOMS

* ★ Reluctance to eat, because it hurts to swallow
* ★ red, raw-looking throat
* ★ an earache (see page 212)
* ★ slightly raised temperature
* ★ swollen glands
* ★ stomach ache in young children.

What can I do?
1 Ask your child to face a bright light and open his mouth. Examine the back of his throat carefully (see page 189). If it is sore, it will look red and raw and you may be able to see cream-colored spots.

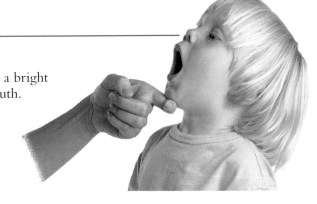

2 Gently feel down each side of your child's neck and just below the angle of his jawbone, checking for tiny lumps under the skin, indicating swollen glands (see page 189).

3 Give your child plenty of cold drinks, and mash solid foods if it hurts him to swallow. Very cold food such as ice cream is less painful to eat than warm food.

4 Take your child's temperature (see page 193), and if it is above normal, give him acetaminophen to bring down his fever.

What might the doctor do?
Most mild sore throats need no treatment, but if the doctor suspects that the infection is caused by bacteria, he will prescribe an antibiotic.

TONSILLITIS

SYMPTOMS

* ★ Very sore throat
* ★ red and enlarged tonsils, possibly covered with creamy spots

* ★ temperature over 38°C (100.4°F)
* ★ swollen glands on the neck.

What is it?
The tonsils are glands at the back of the throat, one on either side, which trap infection and prevent it from spreading. Tonsillitis is an inflammation of the tonsils, causing a very sore throat and other symptoms of illness.

What can I do?
1 Examine your child's tonsils and feel his glands (see page 189). If infected, his tonsils will be large and red, and may have cream-colored spots.

2 Take his temperature (see page 193). Give him acetaminophen to reduce it.

3 Encourage your child to have plenty to drink, especially if he has a fever. Offer him cold drinks and liquid or semi-liquid foods.

What might the doctor do?
Your doctor will examine your child's throat, and may take a throat culture by wiping a sterile swab across it. He will prescribe an antibiotic if the culture shows bacteria.

If your child has recurring bouts of severe tonsillitis your doctor may recommend that he has his tonsils removed. This operation is rarely performed on a child under four years of age.

COUGHS AND CHEST INFECTIONS

Coughs in small children are usually a symptom of a cold or the flu (see pages 200-201), which produces a dry, ticklish cough. A cough may also be a symptom of a chest infection (see pages 216-219) or an early sign of the measles (see page 204). A severe, persistent cough might be whooping cough (see page 207). Your child may get a chest infection after a cold or the flu. He will have other symptoms as well as a cough: he may find breathing difficult, and might cough up mucus. Slightly wheezy breathing is normal for a small child with a cold or the flu, because his airways are very narrow and become even narrower when he is ill, so on its own this may not be a sign of an infection. Occasionally, a chest infection develops as a complication of the measles or whooping cough.

FREQUENT CHEST INFECTIONS

Babies under a year old and children with a long-term chest disorder such as asthma (see page 218) are prone to chest infections. If you smoke, your children are much more likely to develop chest infections than the children of nonsmoking parents.

If your child has frequent chest infections, your doctor may arrange for tests to find the cause.

Breathing
When your child breathes in, air is sucked down his windpipe and bronchi (the airways) into his lungs, where oxygen is absorbed into his bloodstream. His blood then carries the oxygen throughout his body.

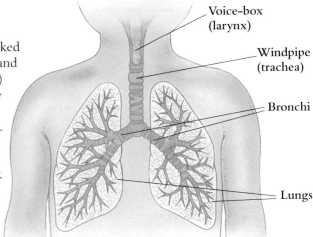

Voice-box (larynx)

Windpipe (trachea)

Bronchi

Lungs

CROUP

What is it?
Croup is an inflammation of the larynx or voice box, which makes it swell, so that your child finds it difficult to breathe. It can become serious, so you must monitor your child carefully.

SYMPTOMS
* Breathing difficulty
* loud, crowing sound as breath is drawn in
* barking cough.

What can I do?
1 Keep calm, and reassure your child. He may be very frightened, but if he panics, it will be even harder for him to breathe.

2 Take your child into the bathroom and create a steamy atmosphere by turning on the hot water full blast. Moist air will help him breathe more easily. Meanwhile put a cold-mist humidifier in his room to moisten the air there, too.

3 Prop your child up on pillows, or sit him on your lap—he will then be able to breathe more easily.

CALL THE DOCTOR
Call your doctor now if your child has difficulty breathing, or if you think he has croup.

4 You can also bundle up your child and take him outside to breathe cold, moist air for five to 10 minutes. This works wonders for croup.

COUGH

What is it?

A cough is a protective reflex action that helps to clear away any irritants or blockages from the airways. It can be either a reaction to irritation in the throat or windpipe, or the result of a chest infection. It may also be caused by an obstruction in the airways. A cough will generally disappear of its own accord. A dry, ticklish cough is rarely serious. It probably means that your child's throat or windpipe is irritated, which may be a by-product of a cold, because mucus dribbles down the throat and irritates it. Her throat might also be irritated by smoke, if she is with adults who smoke. An ear infection can also cause a dry cough.

If your child's cough sounds moist, particularly if she spits up mucus, she probably has a chest infection. While most coughs like this are not serious, they can be a symptom of bronchitis or pneumonia (see pages 218–9).

What the doctor might do

The doctor will listen to your child's breathing. If she has a dry cough, the doctor may prescribe a cough suppressant medication to soothe her throat. If the cough is deep, the doctor may carry out some diagnostic tests. Most coughs and colds are caused by viruses and do not require antibiotics.

What can I do?

1 If your child has a sudden attack of coughing, make sure she hasn't inhaled a small object such as a piece of candy or a button. If she has, try to remove it (see Choking, page 242), but don't put your fingers down her throat to pull it out.

2 If your child has a deep cough, do whatever you can to help her clear the mucus from her chest when she is coughing. Coughing can be distressing for a young child, so hold her on your lap to comfort her during an attack of coughing.

3 Hold a small bowl nearby and encourage her to spit out any mucus that she has coughed up. Productive coughing is nature's way of clearing airways that are clogged by mucus.

Keep your child's head *slightly tipped down*

4 For a dry cough, give a warm drink at bedtime. For a child over 18 months, dissolve a teaspoon of honey in a glass of warm water and add a few drops of fresh lemon juice.

5 Prop your child up with extra pillows in bed at night.

6 Keep her away from cigarette smoke.

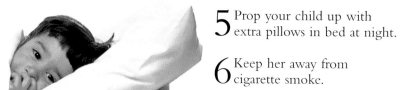

Extra pillows *will prevent mucus from dribbling down her throat at night.*

CALL THE DOCTOR

Call your doctor now if, over about half an hour, your child is breathing faster than usual, or if her breath is labored or very noisy. Call as soon as possible if:
★ your baby is under six months
★ your child cannot sleep
★ the cough is recurrent
★ it lasts more than three days.

BRONCHIOLITIS

What is it?

Bronchiolitis is a common viral illness that causes inflammation of the smallest airways in the lungs, called bronchioles. It occurs during the winter. Those most commonly affected are babies under a year old. The risk of a child getting bronchiolitis increases if his parents are smokers or if he lives in over-crowded accommodation in which viral infections spread more easily.

Your baby may have a runny nose for a day or two, and then suddenly seem much worse, with a fever, dry rasping cough, and rapid or difficult breathing. Mild bronchiolitis usually improves within about a week.

What can I do?

SYMPTOMS

* Runny nose
* fever
* dry, rasping cough
* rapid or difficult breathing
* wheezing
* feeding difficulties.

1 Give your baby plenty of drinks to make sure that he is getting enough fluids.

2 No drug will alter the course of the illness, but children's acetaminophen will help bring down his temperature.

3 Increase the humidity in your child's bedroom using a cool-mist vaporizer. This will help to relieve your child's breathing.

4 Monitor your baby's condition carefully. If you have any concerns about her breathing, do not hesitate to get medical advice.

What might the doctor do?

Antibiotics are not effective because this is a viral infection. In more severe cases your baby may be admitted to hospital where oxygen can be given and the baby can be fed through a tube inserted through the nose and into the stomach or, sometimes, intravenously. Most children are able to return home in 3–10 days, when they are able to feed normally.

The cough may persist for a few weeks longer. Though there are no lasting after-effects of the illness, for the next few years, many children who have had bronchiolitis tend to develop wheezing whenever they have a cold.

CALL THE DOCTOR

Call your doctor now if:
* your baby is breathing faster than usual or his breathing is labored or wheezy
* your baby is having difficulty feeding
* your baby has a blue tinge around the lips.

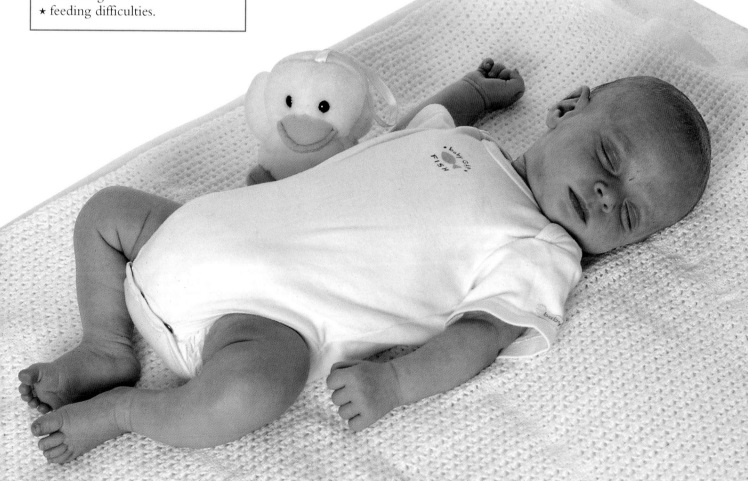

BRONCHITIS

What is it?

Bronchitis is an inflammation of the lining of the main air passages leading to the lungs. It is usually caused by a virus, and may follow a cold, the flu, or a sore throat because the infection has spread downward.

Your child probably won't feel particularly ill, but he may have difficulty sleeping if his cough tends to be worse at night.

SYMPTOMS

- ★ Rattly cough
- ★ slight wheeziness
- ★ slight temperature
- ★ runny nose.

What can I do?

1 Help relieve wheezy breathing and clear your child's lungs during a coughing fit. Sit him on your lap and rub his back. This is comforting as well as therapeutic.

2 Take your child's temperature. If it is raised, give him children's medication with acetaminophen, and plenty to drink.

3 When your child goes to bed, prop him up with extra pillows to prevent mucus from dribbling down his throat (see page 216).

4 Until your child is feeling better, do not allow him to become chilled or damp. Keep him indoors in a warm, but not too hot or stuffy, room.

CALL THE DOCTOR

Call for emergency help immediately if your child shows any of the emergency signs on page 215. Consult your doctor as soon as possible if you think your child has bronchitis, and call him again if he:
- ★ is not better after two days
- ★ coughs up greenish-yellow mucus
- ★ develops a high temperature.

What the doctor might do

Your doctor might prescribe a cough suppressant to help your child sleep and advise you how to humidify your child's bedroom.

ASTHMA

What is it?

Asthma is recurrent episodes of inflammation of the tiny airways leading to the lungs. Breathing, especially exhaling, is difficult. It may be caused by an allergy, but the majority of asthma sufferers do not have allergies. Mild asthma is common, and your child may outgrow it.

SYMPTOMS

- ★ Coughing, particularly at night or after exercise
- ★ slight wheeziness and breathlessness, especially during a cold
- ★ attacks of severe breathlessness, when breathing is shallow and difficult
- ★ feeling of suffocation during an asthma attack
- ★ pale, sweaty skin during an attack
- ★ blue tinge round the lips during a severe attack.

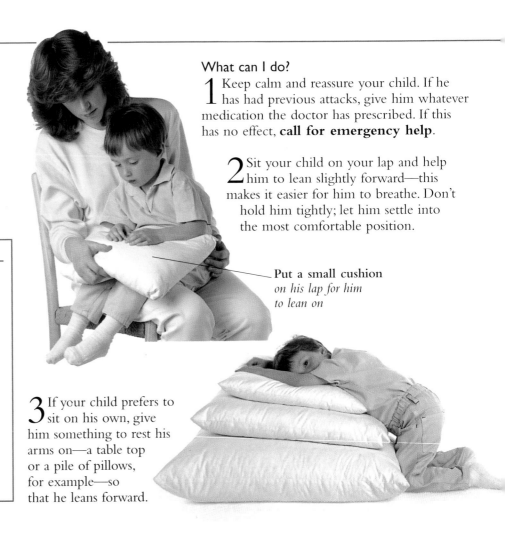

What can I do?

1 Keep calm and reassure your child. If he has had previous attacks, give him whatever medication the doctor has prescribed. If this has no effect, **call for emergency help**.

2 Sit your child on your lap and help him to lean slightly forward—this makes it easier for him to breathe. Don't hold him tightly; let him settle into the most comfortable position.

Put a small cushion *on his lap for him to lean on*

3 If your child prefers to sit on his own, give him something to rest his arms on—a table top or a pile of pillows, for example—so that he leans forward.

PNEUMONIA

What is it?
Pneumonia is an inflammation of the lungs, which causes breathing difficulty. In young children it is nearly always due to the spread of an infection such as a cold or the flu, and is usually caused by a virus, not bacteria. Occasionally pneumonia is the result of a tiny amount of food being inhaled into the lungs which causes a small patch of inflammation and infection to occur.

Pneumonia is a serious disease, but most healthy babies—even those under a year old—recover completely with treatment in about a week.

SYMPTOMS
★ Deterioration in a sick child
★ raised temperature
★ dry cough
★ rapid breathing
★ difficult or noisy breathing.

CALL THE DOCTOR
Call for emergency help immediately if your child develops any of the emergency signs on page 215. Call your doctor now if you think your child has pneumonia.

What can I do?
1 Prop your child up in bed with extra pillows. This will help him breathe more easily.

2 Take your child's temperature and, if it is raised, try to reduce it by giving him acetaminophen (see also page 194).

3 Make sure that your child has plenty to drink, especially if his temperature is raised. Offer your baby cool water.

What the doctor might do
The doctor will advise you on how to care for your child, and, if the infection is bacterial, he may prescribe an antibiotic. If your child is very ill, he might need to be treated in a hospital.

PREVENTING ASTHMA ATTACKS
Try to find out what triggers your child's asthma attacks by keeping a record of when they occur. Vigorous exercise and overexcitement can bring on an attack. Some other common triggers are shown here.

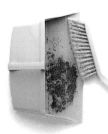

Dust
Reduce dust in your house by vacuuming and damp-mopping, rather than sweeping and dusting. Cover your child's mattress with a plastic sheet.

Animal fur
If you have a pet, let it stay somewhere else for a while, and note whether your child has fewer attacks.

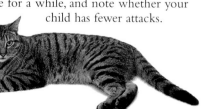

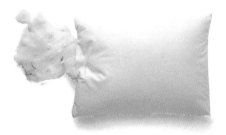

Feather-filled cushions or pillows
Change these for ones with synthetic filling.

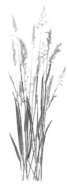

Pollen, especially from grass and trees
Discourage your child from playing in tall grass, and keep him inside when the pollen count is high.

Cigarette smoke
Don't let people smoke near your child or in your house.

EMERGENCY SIGNS
Call for emergency help immediately if your child:
★ has a bluish tinge on his tongue or around his lips
★ is severely breathless
★ does not start to breathe more easily 10 minutes after taking his medication
★ becomes abnormally drowsy.

CALL THE DOCTOR
Call your doctor now if this is your child's first asthma attack. Consult your doctor as soon as possible if you think your child may have asthma.

What the doctor might do
The doctor may prescribe drugs (inhalers) to relieve inflammation and to prevent the wheezing. During a severe attack, he may send your child to the hospital.

STOMACH PAIN

Stomach pain can be a symptom of many disorders, including gastroenteritis and urinary tract infections. It may also be caused by vomiting, and can accompany illnesses such as tonsillitis and measles. Your child may complain of a stomach ache if he feels generally unwell, knows he is about to be sick, or if he has a pain elsewhere but can't quite describe its location.

DEALING WITH A STOMACH ACHE

What causes stomach pain?

Many children have recurrent bouts of stomach pain when something makes them feel anxious or insecure. Provided that your child's pain is not severe and lasts for only an hour or two, you needn't worry; try to find out what is bothering him, and reassure him.

However, if your child is in severe pain for a few hours, you should take it seriously. He might have appendicitis, though this is extremely rare in children under three. Typically, appendicitis pain is felt around the navel for a few hours, then moves to the lower right part of the abdomen.

Waves of severe stomach pain at intervals of about 15 to 20 minutes in a baby or toddler may mean that his bowel has become blocked.

What can I do?

1 Take your child's temperature. If it is slightly raised, he may have appendicitis, especially if the stomach pain is severe or seems to be located around his navel. Don't give him a painkiller to ease it, or anything to reduce his temperature.

2 If you think your child may have appendicitis, don't give him anything to eat or drink. Otherwise, give him some water if he is thirsty, but don't let him eat anything.

3 Comfort your child by giving him hugs and extra attention.

4 If you don't suspect appendicitis, fill a hot water bottle with warm, not hot, water and wrap it in a towel. Let your child lie down with this held against his stomach.

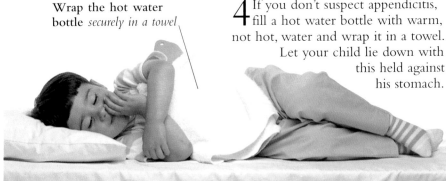

Wrap the hot water bottle *securely in a towel*

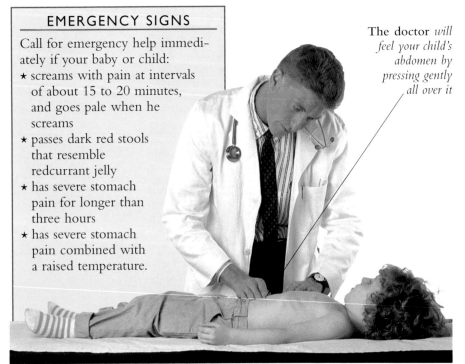

The doctor will feel your child's abdomen by pressing gently all over it

---

EMERGENCY SIGNS

Call for emergency help immediately if your baby or child:

★ screams with pain at intervals of about 15 to 20 minutes, and goes pale when he screams
★ passes dark red stools that resemble redcurrant jelly
★ has severe stomach pain for longer than three hours
★ has severe stomach pain combined with a raised temperature.

CALL THE DOCTOR

Call your doctor now if your child:

★ develops any other symptoms
★ has stomach pain for longer than three hours.

Consult your doctor if your child has frequent stomach pain.

What the doctor might do

The doctor will examine your child to try to find out the cause of his stomach pain. The treatment will depend on his diagnosis, but stomach pain often needs no treatment. If the doctor suspects appendicitis or a blocked bowel, he will arrange for your child to go to the hospital.

CONSTIPATION, VOMITING, AND DIARRHEA

A minor change in diet can cause temporary constipation or diarrhea. Vomiting or diarrhea may accompany almost any illness, and can also be caused by excitement or anxiety. Frequent vomiting or severe diarrhea can quickly make a baby or young child dehydrated. This is a serious condition and must be treated promptly (see page 222).

CONSTIPATION

What is it?
If your child has constipation, she passes stools less frequently than usual, and they are harder than normal. Children's bowel habits vary greatly: some children have a bowel movement twice a day, others go only once every two or three days. Whatever your child's regular pattern, it is quite normal—don't tamper with it. Babies often become slightly constipated when they learn to sit up or crawl, and before they can walk.

CALL THE DOCTOR

Consult your doctor as soon as possible if your child:
★ cries or complains of pain when moving her bowels
★ has streaks of blood in her stools or on her diaper or pants
★ has constipation for more than three to five days.

What can I do?
1 Don't worry if your child is temporarily constipated, it won't do her any harm. Don't give her a laxative, since this will upset the normal action of her bowels, and don't add sugar to her bottle.

2 Give your child plenty of fluids to drink, especially if the weather is hot—this will help to soften her stools. Fruit juice will help ease her constipation.

3 Don't hurry your child when she is sitting on the potty, but, on the other hand, don't let her remain there for too long.

4 Try to include more fiber in your child's diet (see below). This provides the bulk that helps the bowel to grip and move its contents along.

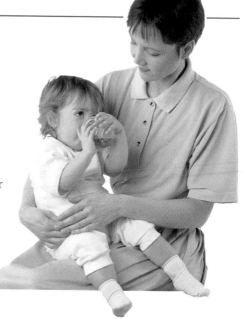

What the doctor might do
The doctor may prescribe a mild laxative and give you some advice on your child's diet. If your child has streaks of blood in her stool, she could have a small tear in the lining of her anus, so the doctor may suggest a lubricant.

GOOD SOURCES OF FIBER
Some examples of foods rich in fiber are shown here. Fresh foods are always best. Wash vegetables and fruit thoroughly, remove ends and stems, and peel for a child under one year. Purée the food for a baby under eight months (see pages 110–11).

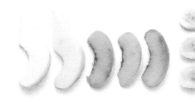

Fresh fruit Offer your child a variety of fruit such as slices of peeled pear, peach, and banana.

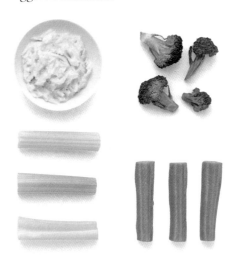

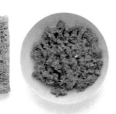

Wholegrain bread　**Wholegrain breakfast cereal**

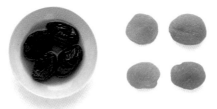

Dried fruit Prunes and apricots are ideal for young children.

Fresh vegetables Mashed potato and lightly cooked broccoli are high in fiber. Celery and carrots can be served raw.

VOMITING

What is it?
When your child vomits, she may throw up most of the contents of her stomach. Babies under about six months old often regurgitate a small amount of their feedings. This is perfectly normal, so don't worry.

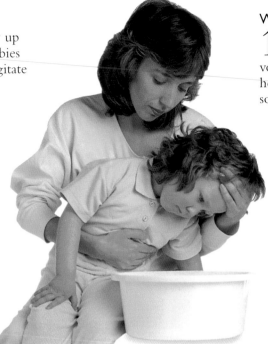

CALL THE DOCTOR

Call the doctor now if your child:
* vomits and seems abnormally drowsy
* throws up green-yellow vomit
* has vomited repeatedly for more than six hours
* shows any signs of dehydration.

What can I do?
1 Hold your child over a bowl and comfort her while she is vomiting (see page 199). Wipe her face afterward and give her some sips of water.

2 Make sure that your child has plenty to drink: she needs 1 to 1½ liters (2 to 3 pints) a day. Use an oral rehydration solution (ORS), available from your pharmacist. If your baby won't take a bottle, try using a teaspoon or a medicine dropper (see page 195) to feed it to her.

IDENTIFYING AND TREATING DEHYDRATION

Your child may be dehydrated if she shows one or more of these symptoms:
* dry mouth and lips
* dark, concentrated urine
* no urine passed for six hours
* sunken eyes
* sunken fontanelle
* abnormal drowsiness or lethargy.

To prevent dehydration, stop regular feedings (other than breast milk) as vomiting starts. Replace with an oral rehydration solution (ORS), found in most pharmacies. Offer a little fluid frequently (every 15 minutes). When vomiting stops, restart feedings in small, frequent amounts. For a baby less than six months, see page 185.

What the doctor might do
The doctor will examine your child to find out what is making her vomit, and will then treat her according to the diagnosis.

If she shows signs of dehydration, the doctor may prescribe an oral rehydration solution for her to drink. If she is very dehydrated, the doctor might arrange for her to be admitted to the hospital, where she can be given fluid intravenously.

GASTROENTERITIS

What is it?
Gastroenteritis is an inflammation in the stomach and intestines that can be caused by a virus infection. It is serious in babies, since it can dehydrate them quickly, but it is rare in breast-fed babies. A mild attack in a child over two is not serious.

SYMPTOMS

* Vomiting and nausea
* diarrhea
* stomach cramps
* loss of appetite
* fever.

What can I do?
1 Make sure that your child drinks plenty of fluids. Follow the instructions in "Treatment of diarrhea" box on page 223.

2 Don't give your child anything to eat until he stops vomiting, then introduce bland foods.

3 If your child has a fever, give him children's medication containing acetaminophen to reduce it.

4 Put a diaper on your child again if he has recently outgrown them.

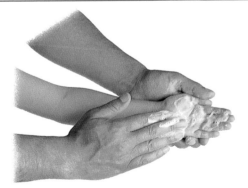

5 Make sure that your child washes his hands after going to the bathroom and before eating. Wash your own hands after changing his diaper and before preparing food.

DIARRHEA

What is it?

If your child has diarrhea, her bowel movements will be watery and more frequent. This has many causes. The most common is viral infection, occasionally contaminated food, and sometimes eating oily or spicy food.

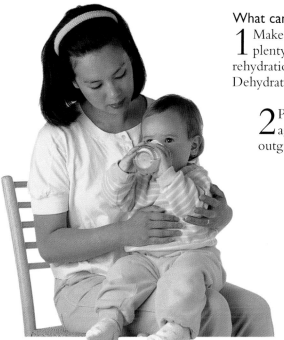

What can I do?

1 Make sure that your child has plenty to drink. An oral rehydration solution (ORS—see Dehydration, page 222) is ideal.

2 Put your child in a diaper again if she has just outgrown them.

3 Pay careful attention to hygiene: wash your hands after changing your baby's diaper and before preparing her food, and make sure that your child always washes her hands after using the toilet and before eating.

CALL THE DOCTOR

Call your doctor now if your child:

★ has had diarrhea for more than six hours

★ has blood in her stool

★ shows any signs of dehydration (see page 222).

TREATMENT OF DIARRHEA

Replace all food and drink (other than breast milk) with an oral rehydration solution (ORS), available from your pharmacist. For a child six to 24 months of age, give 90 to 125ml (3 to 4oz) every hour; if over two years old, give 125 to 250ml (4 to 8oz) every hour. For a baby under six months of age, see page 185. Continue this treatment for the first six hours, then less often over the next 12 hours. When the diarrhea is less frequent, return to the usual formula or whole milk and food, in small, frequent feedings. Do not give your child fruit juices or sugar solutions until the diarrhea stops.

What the doctor might do

The doctor will examine your child to find out the cause of her diarrhea, and will treat her according to the diagnosis. If your child has become dehydrated, the doctor may prescribe an oral rehydration solution for her to drink. If she is very dehydrated, he might arrange for her to be admitted to the hospital, where she can be given the extra liquid she needs intravenously.

CALL THE DOCTOR

Call your doctor now if your child:

★ is under two and may have gastroenteritis

★ is over two and has had symptoms of gastroenteritis for more than two days.

What the doctor might do

The doctor will probably treat your child for dehydration and may advise you to give him only liquids for a few days. He may ask for a sample of your child's stool.

Q&A "What steps can I take to prevent gastroenteritis?"

Clean all your baby's feeding equipment thoroughly for as long as he drinks formula or milk from a bottle (see pages 100–101). Put prepared bottles in the refrigerator —never store them warm in an insulated container, since bacteria thrive in warm conditions.

Pay careful attention to hygiene when preparing food. If you store any cooked food, don't keep it in the refrigerator for longer than two days, and make sure it is thoroughly heated when you serve it, because heat kills the bacteria that could cause gastroenteritis.

Wash dishes and glasses in very hot water. Dry them on paper towels, not a dish towel.

If you are traveling with a baby or a small child in a foreign country, ask your doctor about any precautions you should take, particularly with water, fruit, and salads.

BLADDER, KIDNEY, AND GENITAL PROBLEMS

Most urinary tract infections are caused by bacteria entering the urethra (see diagram below) and spreading up into the bladder. They are reasonably common in young children, and are usually not serious.

Minor abnormalities of the urinary tract make some children prone to such infections. Minor infections of the genitals are also quite common, and are often part of the symptoms of diaper rash (see page 182).

The urinary system
Your child has two kidneys that filter his blood. The clean blood returns to his bloodstream, while the waste product (the urine) drains into his bladder, where it collects until he is ready to urinate.

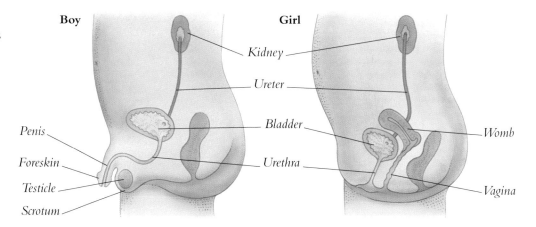

Boy — Penis, Foreskin, Testicle, Scrotum
Girl — Kidney, Ureter, Bladder, Urethra, Womb, Vagina

URINARY TRACT INFECTIONS

What are they?
Any part of the urinary tract—the kidneys, the bladder, and the connecting tubes—can become infected with bacteria. Infections are more common in girls, because the tube from the bladder (the urethra) is shorter in a girl than in a boy, and its opening is nearer to the anus, so germs can spread to it more easily.

What can I do?
1 If your child seems sick, check to see whether her urine looks pink or cloudy. Note whether she is urinating more frequently than usual and whether it seems to hurt when she goes to the bathroom. If your child is in diapers, you won't be able to tell if urination is frequent or painful, but you may notice a change in odor.

2 Make sure that your child has plenty to drink, to keep her kidneys flushed.

3 If your child has a fever, give her a dose of acetaminophen to reduce it.

SYMPTOMS
* Urinating more often than usual
* pain when urinating
* pink, red, or cloudy urine
* change in odor of the urine
* fever
* listlessness
* loss of appetite
* abdominal pain.

CALL THE DOCTOR
Consult your doctor as soon as possible if you think your child has a urinary tract infection.

What the doctor might do
The doctor will examine your child and may ask you to take a sample of her urine (ask your doctor how you should collect this). He may prescribe an antibiotic. Sometimes, special tests are needed to study the urinary tract.

GENITAL PROBLEMS IN GIRLS

What can go wrong?
A little girl's vagina can become sore due to diaper rash (see page 182), an infection such as thrush (see page 213), or pinworms (see page 232). If your daughter has a blood-stained or smelly discharge from her vagina, she may have pushed something into it. Newborn girls often produce a white or blood-stained discharge for a few days, and this is nothing to worry about. After this age until just before puberty, a discharge is abnormal.

What can I do?
1 If your daughter's bottom is sore or red, don't use soap when you wash it—just use water, and dry it thoroughly. Always wipe from the front to back, so that germs can't spread forward from her anus.

2 Don't put rubber pants over your daughter's diapers, since they prevent air from circulating to her bottom. Dress an older child in 100 percent pure cotton underpants.

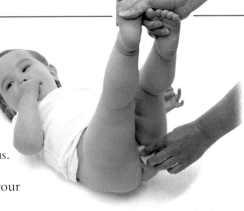

3 If your daughter has a discharge from her vagina, make sure that she hasn't pushed something into it. If she has, **consult your doctor as soon as possible**.

What the doctor might do
The doctor will examine your daughter and may take a sample of the discharge. If she has something lodged in her vagina, he will remove it gently. If she has an infection, he may prescribe antibiotics to be taken by mouth, or a cream to be applied to the affected area, depending on the cause of her symptoms.

SYMPTOMS
* ★ Soreness or itching in or around the vagina
* ★ redness around the vagina
* ★ discharge from the vagina.

CALL THE DOCTOR
Consult your doctor as soon as possible if your daughter:
* ★ has a discharge from her vagina
* ★ still has symptoms after two days of home treatment
* ★ has pushed something into her vagina.

GENITAL PROBLEMS IN BOYS

What can go wrong?
In an uncircumcized boy, the foreskin, which covers the tip of the penis, can become inflamed or infected (balanitis), often as part of diaper rash (see page 182).

If a swelling develops in your son's groin or scrotum, he may have a hernia (intestines bulging through a weak area in the abdomen).

What can I do?
If your son's foreskin is inflamed, wash it without using soap and dry it thoroughly at each diaper change, or at least once a day. Change to a mild laundry soap and rinse his diapers or underpants thoroughly.

How can I prevent inflammation?
Don't try to pull your son's foreskin back—it may not retract until he is three or four. If you force it, you may make his foreskin inflamed.

SYMPTOMS
Inflamed foreskin
* ★ Red, swollen foreskin
* ★ discharge of pus from the penis.

Hernia
* ★ Soft, painless bulge in the groin or scrotum, which may disappear when your child lies down and get bigger when he coughs, sneezes, or cries.

What the doctor might do
If your son's foreskin is inflamed, the doctor may prescribe an antibiotic cream. If he has a hernia, your doctor will recommend surgery to repair the hernia in his groin or scrotum.

CALL THE DOCTOR
Consult your doctor as soon as possible if:
* ★ your son's foreskin looks red or swollen, or if there is any discharge
* ★ your son's hernia becomes painful, or changes in any other way.

Consult your doctor if you think your son may have a hernia.

CIRCUMCISION
This is a surgical procedure to remove the foreskin. If you want your son circumcized, discuss it with your doctor. Once routine for newborn boys, it is now done only for religious or specific medical reasons.

SKIN PROBLEMS

Minor skin problems are common in childhood. Most clear up quickly, but some are very contagious, and must be treated promptly.

If your child has a rash combined with other signs of illness, he may have an infectious illness (see pages 203–8). For other problems, see below.

QUICK DIAGNOSIS GUIDE
One or more red spots, or a rash, see Spots and boils, Hives, Heat rash (below and opposite), Insect stings (page 252) or, if dry and scaly, see Eczema (page 228).
Raw, cracked areas, usually on or around the lips, or on the cheeks and hands, see Chapped skin (page 229).
Small blisters or crusty patches on or around the mouth, see Cold sores and Impetigo (pages 230–31).
Hard lump of skin, usually on the hands or feet, see Warts (page 230).
Itchy head, see Lice and nits (page 232).
Intense itching around the anus, see Pinworms (page 232).

DEALING WITH ITCHING
Many skin problems cause itching, and since scratching can make the skin infected, it is important to relieve your child's itchiness.
★ Dress him in cotton clothes, since cotton is less irritating to the skin than wool or other fabrics.
★ Gently dab the area with cotton balls soaked in calamine lotion, to soothe inflamed or irritated skin.
★ Dissolve a handful of baking soda in your child's bathwater.
★ Put socks on his hands when he is in bed.

SPOTS AND BOILS

What are they?
A spot is a small red swelling (pimple), usually on the face. A boil is an infection in the skin that causes a large, painful lump, which then festers to produce a head of pus in the middle. Boils are most likely to occur on the face or on pressure points such as the buttocks, but they can appear anywhere on the body.

Don't worry if your child gets occasional spots, but recurrent boils may be a sign of illness.

SYMPTOMS

Spot
★ Small, red, painless lump.

Boil
★ Painful, red lump that gradually gets larger
★ white or yellow center of pus appearing after a day or two.

CALL THE DOCTOR
Consult your doctor as soon as possible if:
★ your child has a spot that looks inflamed
★ your child has a boil in an awkward or painful place
★ the center of pus does not appear three days after the boil first developed
★ red streaks spread out from the boil.
Consult your doctor if your child often gets boils.

What can I do?
1 If your child gets occasional spots, simply ignore them. They will clear up in a few days without treatment. If she tends to drool, and the spots appear around her mouth, smear a barrier cream over the area.

2 If your child has a boil, or a spot that looks inflamed, gently clean it, and the skin around it, with a cotton ball dipped in antiseptic.

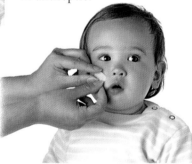

3 Cover it with an adhesive bandage. If it is rubbed by clothing, or is in a painful place such as on the buttocks, pad it with a gauze pad and then put adhesive bandage over it.

4 The boil will come to a head and burst of its own accord in a few days. Don't squeeze it—this may spread the infection. After it has burst, clean it gently with a cotton ball dipped in antiseptic, and keep it covered with a bandage until it has healed.

What might the doctor do?
The doctor may lance the boil and drain away the pus, to reduce the pain and swelling, and might prescribe a cream. If your child has a lot of boils, or if they keep recurring, the doctor may prescribe a course of antibiotics.

HIVES

What is it?
Hives (also known as urticaria) is an intensely itchy rash of red patches. The patches usually fade after a few hours, but new ones may appear. It can be caused by strong sunshine or by an allergy to certain foods (for example, milk or a citrus fruit) or drugs (for instance, penicillin).

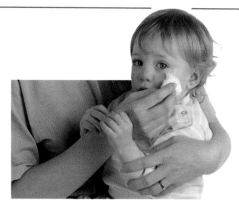

SYMPTOMS

* Itchy rash of raised red patches (welts), sometimes with a pale center
* welts varying in length from 1mm to 1cm (¹⁄₁₆ to ½in)
* larger welts joining together.

What can I do?
1 Dab your child's rash with cotton balls dipped in calamine lotion.

2 If the rash is caused by an allergy, try to find out what your child is allergic to, so that you can help her avoid it in future. The rash usually develops a few hours after contact with an allergen, so try to remember whether, for example, she has recently eaten a new food.

CALL THE DOCTOR
Call your doctor now if your child's face or neck is swollen, or if she is wheezing.
Consult your doctor as soon as possible if:
★ the rash does not disappear within four hours
★ your child has frequent attacks of hives.

What the doctor might do
The doctor may prescribe an antihistamine medication. He might also carry out tests to discover the cause of your child's allergy. If your child's face, tongue, or throat is swollen, she might need an injection to reduce the swelling.

HEAT RASH

What is it?
Heat rash is a faint rash caused by overheating. It is more common in babies than in children, and usually appears on the face or in skin creases, where sweat can gather. It is not a serious disorder, and you can treat it yourself at home.

SYMPTOMS
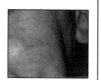

* Pink rash on the face or in skin creases.

CALL THE DOCTOR
Consult your doctor as soon as possible if the rash has not faded 12 hours after your child cools down.

What can I do?
1 Take off any heavy bedding and remove a layer of your baby's clothing. Let him sleep dressed in just an undershirt and diaper.

2 Give him a bath in luke-warm water. Pat his skin dry gently, leaving it slightly damp so that he cools down as his skin dries. When he is dry, apply a little baby powder to absorb new sweat.

3 Take your baby's temperature and, if it is raised, give him the recommended dose of acetaminophen.

How can I prevent heat rash?
Dress your baby in light clothes when the weather is hot, with cotton next to his skin, rather than wool or a manmade fiber. Make sure he is well protected from the sun.

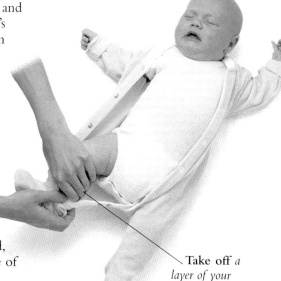

Take off *a layer of your baby's clothing*

What the doctor might do
The doctor will check that the rash is just a heat rash. If it is, your baby needs no medical treatment. If the rash has another cause, the doctor will treat that.

ECZEMA

What is it?

Eczema is an allergy or irritation resulting in areas of itchy, red, scaly skin. It most commonly affects the face and skin creases such as the inside of the elbows and the back of the knees, but it can be more widespread.

It usually first appears between the ages of three months and two years, then improves as the child grows older. About half of all children with eczema grow out of it by the age of six, and nearly all of them grow out of it by puberty. Your child is more likely to develop eczema if other people in the family suffer from conditions such as eczema, asthma, and hay fever.

SYMPTOMS

* Itchy, red, scaly, dry patches, usually on the face or in skin creases
* clear fluid oozing from the affected areas.

What can I do?

1 When you give your child a bath, clean the affected areas by wiping them with baby oil. Avoid soaps. Rinse the oil off with plenty of water.

Use cotton balls *to apply the baby oil*

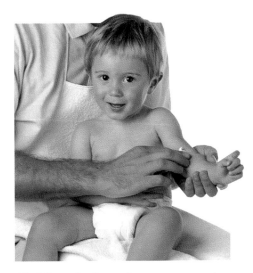

2 After a bath, apply an unscented moisturizing cream to your child's skin, since it may be very dry.

3 Dress your child in cotton, rather than wool. In cold weather, put cotton clothing under warmer layers.

4 Try to stop your child from scratching the affected areas— put cotton socks on his hands at night and keep his fingernails short.

5 Try to discover a possible cause of allergy. Common allergens include foods (especially dairy products and wheat), animal fur, woolen clothes, and laundry detergents. Anxiety can also trigger eczema.

6 When your child's eczema is bad, keep him from anyone with chicken pox or cold sores because of a greater infection risk.

CALL THE DOCTOR

Consult your doctor as soon as possible if:
* your child's eczema is very widespread or very itchy
* fluid is oozing from the eczema.

Consult your doctor if you think your child has eczema.

What the doctor might do

The doctor may prescribe a cream, and if the area is infected, an antibiotic. Most importantly, he'll try to determine a possible allergen and advise you on how to eliminate it from your child's daily environment, if at all possible.

SUNBURN

What is it?
Sunburn is sore or reddened skin caused by exposure to the sun. Babies and young children have very sensitive skin, so they are particularly vulnerable to it. Too much exposure to the sun can cause skin cancer later in life.

SYMPTOMS

* Red, sore areas of skin
* blisters appearing on badly affected areas
* flaking or peeling skin a day or two later.

What can I do?
1 Take your child inside or into the shade as soon as her skin begins to look red. Bear in mind that the worst symptoms of sunburn are likely to be delayed for a few hours.

2 Cool any reddened areas with cold water, then apply a soothing lotion or dab on some calamine lotion. Avoid lotions with topical anesthetics.

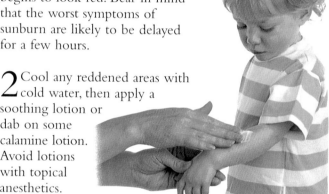

PREVENTING SUNBURN
Until your child is one, always keep her covered up when she is in the sun. Try to minimize the amount of time an older child spends playing in the sun. Apply a sunscreen or block with a sun-protection factor of at least 15 every few hours. Dress her in a T-shirt and a sun hat. Keep the T-shirt on her when she is swimming or near water. Remember a child can still get sunburn, even through a shirt!

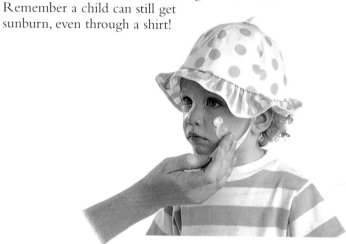

CALL THE DOCTOR

Consult your doctor as soon as possible if:
* your child has a fever and seems sick
* blisters appear over a large area.

What the doctor might do
The doctor may prescribe a soothing and healing cream.

CHAPPED SKIN

What is it?
Chaps are small cracks in the skin that occur when the skin becomes dry after being exposed to cold or hot, dry air. Chapping is not serious, but it can be painful.

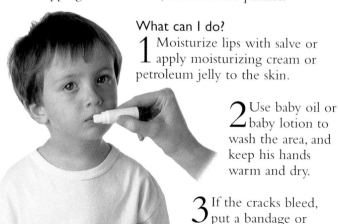

What can I do?
1 Moisturize lips with salve or apply moisturizing cream or petroleum jelly to the skin.

2 Use baby oil or baby lotion to wash the area, and keep his hands warm and dry.

3 If the cracks bleed, put a bandage or gauze pad over them.

SYMPTOMS

* Tiny cracks in the skin, usually on or around the lips or on the cheeks or hands
* bleeding if the cracks are deep.

CALL THE DOCTOR

Consult your doctor as soon as possible if:
* the cracks do not heal after three days
* the cracks become red, sore, or pus-filled.

What the doctor might do
If the area is infected, the doctor may prescribe an antibiotic. Otherwise, just protect it from further irritants.

COLD SORES

What are they?

Cold sores are small blisters, usually on or around the lips but they sometimes develop inside the mouth or elsewhere on the face.

They are caused by a virus which, once it has infected a child, lies dormant in the skin and tends to flare up occasionally, so if your child has had a cold sore, he is liable to get others in the future. Strong sunlight can trigger a recurrence, and so can a minor illness, such as a cold (which is why they are called cold sores).

SYMPTOMS
★ Raised, red area that tingles or itches, usually around the mouth
★ small, painful yellow blisters forming about a day later
★ blisters crusting over after a day or two
★ fever and general illness during the first attack.

What can I do?

1 At the first sign of a cold sore, hold an ice cube wrapped in cloth against the affected area for 10 minutes. This may prevent the blister from developing.

2 Keep his hands clean, and stop him from touching the sore, which could spread infection.

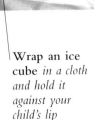

3 Since cold sores are very contagious, don't let your child kiss other people, and if he tends to put toys into his mouth, don't let him share them with other children until the sore has gone.

Wrap an ice cube *in a cloth and hold it against your child's lip*

4 If your child has ever had a cold sore, protect his lips from strong sunlight with a sunscreen, because sunlight can trigger a recurrence.

CALL THE DOCTOR
Consult your doctor as soon as possible if:
★ your child has a cold sore for the first time
★ your child's cold sore starts to ooze or spread
★ your child has a cold sore near his eyes.

What the doctor might do

The doctor may prescribe a cream to be spread over the affected area several times a day, in which case the treatment will help the blister to heal.

WARTS

What are they?

A wart is a lump of hard, dry skin; a plantar wart (verruca) is a wart on the sole of the foot. Warts are caused by a virus that invades the skin, and most children get them occasionally.

Warts are not painful, and disappear spontaneously, usually after a few months, so treatment is not necessary. Plantar warts are painful because of the pressure put on them whenever your child walks or wears shoes, so they should be treated promptly.

SYMPTOMS
Wart
★ Hard lump of dry skin.
Plantar wart (verruca)
★ Hard, painful area on the sole of the foot, perhaps with a tiny black center.

What can I do?

1 If your child has a wart, simply ignore it, unless it is on his genitals or near his anus; in that case call your doctor. It will disappear on its own after a few months, although some last for a year or more.

IMPETIGO

What is it?

Impetigo is a bacterial skin infection that may develop when a rash such as eczema, or a cold sore becomes infected, although healthy skin can sometimes become infected with impetigo. It usually affects the skin around the mouth and nose, but it can occur anywhere on the body. Impetigo isn't a serious disorder in children, but in a young baby it can spread over a large area and make him seriously ill. It is very contagious, so it is important to have it treated promptly.

SYMPTOMS

- ★ Rash of small red spots
- ★ blisters forming over the spots
- ★ the spots burst, then form large brownish-yellow scabs
- ★ fever and general malaise in a young baby.

What can I do?

1 Keep your child's washcloth and towel separate from those of the rest of the family, and wash them frequently, so the infection doesn't spread.

2 Try to keep your child from touching the affected area—don't let him suck his thumb or pick his nose, because this could spread the infection.

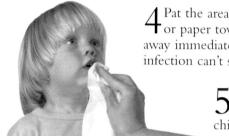

3 Gently remove the scabs each day by wiping them with warm, soapy cotton balls. Don't rub hard, but persevere until they loosen.

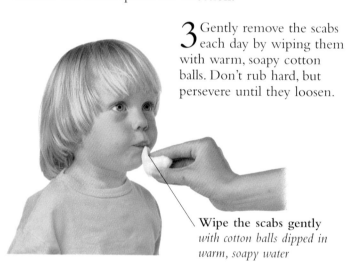

Wipe the scabs gently *with cotton balls dipped in warm, soapy water*

4 Pat the area dry with a tissue or paper towel and throw it away immediately, so that the infection can't spread.

5 Keep your child away from other children, especially young babies, until he is better.

CALL THE DOCTOR

Call your doctor now if your baby is under three months old and suddenly develops widespread impetigo. Consult your doctor as soon as possible if you think your child has impetigo.

What the doctor might do

The doctor may prescribe a cream and tell you to wipe the scabs away (see left) before applying it. If the infection is widespread, he may prescribe an antibiotic.

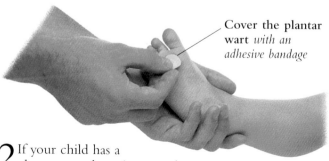

Cover the plantar wart *with an adhesive bandage*

2 If your child has a plantar wart, keep it covered with an adhesive bandage and don't let him go barefoot until it has cleared up. It may disappear spontaneously. Keep his towel and washcloth separate.

CALL THE DOCTOR

Consult your doctor if:
- ★ your child's warts multiply
- ★ your child has a wart on his genitals or anus
- ★ your child has a plantar wart, or verruca.

What the doctor might do

Your doctor may prescribe a lotion to be applied regularly to the wart until it gradually disappears. Alternatively, he may refer your child to a dermatologist.

HEAD LICE

What are they?
Head lice are tiny insects that infest the hair, and make the child's head itchy. Their minute white eggs (nits) cling to his hair roots. Head lice spread very easily from one head to another, so treat the whole family if your child picks up lice. Tell your friends to check their children's heads, and tell the staff at your child's toddler group or day care, or nursery school. Keep him at home until he is treated.

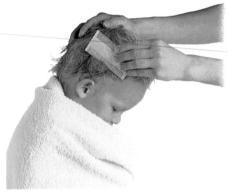

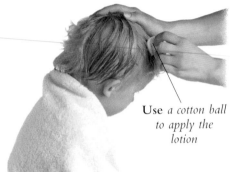

Use a cotton ball to apply the lotion

SYMPTOMS

★ Itchy head
★ tiny white grains firmly attached to the hairs near the roots
★ red bite marks under the hair.

What can I do?
1 Ask your pharmacist for a lotion or shampoo to kill the lice and nits. Also buy a special fine comb to remove the dead lice and nits after treatment.

2 Apply lotion or shampoo all over your child's head, and leave it on his hair for as long as the insructions specify. Wash and rinse his hair, then comb it thoroughly with the special comb.

3 Seal your child's hats, brush, and comb in a plastic bag and leave for at least ten days—the nits will die.

4 As an alternative to wet-combing, ask your healthcare provider to suggest a lotion you can use that will kill the lice and nits. You can then comb them off. If you use this method follow the instructions carefully. You can also use the lotion to clean your child's brush and comb.

PINWORMS

What are they?
Pinworms are tiny, white threadlike worms, about 1cm (½in) long. They can enter the body in contaminated food, and then live in the bowels, coming out at night to lay eggs around the anus, and causing intense itchiness. They are common in children, and are harmless, although the itching may be extremely uncomfortable. In little girls, the worms may crawl forward to the vagina.

SYMPTOMS

★ Intense itching around the anus, which is usually worse at night
★ intense itching around the vagina
★ tiny white worms in the stool or around the anus.

What can I do?
1 Try to prevent your child from scratching, since she might inflame the skin around her anus or vagina.

2 Keep her fingernails short so that if she scratches, she doesn't pick up any eggs under her nails, which could reinfect her or other people.

3 Make sure that the whole family washes their hands thoroughly after going to the lavatory and before eating. Use a nail brush to clean the nails properly.

CALL THE DOCTOR

Consult your doctor as soon as possible if you think your child has pinworms.

4 If your child no longer wears diapers, make sure she wears pajamas, or cotton underpants under a nightgown. Change her underpants and pajama pants every day and sterilize them in boiling water to kill any worms or eggs on them. Change her bedlinen every day and wash and rinse it thoroughly in very hot water.

5 When she feels itchy, lay her across your lap and look for tiny white worms near her anus. Remove any you see with a wad of damp toilet paper and flush them away.

What might the doctor do?
The doctor will probably prescribe a medicine for the whole family, which will kill the worms. He may also prescribe a cream for your child to soothe any inflammation around the anus or vagina.

EPILEPSY

Epilepsy, which causes recurrent seizures, affects many people, including children. A seizure is caused by excessive electrical discharges by brain cells. The most common cause of seizures in children is a high fever (see page 194). This is not considered to be a form of epilepsy. A single seizure does not mean your child has epilepsy.

EPILEPSY

What is it?
Epilepsy is a tendency to have seizures (also called fits or convulsions), which are bursts of abnormal electrical activity in the brain. With treatment, most children grow out of it by adolescence. There are several different types of epilepsy; two common forms in childhood are absence seizures and tonic-clonic seizures (see symptoms box).

What can I do?
1 Put your child on her side on the floor during a seizure. Stay with her to make sure she doesn't injure herself, but don't try to restrain her.

2 After a major seizure, put your child into the recovery position (see page 241). Don't wake her if she falls asleep, but make sure that she is breathing properly (see page 238).

3 Try to avoid letting your child get into situations that could be dangerous if she has a seizure—for example, put a guard at the top of the stairs, and don't leave her alone in the bath. But don't be overprotective—she shouldn't feel that her epilepsy makes her abnormal.

What might the doctor do?
The doctor may send your child to hospital for tests. He may also prescribe a drug to help control the seizures; if so, tell the doctor if your child's behavior changes in any way, but don't stop giving her the drug.

As you roll *the child over, keep her hand held against her cheek*

The recovery position
If your child has a seizure, place her in the recovery position and ensure that she is breathing properly. Leave her in this position until she regains consciousness. If she falls asleep, let her wake naturally.

SYMPTOMS

Absence seizures (petit mal seizures)
★ Sudden lack of movement
★ dazed expression
★ complete recovery in a few seconds.

Tonic-clonic seizures (grand mal seizures)
★ Sudden unconsciousness, so that your child falls down
★ stiff arms and legs
★ twitching or jerky movements
★ urination
★ sleeping, or gradual return to consciousness, when the twitching movements stop.

CALL THE DOCTOR

Call your doctor now if your child has:
★ a tonic-clonic seizure for the first time
★ a tonic-clonic seizure lasting more than three minutes
★ a series of seizures in rapid succession.
Consult your doctor if you think your child has absence seizures.

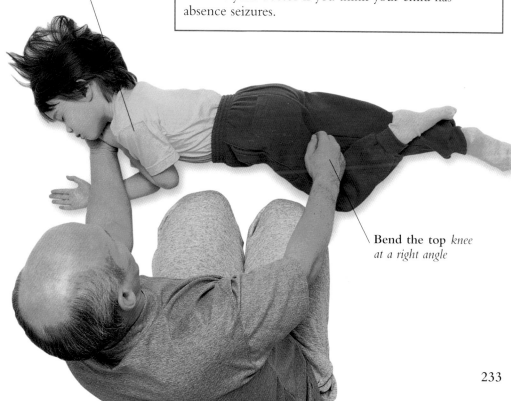

Bend the top *knee at a right angle*

YOUR CHILD'S SAFETY

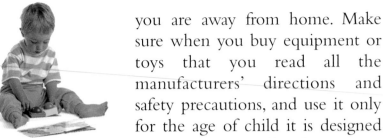

About a quarter of all the injuries that happen in the home involve children under four, but there are a number of ways you can make your home safer. Best of all, keep your child under your own watchful eye. The chances of an injury happening are greatest when your child is tired, hungry, or unwell, or when you are busy or worried. The risks are also high when you are away from home. Make sure when you buy equipment or toys that you read all the manufacturers' directions and safety precautions, and use it only for the age of child it is designed for. Buy new if possible. Secondhand items may not comply with safety regulations or may have been damaged or worn beyond safe limits, and instructions about their use may be missing.

SAFETY IN YOUR HOME

All children are injury prone, because their desire to explore and experiment far outstrips their common sense and forethought. Many injuries can easily be prevented, and it is your responsibility to make sure that your child can't injure himself. However, keeping him safe should not mean restricting his activities, but simply making sure that his world is safe for him to play in and explore.

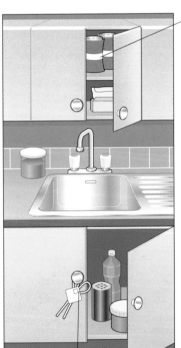

Store *plastic bags and plastic wrap out of your child's reach*

Buy *coiled electrical cords or make sure cords are short*

Push *hot drinks to the back of kitchen surfaces*

Keep sharp *utensils such as kitchen knives in a drawer with a child-resistant catch*

Fit a guard *round your stove and turn your saucepan handles away from the front. Use the back burners rather than the front ones*

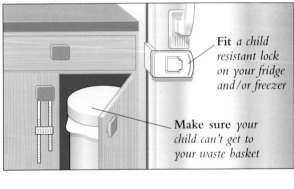

Fit *a child resistant lock on your fridge and/or freezer*

Make sure *your child can't get to your waste basket*

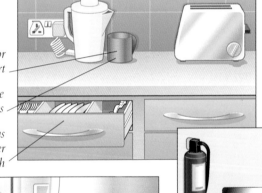

Keep *a child-resistant catch on all your kitchen cupboards*

KITCHEN
Your kitchen is full of potential hazards for a child and these dangers are increased if you are busy. Keep him away from the cooking area when you are cooking—an infant seat or a playpen is ideal. Don't forget that stove burners, kettles, and irons stay hot long after you have switched them off. At mealtimes, keep hot food near the center of the table, so that your child can't grab it. Don't use a tablecloth, since he could pull it and spill hot things over himself.

Don't let *your child touch the oven door while it is hot*

KEEPING YOUR BABY SAFE

With each new skill he develops, your baby will find ways of running into danger, so you must think ahead to avoid hazards. He will learn to roll over when he is very young, so if you need to lay him down for even a moment, put him on the floor. He will soon grab things so make sure that anything he can reach is safe to handle and too large to swallow or choke on. Don't eat or drink, or carry anything hot while you are holding your baby. Never leave him alone with a bottle—he could choke. Always use safety straps on his carriage and highchair. Don't put him in an infant seat on a high surface—it could easily fall off. Don't leave a young child alone with your baby: he might pick him up and drop him, or give him dangerous objects to play with.

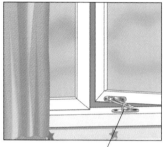

Fix *locks on the windows, so that they can be opened only a little way. Open sash windows from the top*

BEDROOM

Your child will spend a lot of time in his bedroom. Don't put a pillow in his crib until he is at least two, and don't use loose plastic sheeting as a waterproof mattress cover. Never attach his toys to the crib with cords—they might wind round his neck. Keep large toys and bumper pads out of the crib—your child could use them as stepping stones to climb out—and don't string toys across the crib once he can sit up. His toys should be non-toxic and non-flammable, and must have no sharp edges or pieces small enough to swallow. Choose furniture carefully and never place it under a window—your child may climb up on it.

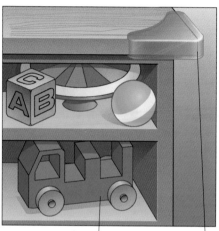

Store *toys in a low cupboard or shelf, so your child can reach them without climbing*

Make *sure that your furniture is sturdy and has rounded edges.*

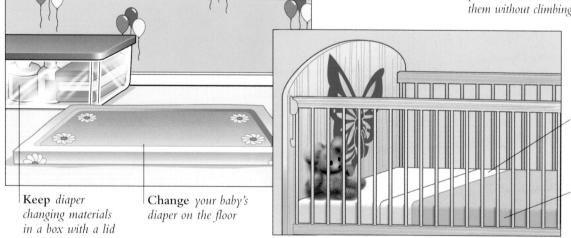

Keep *diaper changing materials in a box with a lid*

Change *your baby's diaper on the floor*

Use flame-resistant *bedding and sleepwear*

Set *the crib mattress to its lowest position before your baby can pull himself to standing*

BATHROOM

Never leave a child under four alone in the bath, or in the bathroom if the bathtub is full, even for a few seconds. Use a non-slip bath mat. Set your water heater lower than 55°C (130°F), and run the cold water into your child's bath first. Test the temperature before putting your child in. Other injuries that may occur in the bathroom can easily be prevented:
★ Keep all medicines out of your child's reach in a cabinet with a lock or a child-resistant catch.
★ Put razors and cosmetics out of your child's reach.
★ Keep cleaning chemicals out of sight and out of reach.
★ A portable electric heater should be not be used anywhere that your baby might reach it.
★ Keep the toilet brush in a cupboard with a child-resistant catch.
★ If you have a shower with a glass screen, you should replace the screen with a curtain or install safety glass instead.

IN THE YARD

Keep an eye on your child when he is playing in the yard, and if you put your baby to sleep outside, have a mosquito net handy to slip over the carriage. Never let your child play in or near a wading pool without an adult supervising him, and empty the pool after use. If you are near a stream or a pond, fence your yard securely. Keep all your walks in good condition—remove weeds regularly so that they don't become slippery in wet weather, and repair walks if they are uneven.

Lock away *all your gardening tools and equipment, weed-killer, fertilizer, and pesticide*

Keep *a garden pond covered with wire netting or surround it with a sturdy fence. Your child could drown in just a few centimeters of water*

Make sure *that the sand in your child's sandbox is too shallow for him to bury himself and teach him not to throw sand. Cover the sandbox when he is not playing in it*

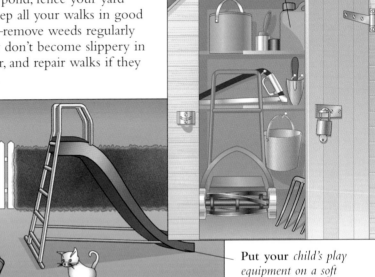

Put your *child's play equipment on a soft surface, preferably sand or woodchips*

LIVING ROOM

When you buy upholstered furniture, ask the salesperson about the fabric content. You don't want it to give off any toxic fumes if you have a fire. Always use a fireplace screen. Don't let your child touch the back of your television.

Don't leave cigarettes, matches, alcohol, sewing equipment, or coins lying around. Keep indoor plants out of his reach, since some are poisonous.

If you have low glass panels in doors or windows, use toughened, laminated, or wire-net glass, apply a transparent safety film, or put colored stickers on them, so that your child can see where the glass is. Avoid glass-topped tables.

HALL AND STAIRS

Put safety gates at the top and bottom of the stairs before your child can crawl or climb. Make sure that

ELECTRICITY

Electric shocks from any power source can be very serious, so minimize the chances of your child receiving a shock:
★ Turn off electrical appliances when you are not using them.
★ Cover unused sockets with childproof socket covers, or mask them with heavy insulating tape.
★ Check electrical cords regularly, and repair any with exposed wires.
★ Don't let your child play with electrically powered toys until he is at least four.

the hall, stairs, and landings are well lit, and that your banisters aren't too wide apart. Don't leave toys, piles of laundry, or anything else on steps.

Make sure that the door knobs and locks are out of his reach or not easily opened. Install smoke detectors.

Repair loose tiles or tears in rugs or flooring, and put a nonslip backing on any rugs. On polished floors, don't let your child wear socks without shoes, and if you let him go barefoot, watch out for splinters.

CARS

Your child should always travel in a car seat that is officially approved for his age and weight. Use the locks on car doors and when driving don't let your child lean out of the window or put his hand out. Never leave your child alone in the car.

Be extra cautious when he is playing outside in the yard. Check where your child is before you close the car door, and when backing out of a driveway. If he is just behind the car, you won't see him in the rearview mirror.

FIRST AID

If your child is injured, always treat the most serious injury first. If he is unconscious, check his breathing, and resuscitate him if necessary (see page 238), before giving first aid for any other injury. If he is breathing, first treat anything that might prevent him from breathing properly, such as choking, suffocation, or drowning (see pages 242–43), then control any heavy bleeding (see page 246). If your child is badly injured or in shock, he will need urgent medical treatment, but you should give first aid before calling for medical help. But check this page for occasions when improper movements pose serious risks; then you must call an ambulance. Most urban areas in Canada are served by the 911 emergency service.

GETTING YOUR CHILD TO A HOSPITAL

Call for an ambulance, or ask someone else to phone if:
★ you think your child might have a spinal injury
★ you think he'll need special treatment on the way to the hospital.
★ If you have to take your child to the hospital yourself, have someone else drive while you sit with your child and continue to give first aid.

If your child is unconscious, don't leave him alone for more than a minute or so while you call for help. If he is not breathing, resuscitate him before phoning for an ambulance. Don't stop until he is breathing again, but shout to other people between breaths if necessary.

WARNING

If there is a chance that your child has injured his neck or spine—for example, after a bad fall—don't move him unless it is absolutely essential. Leave him in whatever position you found him while you check to see if he is breathing. If you need to perform artificial respiration, get someone to help you if possible. Turn your child on his back very gently without twisting his spine—try to hold his head, shoulders, and hips so that his body turns as a single unit.

FIRST AID KIT

Keep a supply of first aid equipment in a clean, dry container, and replace anything you use as soon as possible. Take some antiseptic wipes with you on outings, to clean cuts and scrapes.

Surgical tape *This is useful for sticking on bandages, and drawing together the edges of large cuts.*

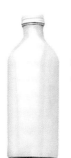

Calamine lotion *Soothes insect bites*

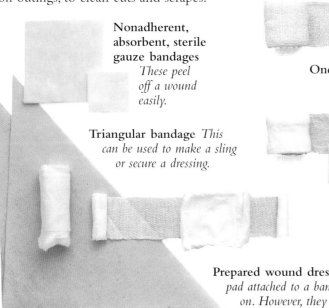

Nonadherent, absorbent, sterile gauze bandages *These peel off a wound easily.*

Triangular bandage *This can be used to make a sling or secure a dressing.*

One elastic bandage

Gauze bandage rolls

Scissors

Tweezers

Safety pins

Assorted adhesive bandages *Use these for dressing minor cuts and scrapes.*

Prepared wound dressings *These consist of a pad attached to a bandage, and are easy to put on. However, they are expensive and only available from medical suppliers.*

LIFESAVING TECHNIQUES

Familiarize yourself with lifesaving skills so that you can act quickly in an emergency. Every second counts. If your child seems to be unconscious, follow these procedures before treating any injuries. If he has stopped breathing, it is vital to get air into his lungs quickly, so that he doesn't suffer brain damage. You can prevent this, and revive your child by breathing your own air into his lungs. If his heart has stopped beating, you can pump it manually to keep his blood circulating through his body. Don't give up—children have been revived after several hours of resuscitation.

WARNING

This section is not meant to replace a CPR/Lifesaver course. If possible, take a course. It could save your child's life.

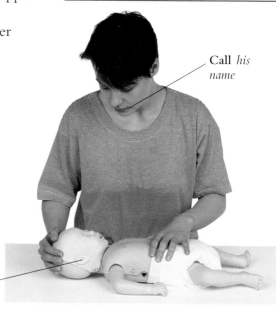

Call *his name*

Assess *your baby's condition*

CHECKING FOR UNCONSCIOUSNESS

Gently tap your child's shoulders. Call his name, and note whether he responds. **Don't** shake him, since this could make any injuries he may have worse. Always be aware of possible spinal injuries.

+ If he doesn't respond, he is unconscious, so check his breathing immediately and call an ambulance.

+ If he responds, check for injury and treat any that he has (see pages 244–53).

CHECKING BREATHING

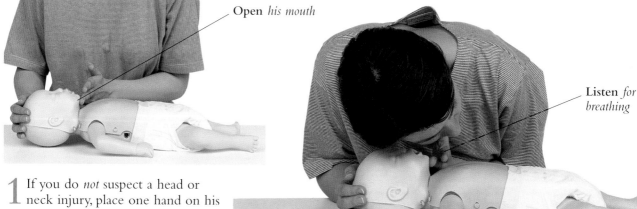

Open *his mouth*

Listen *for breathing*

1 If you do *not* suspect a head or neck injury, place one hand on his forehead and press gently to tilt his head back slightly. Open his mouth.

+ If there are no signs of breathing, check if there is something in the child's mouth, which has obstructed breathing. You should be able to see an object before attempting to remove it. Be very careful not to push anything down his throat. Check again for any signs of breathing.

2 Place your ear close to his mouth and nose, looking toward his feet. Listen for any sound of breathing, note whether you can feel any breath against your ear, and watch his chest to see whether it rises and falls as he breathes.

+ If there is still no sign of breathing, start artificial respiration right away (opposite).

+ If your child is breathing, put him on his side in the recovery position (see page 241) and call for emergency help immediately.

ARTIFICIAL RESPIRATION FOR A BABY

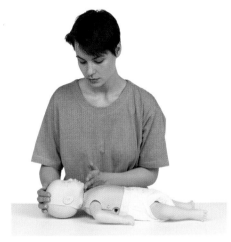

1 Lift your baby's chin to pull his jaw forward. Cup your baby's forehead to support him and keep his head tilted back.

2 Take a deep breath, place your lips around your baby's mouth and nose, making as good a seal as you can, then breathe out gently.

3 Watch your baby's chest to see whether it rises as you breathe out.

✚ **If his chest doesn't rise,** change the tilt of his head and jaw and try again. If there is still no air entry, treat him for choking (see page 242).

✚ **If his chest rises,** remove your mouth from his face and let his chest fall. Give two gentle breaths, then check for signs of circulation (see next page).

ARTIFICIAL RESPIRATION FOR A CHILD

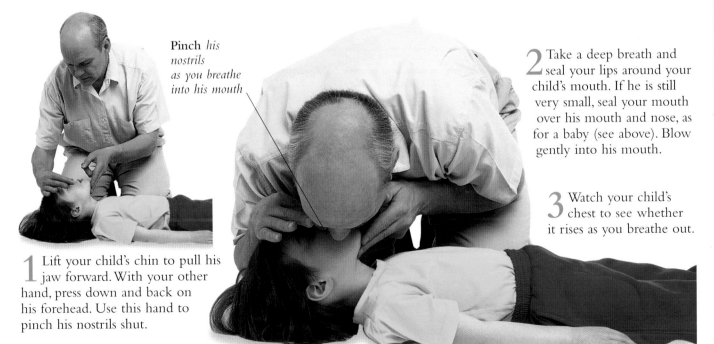

Pinch *his nostrils as you breathe into his mouth*

1 Lift your child's chin to pull his jaw forward. With your other hand, press down and back on his forehead. Use this hand to pinch his nostrils shut.

2 Take a deep breath and seal your lips around your child's mouth. If he is still very small, seal your mouth over his mouth and nose, as for a baby (see above). Blow gently into his mouth.

3 Watch your child's chest to see whether it rises as you breathe out.

✚ **If his chest doesn't rise,** reposition his head and jaw and try again. If there is still no air entry, treat him for choking (see page 242).

✚ **If his chest rises,** remove your mouth from his face and let his chest fall. Give two breaths, then check for signs of circulation (see next page).

LIFESAVING TECHNIQUES *continued*

CHECKING FOR (SIGNS OF) CIRCULATION

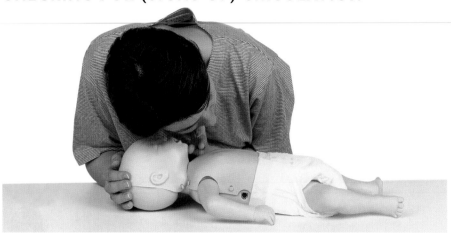

Look for signs of circulation in the baby or child, such as breathing (see page 238), any movement, a return of color to the skin, swallowing or coughing. Be aware that pulses may be hard to find.

FOR A BABY OR A CHILD
✚ If there are no signs of circulation, his heart may have stopped. Start external chest compression immediately (see below).

✚ If there are signs of circulation (for example, the skin retains its normal color), but the child is not breathing, continue breathing gently into his lungs at a rate of about one breath every three seconds, until he starts to breathe on his own, or until emergency help arrives. As soon as he starts to breathe again, turn him on his side in the recovery position (see opposite).

CARDIOPULMONARY RESUSCITATION (CPR)

FOR A BABY

1 Place your baby on a firm surface. With one hand on the baby's head, position the tips of two fingers on the lower breastbone just below the nipple line.

2 Press straight down to a depth of about 1.5–2cm (½–1in). Do this five times at a rate of two compressions per second.

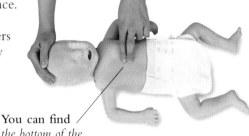

You can find *the bottom of the breastbone by feeling where the rib cage forms an inverted V-shape*

3 Give one full breath of artificial ventilation. Continue the cycle of five chest compressions to one breath of artificial ventilation for about a minute, checking for signs of circulation between each cycle.

4 Once the cycle has been continued for about a minute, call an ambulance, and continue giving CPR until help arrives.

FOR A CHILD OVER ONE

1 Place your child on her back on a firm surface. Tilt the head back slightly.

2 Move your middle finger along the ribs to where they meet the breastbone. Place your index finger next to it and note this spot.

3 Place the heel of the same hand on the spot you have just noted. Press down to a depth of about 2.5–3.8cm (1–1½in) then release the pressure. Do this five times at a rate of about 100 compressions a minute (about two compressions per second).

4 Give one full breath of artificial ventilation. Continue the cycle of five chest compressions to one breath, checking for signs of circulation every few minutes. Call an ambulance and continue CPR until the child recovers or the ambulance personnel can take over.

Locate *the correct hand position by feeling for the bottom of the breastbone*

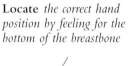

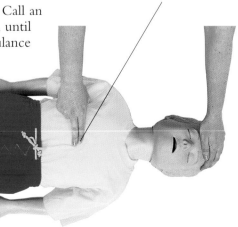

THE RECOVERY POSITION

Put your child into this position if he is unconscious, but breathing. This is the safest position because it prevents his tongue from falling back into his throat and obstructing his airway, and avoids the risk of him choking if he vomits. For a baby, see right.

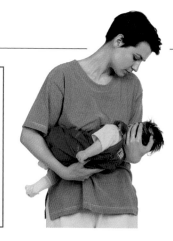

RECOVERY POSITION FOR A BABY
A baby or child under the age of two should be cradled in your arms with his head tilted down to avoid obstruction of his airway.

FOR A CHILD OVER TWO

1 Kneel beside your child. Tilt her head back and lift her chin forward. This keeps her air passages open while you put her in the recovery position.

Her head *must be tilted well back with the chin jutting forward*

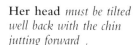

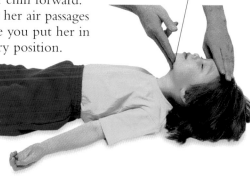

2 If necessary, straighten her legs. Bend the arm nearest to you so that it makes a right angle and lay it on the ground, with the palm of the hand upward.

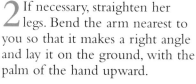

Bend *top leg into a right angle to prevent her rolling forward*

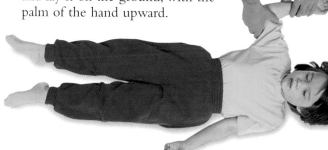

3 Bring her other arm across her chest. Hold the back of her hand against her opposite cheek.

Move *furthest arm across her chest and bend it*

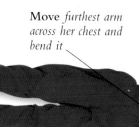

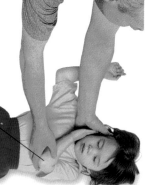

4 Use your free hand to clasp gently under the thigh furthest from you. Leaving the foot flat on the ground, carefully pull the knee up to bend the leg. Keeping your child's hand against her cheek to support her head, pull on the thigh of the bent leg to roll her toward you and onto her side.

5 Adjust her arm and leg so she cannot fall forward, and tilt her head. Call an ambulance.

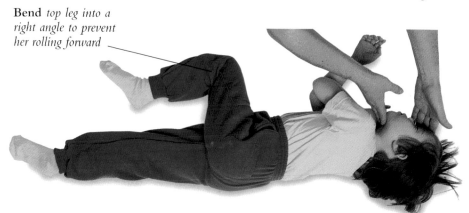

CHOKING

This happens when a small object or piece of food gets lodged in the windpipe, causing a coughing fit. It is important to dislodge the object quickly, so that your child can breathe properly again. If a child is unable to cry, talk, or cough forcefully, follow these steps:

EMERGENCY

✚ Call for emergency help immediately if:
 ★ your child stops breathing
 ★ you cannot remove the blockage
 ★ your child continues to choke after you have removed the blockage.

HELPING A BABY

1 Hold your baby face down with his head low along your forearm. Support his head and shoulders on your hand. Give five sharp slaps to the upper part of his back.

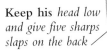

Keep his *head low and give five sharps slaps on the back*

2 If he is still choking, turn him over and do five quick chest thrusts using as for chest compressions (see page 240). Repeat back blows and chest compressions alternately until blockage is removed.

Turn him *on to his back along your other arm*

3 If your baby does not start breathing normally when the blockage is removed, carry out artificial respiration immediately (see pages 238–39).

4 If the blockage hasn't cleared, call an ambulance and repeat steps 1–2 until medical help arrives or the baby starts to breathe.

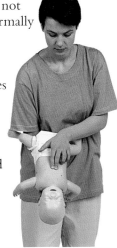

HELPING A CHILD

1 Stay with your child and encourage him to cough up the obstruction. Do not interfere unless his cough becomes weak, or he emits a high-pitched crowing noise when he breathes. If that happens, tell him that you are going to help him.

2 Stand behind him, or in the case of a small child, kneel behind him and wrap your arms around his waist. Make a fist and place it, thumb side in, against his stomach, above the navel (but well below the breastbone), and using your other hand to exert pressure, quickly press your fist inward and upward into his abdomen.

3 If he does not start breathing normally once the blockage has been removed from his windpipe, carry out artificial respiration (see page 239).

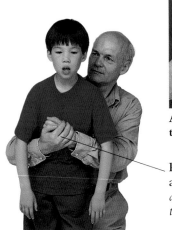

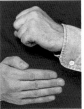

Abdominal thrust

Place a fist against *the upper abdomen below the rib cage*

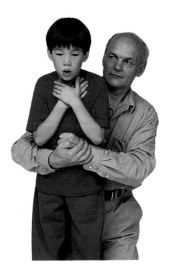

4 If the abdominal thrusts fail to dislodge the object, call an ambulance. Continue the above cycle until help arrives, or your attempts to dislodge the object are successful.

SUFFOCATION

Anything lying across your child's face may block his mouth and nose and prevent him from breathing.

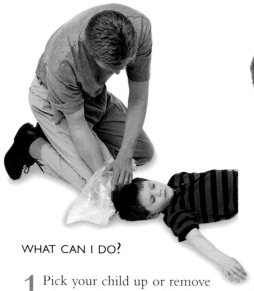

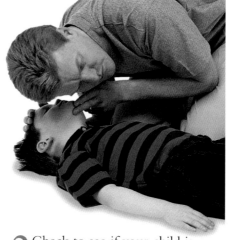

WHAT CAN I DO?

1 Pick your child up or remove whatever is covering his face.

2 Check to see if your child is conscious and breathing (see page 238).

(see page 238)

EMERGENCY

✚ Call for emergency help immediately if your child:
★ becomes unconscious
★ stops breathing, even if only for a few seconds
★ shows any symptoms that worry you.

✚ **If he is not breathing,** start artificial respiration immediately (see page 238) and ask someone to call for emergency help.

✚ **If he is breathing but unconscious,** place him in the recovery position (see page 241), then call for emergency help.

✚ **If he is conscious,** simply comfort and reassure him.

DROWNING

Babies and children can drown in very shallow water. This is one reason why they should never be left unattended in a bathtub or backyard wading pool containing even a small amount of water. When a young child's face is submerged, his automatic reaction is to take a deep breath to scream, rather than to lift his face up out of the water. As the child struggles for breath, water enters the airway.

✚ **If she is not breathing,** don't waste time draining water from her lungs. Clear any debris from her mouth and start artificial respiration (see page 238)—if possible while she is still being carried from the water—and **call for emergency help.** Continue artificial respiration until help arrives or until she starts to breathe. If she is breathing, put her in the recovery position (see page 241).

EMERGENCY

✚ **Call for emergency help immediately** if your child was rescued from drowning, even if she didn't become unconscious.

✚ **If she is conscious,** simply comfort and reassure her, and make sure she keeps warm until help arrives.

✚ **If she is breathing but unconscious,** place her in the recovery position (see page 241). Cover her with a coat or blanket to keep her warm. Get her to a warm room as soon as you can, because she may have become dangerously chilled after even a short period of immersion in cold water. Young children lose their body heat much more quickly than adults. Monitor her breathing closely. If she vomits, put her on her side.

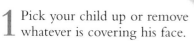

Tilt her head back and begin artificial respiration

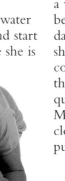

SHOCK

A life-threatening state of collapse, when blood pressure falls dangerously low, shock is a reaction to any severe injury, especially one in which your child has been badly burned or suffered heavy bleeding.

SYMPTOMS

* Pale, cold, sweaty skin
* blue or grayish tinge inside the lips or under the fingernails
* rapid and shallow breathing
* restlessness
* drowsiness or confusion
* unconsciousness.

EMERGENCY

✚ Call for emergency help immediately if your child is in shock.

WHAT CAN I DO?

1 Lay your child down on his back, if possible on a coat or blanket. Turn his head to one side, then raise his feet about 30cm (12in) and rest them on something, such as a pile of clothes or a bag. **Don't** raise his legs if he has a broken leg.

2 Cover him with a blanket or coat, or hug him, to keep him warm. **Don't** try to warm him up with a hot water bottle or an electric blanket—this only draws blood away from the vital body organs to the skin.

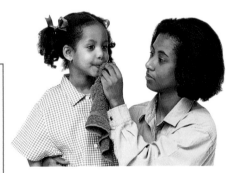

3 If he complains of thirst, moisten his lips with a damp cloth. **Don't** give him anything to eat or drink, as this might cause delays in administering an anesthetic to your child at the hospital.

4 If he becomes unconscious, check his breathing (see page 238).

✚ If the child is not breathing, start artificial respiration (see page 239).

✚ If the child is breathing, put him into the recovery position (see page 241).

POISONING

Poisoning is one of the most common emergencies in children. Post the number of the nearest Poison Control Center by your telephone.

SYMPTOMS

Your child's symptoms will depend on the type of poison he has swallowed. You may notice any of these signs:
* stomach pain
* vomiting
* symptoms of shock (see above)
* seizures
* drowsiness
* unconsciousness
* burns or discoloration around the mouth if your child has swallowed a corrosive poison
* poison or empty container nearby.

WHAT CAN I DO?

1 If your child is unconscious, check her breathing (see page 238).

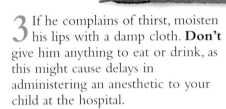

✚ If she is not breathing, start artificial respiration immediately (see page 239), but wipe her face first or place a fine cloth over her mouth and breathe through that, to avoid getting any poison into your own mouth.

✚ If she is breathing, put her into the recovery position (see page 241).

EMERGENCY

✚ Call for emergency help immediately if you think your child has swallowed something poisonous.

2 If you see signs of burning around your child's mouth, or think she has swallowed a chemical product, wash her skin and lips with water. Try to find out what she has taken, and when.

3 Induce vomiting only on your doctor's or Poison Control Center's advice. This includes the use of ipecac syrup. Vomiting may make some situations worse.

4 If your child vomits, save a sample for medical personnel.

5 Save any containers that might have held poison. Take them to the emergency department with you.

BURNS AND SCALDS

A burn that causes reddening of the skin over an area of about 2–3cm (1in) is a minor burn, and can safely be treated at home. A burn affecting an area greater than this is a major burn, and is dangerous, since infection can enter it. For sunburn, see page 229.

MINOR BURNS
WHAT CAN I DO?

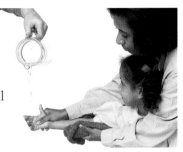

1 Cool the burn immediately, by holding it under cold, slowly running water until the pain decreases. This will help to prevent blisters from developing.

2 If a blister develops, put a pad of clean, non-fluffy material over it and hold it in place with adhesive bandages or surgical tape.
Don't burst the blister—it protects the damaged area underneath while the new skin is growing.
Don't put any cream or lotion on the burn.

BURNING CLOTHES
WHAT CAN I DO?

1 Stop the child from moving since movement will fan the flames. Lay your child on the ground with the burning area up.

2 Put out the fire by throwing water on it or smothering the flames with a rug, blanket, or heavy curtain, keeping this away from your child's head, if possible.
Don't throw water over him if he is near an electrical appliance that is turned on.
Don't try to smother the flames with nylon or any other flammable fabric.

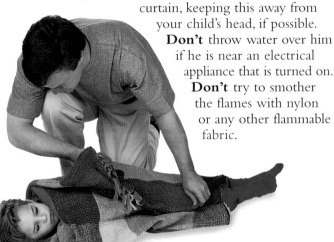

3 When the flames are out, treat your child for a major burn (see right).

✚ Get your child professional medical help as soon as you have given first aid if:
✶ the burn covers an area of more than about 2 to 3cm (1in)
✶ the burn was caused by an electric shock (see page 251).

MAJOR BURNS
WHAT CAN I DO?

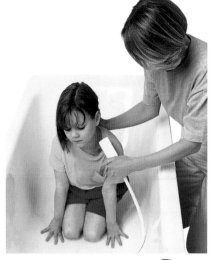

1 Cool the burn immediately by drenching it with cool water: either in the shower, or in a cool bath. **Don't** rub her skin.

✚ **If chemicals have burned her skin,** wash them off with plenty of water, but **don't** let it run onto unharmed areas.

2 Remove any clothing that has been soaked in boiling water, fat, or corrosive chemicals, taking care not to let it touch her skin anywhere else. Cut clothes off rather than pulling them over her face. **Don't** remove dry, burned clothing, or clothing that is sticking to the burned area.

3 Cover the area very loosely with a clean, non-fluffy material. If you don't have a sterile dressing, a clean handkerchief or pillowcase will do.

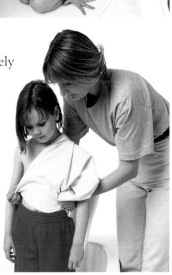

4 Check for symptoms of shock, and treat your child for this if necessary (see opposite). If she complains of thirst, moisten her lips with a damp cloth.

HEAVY BLEEDING

If blood spurts forcefully from a wound, or bleeding continues despite steady direct pressure on the wound, try these added measures to stem the flow.

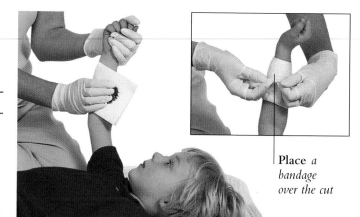

EMERGENCY

✚ Get your child professional medical help as soon as you have given first aid if he's been bleeding heavily.

WHAT CAN I DO?

1 Raise the injured part above the level of your child's heart, to reduce the amount of blood flowing through it. Check for embedded objects; if there are any, treat them as described below.

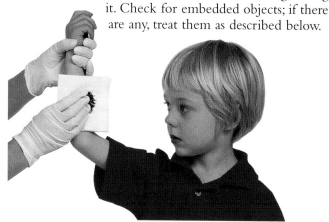

Place *a bandage over the cut*

2 Place a pad of clean, non-fluffy material over the wound—a clean handkerchief or dishtowel is ideal—then press hard on it for about 10 minutes. If there is no clean material available, press with your fingers, drawing the edges of the cut firmly together.

3 Leaving the original pad in place, bind a clean pad or dressing firmly over the wound so that the pressure is maintained. If this becomes soaked with blood, don't remove it, just bandage another pad over it, maintaining the pressure all the time.

4 Check for symptoms of shock (see page 244), and treat your child for this if necessary.

EMBEDDED OBJECTS

Small pieces of dirt in a cut will probably be washed out by bleeding, and larger pieces may wipe easily off the surface of the wound. If your child has something embedded in a wound, treat it as shown below.

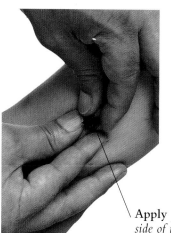

WHAT CAN I DO?

1 Help your child rest. Apply pressure on either side of the object and raise the injured part above the level of your child's heart. **Don't** try to remove any objects that are embedded in a wound as you may cause further damage and bleeding.

Apply *pressure either side of the wound*

EMERGENCY

✚ Get your child professional medical help as soon as you have given first aid if he has an embedded object.

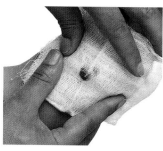

1 Place a piece of gauze over the wound and object to minimize the risk of infection.

2 Use spare bandage rolls to build up padding to the same height as the embedded object.

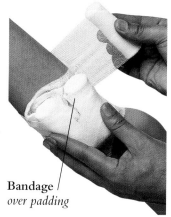

Bandage *over padding*

3 Secure the padding by bandaging over it, being careful not to press on the embedded object. Take your child to the hospital.

CUTS AND SCRAPES

Cuts and scrapes are common throughout childhood, and you can treat most of them yourself at home. Keep your child's tetanus injections up to date (see page 202), since tetanus can result from dirt entering a wound. Treat an animal bite as a cut.

EMERGENCY

✚ Call your doctor and get your child professional medical help as soon as you have given first aid if:

★ the cut is large or deep
★ the cut has gaping edges
★ your child has cut his face badly
★ the cut or scrape is very dirty
★ your child has a puncture wound (a deep cut with only a small opening in the skin) caused by something like a rusty nail or animal's tooth.

CALL THE DOCTOR

☎ Consult your doctor as soon as possible if the area around the wound later becomes tender and red—it may be infected.

WHAT CAN I DO?

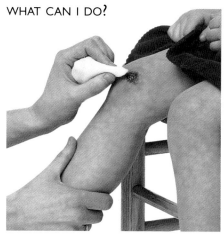

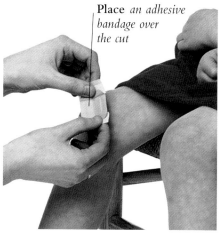

Place *an adhesive bandage over the cut*

1 Wash your hands first, if possible. Clean the cut by holding it under running water, or wiping gently around it with an antiseptic swab or cotton soaked in warm water. Use a clean ball or piece of cotton for each stroke. **Don't** remove anything that is embedded in the cut (see opposite).

✚ **If your child has been bitten by an animal,** or if there is any risk of rabies, contact your doctor.

2 If the cut is still bleeding after five minutes, press a pad such as a clean handkerchief firmly on it for a few minutes.

3 Put an adhesive bandage or dressing over it, to help protect it and keep it clean. **Don't** put any antiseptic ointment on your child's cut, unless it is suggested by your physician.

4 Keep the cut covered with an adhesive bandage or a dressing until it has healed completely. This ensures that the area stays clean and helps the cut to heal quickly. Change the bandage every day.

NOSEBLEEDS

Nosebleeds can result from a bump on the nose, nose-picking, or excessive nose-blowing. A few children seem prone to nosebleeds, probably because they have fragile blood vessels in their noses.

CALL THE DOCTOR

☎ Call your doctor now if your child's nose is still bleeding just as badly after half an hour. Consult your doctor if your child has frequent, severe nosebleeds.

WHAT CAN I DO?

1 Help your child lean forward over a bowl or sink, and pinch her nostrils firmly together for about 10 minutes. Try to stop her from sniffing or swallowing the blood —encourage her to spit it out into the bowl instead.

2 After 10 minutes, release the nostrils gradually. If the bleeding has stopped, have your child sit quietly. If it has not, squeeze the nostrils for another 10 minutes.

3 Don't have your child blow her nose for about four hours after the bleeding has stopped.

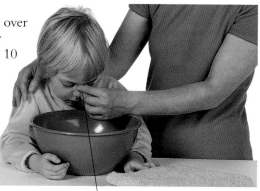

Pinch *your child's nostrils firmly*

HEAD AND FACE INJURY

Bumps on the head are common in young children, but are seldom serious. A cut on the forehead or scalp, even a small one, is likely to bleed profusely. If your child has had a severe blow to her head, she may have a concussion, which results when the brain is shaken within the skull, or from bleeding inside the skull—this may not be apparent for some hours.

WHAT CAN I DO?

1 If your child's head is bruised, hold a cloth wrung out in very cold water, or an ice pack wrapped in a damp cloth, over the bruise. This may stop it from swelling up. Check the skin underneath the pack every minute, and remove the pack if a red patch with a white waxy center develops.

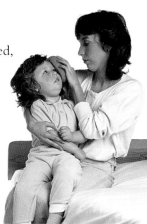

2 If your child's head is bleeding, place a clean cloth over the cut and press on the wound, just as you would for bleeding anywhere else on the body (see page 246).

BROKEN TEETH

If your child has broken a tooth, or one has become dislodged, cover the tooth or broken piece with milk, and take your child and her tooth to your dentist or to hospital immediately.

EMERGENCY

✚ Call for emergency help immediately if your child has injured her head and shows any unusual behavior or has any of these symptoms up to 24 hours later:
* ★ unconsciousness, however brief
* ★ vomiting
* ★ noisy breathing or snoring, if your child doesn't normally snore
* ★ difficulty in waking, or abnormal drowsiness
* ★ discharge of clear or bloodstained fluid from her nose or ear
* ★ unusual crying
* ★ severe headache
* ★ dislike of bright light.

3 Watch your child carefully for the next 24 hours, in case she develops any of the emergency signs listed above. If she bumped her head badly, wake her every three hours—**if she won't wake up, call for emergency help immediately.**

If a discharge of clear or bloodstained fluid trickles from your child's nose or ear (and there is no chance of a spinal injury), put her into the recovery position with a pad of clean material placed under her nose or ear. If she deteriorates or loses consciousness, assess her condition (see page 238). Be prepared to resuscitate (see page 239). **Call an ambulance.**

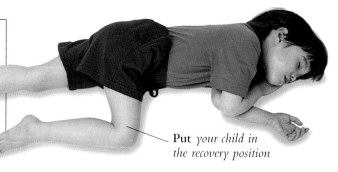

Put *your child in the recovery position*

BRUISES AND SWELLING

A bruise appears when a fall or blow causes bleeding into the tissues beneath the skin, which produces swelling and discoloration.

CRUSHED FINGERS AND TOES

If your child has crushed his fingers in a door or window, or dropped something heavy on his foot, hold the injured area under cold running water for a few minutes. If it is very swollen, or still painful after about half an hour, seek medical care.

WHAT CAN I DO?

1 Hold a pad wrung out in very cold water, or an ice pack wrapped in a damp cloth, over the bruise for about half an hour. This should help to reduce pain and swelling.

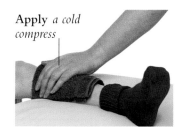

Apply *a cold compress*

2 If your child seems to be in great pain or if it hurts him to use a bruised limb, especially if the swelling is severe, check for any signs of a sprained joint or a broken bone (see opposite).

SPRAINED JOINTS

When a joint is sprained, the ligaments are damaged. This can cause symptoms very similar to those of a broken bone: if you are not sure which it is, treat it as a broken bone (see below).

WHAT CAN I DO?

1 Taking care not to pull or twist the injured joint, gently take off your child's shoe and sock, or any other items that might constrict swelling around the injury.

2 Support the injured joint in the most comfortable position for your child, then hold a cloth wrung out in ice cold water, or an ice pack wrapped in a damp cloth, on the joint, to reduce swelling and pain.

EMERGENCY

✚ Get professional medical help as soon as you have given first aid.

3 Wrap a thick layer of cotton around the joint, then bandage it firmly, but not so tightly that the beds of her toenails (or fingernails if you have bandaged her wrist or elbow) turn white or pale blue.

SYMPTOMS

★ Pain in the injured area
★ swelling and, later, bruising
★ difficulty moving the joint.

FRACTURES AND DISLOCATED JOINTS

Broken bones are unusual in young children—their bones have not hardened, so they are flexible and tend to bend rather than break. Sometimes there may be a partial break, which mends easily. A joint is dislocated if one or more bones slip out of place.

SYMPTOMS

★ Severe pain in the injured area
★ swelling and, later, bruising
★ difficulty moving the injured part
★ misshapen appearance to the injured part—a limb may be bent in an odd way, or may look shorter than the uninjured limb.

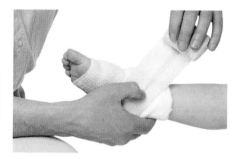

Tie *the bandages on the uninjured side*

WHAT CAN I DO?

1 If you think your child's back or neck might be injured, do not move him or change his position unless he is in danger (see page 237).

2 Support an injured arm in the most comfortable position for your child. For a broken wrist, arm, or collarbone, put padding around the injured area and, if your child will let you, gently fold his arm across his chest, then support it in an arm sling, fastening the bandage with a reef knot tied just below the shoulder. Don't try to force his arm

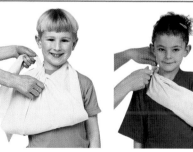

Arm sling   **Elevation sling**

into this position. If there is bleeding or swelling that needs to be reduced, the arm should be raised in an elevation sling. The fingertips are brought up to the level of the opposite shoulder, the sling is wrapped around the arm, passed from the elbow across the back, and then tied at the shoulder.

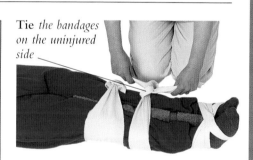

For a broken leg or ankle, you may need to splint the injury if help is not available. Lay your child down and pad the injured area and between his knees and ankles. Bandage the injured leg to the other one, securing it above and below the injury. Pad under the knots.

3 Check for symptoms of shock and treat him for this if necessary (see page 244). If you think he has a broken leg, don't raise his legs.

EMERGENCY

✚ Call for emergency help as soon as you have given first aid.

FOREIGN BODY IN THE EYE

Eyelashes or particles of dust can easily get into the eye. If your child's eye seems irritated but you can't see anything in it, she may have an eye infection (see page 209).

SYMPTOMS

★ Pain in the eye
★ red, watering eye
★ your child may rub her eye.

CHEMICALS IN THE EYE

If your child has splashed any chemicals or corrosive fluids in her eyes, wash her eyes out immediately under cold running water, keeping her eyelids apart with your fingers. If only one eye is affected, tilt her head so that the injured eye is lower, and the chemical cannot wash over into the uninjured one. Then cover the eye with a pad and take your child to a hospital. If possible, take the chemical bottle with you.

WHAT CAN I DO?

1 Wait a few minutes to see if the natural watering of the eye washes the foreign body away. Try to stop your child from rubbing her eye.

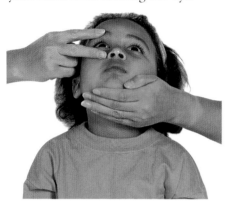

2 Sit your child down, facing the light. Separate the eyelids. Ask her to look right, left, up, and down. Make sure that you examine all of the eye.

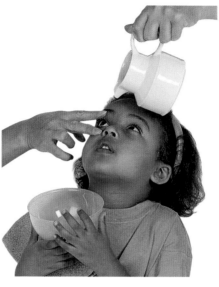

3 If you can see the object on the white part of the eye, wash it out using clean water. Aim for the inner corner and be very gentle. Or, use a damp hankerchief to lift it off.

4 If an object is under the eyelid, you can ask an older child to clear it by lifting the upper eyelid over the lower. If the eye is still red or sore once the object has been removed, take her to the hospital.

A FOREIGN BODY THAT CANNOT BE REMOVED

Cover the eye with a sterile dressing. Reassure the child and take her to the hospital.

FOREIGN BODY IN THE EAR

Insects may crawl into your child's ear, and children may push small objects into their ears. Don't let your child play with beads or similar small objects until he is old enough to understand that they should not be put into his ears.

SYMPTOMS

★ Tickling in the ear
★ partial deafness
★ your child may rub or tug at his ear.

WHAT CAN I DO?

1 If your child has an insect in her ear, she may be very alarmed. Sit her down and support her head with the affected ear uppermost. Gently flood the ear with tepid water so that the insect floats out. If you can't remove the insect, take your child to hospital.

2 Children often push things into their ears. A hard object may become stuck. This may result in pain and temporary deafness; it may damage the eardrum. Do not attempt to remove the object, even if you can see it. Reassure your child and ask her what she put into her ear. Take your child to hospital.

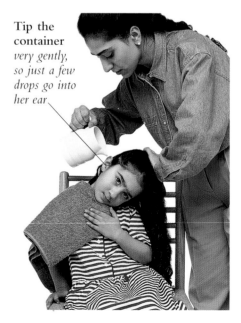

Tip the container *very gently, so just a few drops go into her ear.*

FOREIGN BODY IN THE NOSE

Children sometimes stuff small pieces of food or other objects such as beads or marbles up their noses.

SYMPTOMS

★ Smelly, blood-stained discharge from the nose.

WHAT CAN I DO?

If your child can blow his nose, help him to blow it, one nostril at a time. If this does not dislodge the object, don't try to remove it yourself—take your child to the hospital straight away.

ELECTRIC SHOCK

A mild electrical shock gives only a brief pins and needles sensation. A severe one can knock your child down, render her unconscious and stop both breathing and heartbeat. Electric current can also burn.

EMERGENCY

✚ Take your child to the hospital as soon as you have given first aid if:
  ★ he was unconscious, even if only for a few seconds
  ★ he has any electrical burns.

WHAT CAN I DO?

1 Switch off the electricity, at the source if possible.

✚ **If you can't do this,** stand on an insulating material—such as a rubber mat or a pile of dry newspapers. Separate your child from the electrical source by pushing the cable or your child away, using some dry, nonconducting object such as a wooden chair or broom handle.

Move *the cable rather than your child's arm*

ELECTRICAL BURNS

Electricity can burn where the current enters the body and where it leaves, so your child may have burns where he touched the electrical source and anywhere that was in contact with the ground. Although these burns may look small, they are often very deep.

---

2 Check to see if your child is conscious (see page 238).

✚ **If he is unconscious,** check his breathing: start artificial respiration immediately if necessary (see page 239). If he is breathing, put him in the recovery position (see page 241).

✚ **If he is conscious,** comfort and reassure him. Look for symptoms of shock (see page 244).

3 Examine him for any burns: check areas that were in contact with the electrical source or the ground (burns will look red or scorched, and may swell up). If you find any, treat them as major burns (see page 245).

INSECT BITES AND STINGS

Most plants and insects cause only minor stings which, while they may be painful, are not dangerous for your child. However, a few people develop a serious allergic reaction to stings, and therefore need urgent medical treatment.

SYMPTOMS

* ★ Sharp pain
* ★ redness
* ★ slight swelling
* ★ itching.

EMERGENCY

✚ Take your child to a hospital emergency room as soon as you have given first aid if he:
* ★ has difficulty breathing
* ★ develops a widespread rash with welts
* ★ feels dizzy or faints
* ★ develops symptoms of shock (see page 244)
* ★ has been stung inside his mouth.

WHAT CAN I DO?

1 If your child has been stung by a bee, see if the stinger has been left in the skin. Scrape it off with your fingernail, or a credit card. If the tiny sac of poison is visible and still intact, try not to squeeze it.

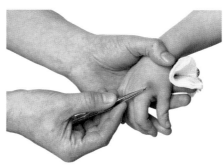

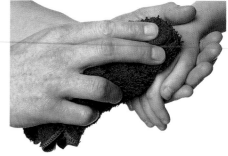

2 Hold a cloth wrung out in ice cold water over the sting.

3 Soothe the area around the sting, which will quickly become red, swollen and itchy, by dabbing it gently with cotton balls dipped in baking soda and water. Don't use antihistamine ointment, or combinations of calamine lotion and antihistamine.

If he has been stung in his mouth, give him a cold drink or, if he is over two, let him suck an ice cube and call for emergency help.

SNAKE AND SPIDER BITES, SCORPION STINGS

Bites from snakes and poisonous spiders are serious for young children. Snake bites carry a risk of tetanus, but your child can be vaccinated against this. Ask your physician about local varieties of snakes and spiders.

SYMPTOMS

Your child's symptoms will depend on what has bitten or stung her; some symptoms may not appear for a few hours:
* ★ severe pain
* ★ one or two puncture marks
* ★ swelling
* ★ nausea or vomiting
* ★ difficulty breathing
* ★ shock (see page 244)
* ★ convulsions
* ★ drowsiness
* ★ unconsciousness.

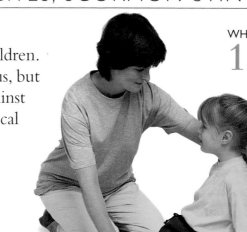

Keep *the bitten part lower than her heart*

EMERGENCY

✚ Take your child to a hospital as soon as you have given first aid if she has been bitten by a snake or spider, or stung by a scorpion.

WHAT CAN I DO?

1 Calm your child, and help her to sit or lie down. Keep the bitten or stung part still, and position it below the level of her heart.

2 Wash the area, but **don't** suck out any poison.

3 Check for shock, and treat your child for this if necessary (see page 244). If she was bitten or stung on the leg or foot, don't raise her legs.

4 If she becomes unconscious, check her breathing (see page 238).

✚ **If she is not breathing,** begin artificial respiration (see page 239).

✚ **If she is breathing,** put her into the recovery position (see page 241).

FROSTBITE

Frostbite is damage to tissue, usually the fingers, toes, or ears, due to exposure to cold.

SYMPTOMS
★ Skin is cold, hard, and white ★ fingers, toes, or ears become red, and painful when warmed.

WHAT CAN I DO?

1 Put the frozen part of your child's body under your arm.

2 If frostbite is severe, and medical help is not available, immerse affected area in warm water.

3 If there is tissue damage, take the child to your physician.

HYPOTHERMIA

Hypothermia is a fall in body temperature due to exposure to cold, wind, or rain. Small children may be susceptible to hypothermia.

SYMPTOMS
★ Pale skin color ★ listlessness or disorientation ★ body temperature below normal.

WHAT CAN I DO?

1 Place child in warm room.

2 Wrap child in blanket.

3 If you take child to hospital, be sure to keep her warm.

THORNS AND SPLINTERS

Thorns or tiny splinters will often become embedded in a child's hands or feet. Splinters in the fingertips will hurt more than those in the feet.

CALL THE DOCTOR

☎ Consult your doctor as soon as possible if:
★ the area around a splinter becomes red, swollen, or tender up to 48 hours later
★ you cannot remove a large or painful splinter
★ your child has a splinter of glass or metal.

WHAT CAN I DO?

1 If the end of the splinter is sticking out, use a pair of clean tweezers to pull the splinter straight out gently. Wash the area thoroughly with soap and water.

2 If there is no loose end, but you can see the splinter clearly, it is probably lying just below the surface of the skin. Sterilize a needle in a flame and let it cool. Then, starting where the splinter entered, gently tear the skin a little way along the line of the splinter. Carefully lift up the end of the splinter with the needle point and pull it out with tweezers, then wash the area thoroughly with soap and water.

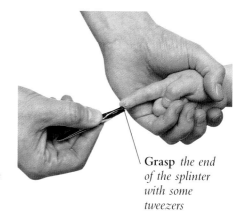

Grasp *the end of the splinter with some tweezers*

3 If a small thorn or splinter has gone straight down into the skin, and is not painful, it is best to leave it alone. It will probably work its own way out.

BLISTERS

Blisters form when burns, scalds, or friction damage the skin. The fluid-filled blister protects the new skin forming underneath.

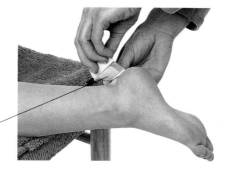

Cover the blister *with an adhesive bandage to prevent your child's shoe from rubbing it*

WHAT CAN I DO?

1 Don't burst or prick the blister or try to remove the top layer of skin. This will leave the raw skin open to infection. Dress your child in clothes that will not rub against it.

2 If the blister bursts, cover it with an adhesive bandage with a pad large enough to cover the blister.

GROWTH CHARTS: GIRLS

The charts below show average growth in girls (the solid line), and the range of normal measurements. Your doctor will check your baby's progress by weighing and measuring her regularly and marking in her own growth curves on similar charts. The shape of her curve should match closely the shape of the "average" curve: this shows a healthy rate of growth.

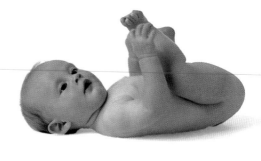

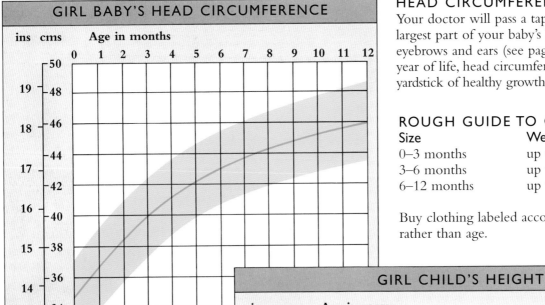

GIRL BABY'S HEAD CIRCUMFERENCE

HEAD CIRCUMFERENCE

Your doctor will pass a tape measure round the largest part of your baby's head, just above her eyebrows and ears (see page 81). During the first year of life, head circumference is an easier yardstick of healthy growth to measure than length.

ROUGH GUIDE TO CLOTHES SIZES

Size	Weight
0–3 months	up to 5kg (13lbs)
3–6 months	up to 6–8kg (14–18lbs)
6–12 months	up to 8–10kg (18–22lbs)

Buy clothing labeled according to weight, rather than age.

⎯ average

▨ range of measurements likely in a normal child; 94 percent of girls fall within this area

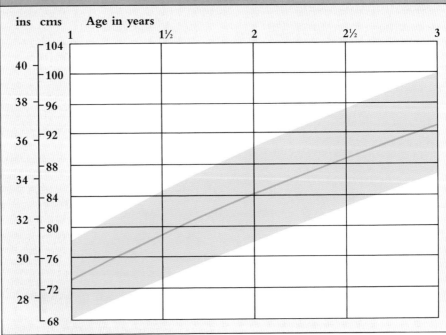

GIRL CHILD'S HEIGHT

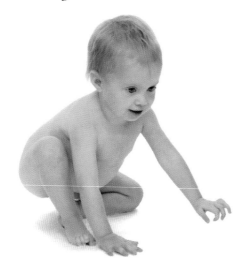

YOUR CHILD'S HEIGHT

About every six months measure your child standing up against the same wall. She should stand close to it, feet together, and without shoes. Use a ruler at right angles to the wall to mark her height, then measure the distance from mark to floor. Don't worry if your child has periods of slow growth interspersed with spurts; but if two consecutive measurements seem very low, consult your doctor.

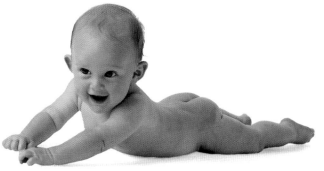

GIRL BABY'S WEIGHT

1bs	kgs	Age in months

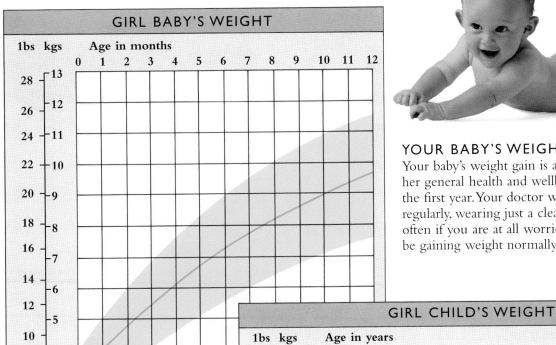

YOUR BABY'S WEIGHT

Your baby's weight gain is a vital indicator of her general health and wellbeing throughout the first year. Your doctor will weigh her regularly, wearing just a clean diaper, and more often if you are at all worried that she might not be gaining weight normally.

GIRL CHILD'S WEIGHT

1bs	kgs	Age in years

YOUR CHILD'S WEIGHT

After her first birthday, your child won't put weight on steadily, but the periods of slow and rapid growth will gradually balance out. She shouldn't lose weight: even if she seems very chubby to you, she only needs to mark time until her height catches up. Seek your doctor's advice if her weight drops, or if two consecutive measurements are less than you would expect.

GROWTH CHARTS: BOYS

The charts below show average growth in boys (the solid line), and the range of normal measurements. Your doctor will check your baby's progress by weighing and measuring him regularly and marking in his own growth curves on similar charts. The shape of his curve should match closely the shape of the "average" curve: this shows a healthy rate of growth.

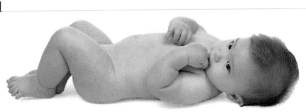

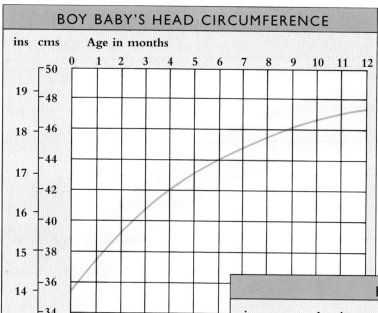

BOY BABY'S HEAD CIRCUMFERENCE

HEAD CIRCUMFERENCE

Your doctor will pass a tape measure round the largest part of your baby's head, just above his eyebrows and ears (see page 81). During the first year of life, head circumference is an easier yardstick of healthy growth to measure than length.

ROUGH GUIDE TO CLOTHES SIZES

Size	Weight
0–3 months,	up to 5kg (13lbs)
3–6 months	up to 6–8kg (14–18lbs)
6–12 months	up to 8–10kg (18–22lbs)

Buy clothing labeled according to weight, rather than age.

⟋ average

range of measurements likely in a normal child; 94 percent of boys fall within this area

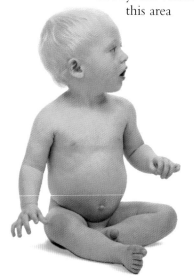

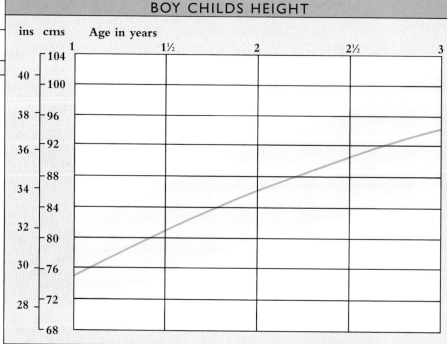

BOY CHILDS HEIGHT

YOUR CHILD'S HEIGHT

About every six months measure your child standing up against the same wall. He should stand close to it, feet together, and without shoes. Use a ruler at right angles to the wall to mark his height, then measure the distance from mark to floor. Don't worry if your child has periods of slow growth interspersed with spurts; but if two consecutive measurements seem very low, consult your doctor.

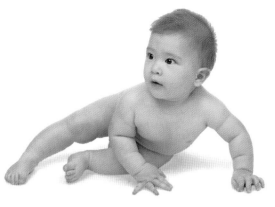

BOY BABY'S WEIGHT

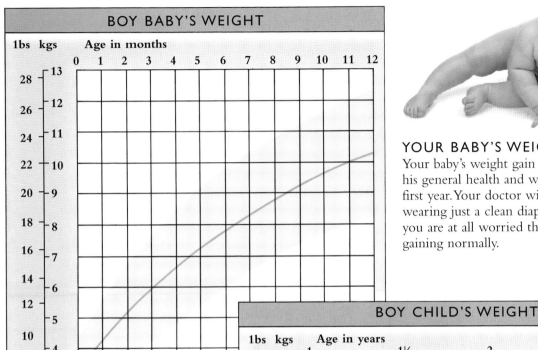

1bs	kgs	Age in months

YOUR BABY'S WEIGHT

Your baby's weight gain is a vital indicator of his general health and wellbeing throughout the first year. Your doctor will weigh him regularly, wearing just a clean diaper, and more often if you are at all worried that he might not be gaining normally.

BOY CHILD'S WEIGHT

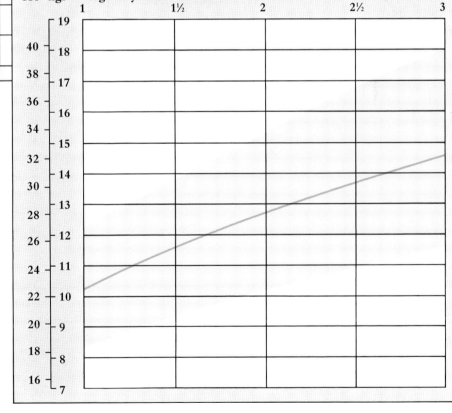

1bs	kgs	Age in years

YOUR CHILD'S WEIGHT

After his first birthday, your child won't put weight on steadily, but the periods of slow and rapid growth will gradually balance out. He shouldn't lose weight: even if he seems very chubby to you, he only needs to mark time until his height catches up. Seek your doctor's advice if his weight drops, or if two consecutive measurements are less than you would expect.

USEFUL ADDRESSES

PRENATAL SUPPORT

Healthy Pregnancy—National Women's Health Information Center
US Department of Health and Human Services,
Suite 300, 8550 Arlington Blvd.,
Fairfax, VA 22031
Web: www.4woman.org/Pregnancy

Motherisk
Alcohol and Substance Use
Helpline: 1-877-327-4636
Nausea and Vomiting of Pregnancy
Helpline: 1-800-436-8477
HIV and HIV Treatment in Pregnancy
Tel: 1-888-246-5840
Motherisk's Home Line
Tel: (416) 813-6780
Web: www.motherisk.org

Nutrition for a Healthy Pregnancy
Health Canada
Web: www.hc- sc.gc.ca/hppb/nutrition/
pube/pregnancy/e_index.html

Pregnancy and Birth
Society of Obstetricians and
Gynaecologists of Canada
Web: sogc.medical.org/SOGCnet/
sogc_docs/common/pub_ed/topic
_preg_e.shtml

Pregnancy Health Center—Women's Health Matters
Sunnybrook and Women's College
Health Sciences Center
Web: www.womenshealthmatters.ca/
centres/pregnancy

POSTNATAL SUPPORT

La Leche League Canada
18C Industrial Drive,
PO Box 29,
Chesterville, ON K0C 1H0
Tel: (613) 448-1842
Fax: (613) 448-1845
Web: www.lalecheleaguecanada.ca

PASS-CAN—Postpartum Adjustment Support Services Canada
#3, 460 Woody Road,
Oakville, ON L6K 3T6
Tel: (905) 844-9009
Fax: (905) 844-5973
Web: www.passcan.ca

PARENTS' GROUPS

Canadian Foundation for the Study of Infant Deaths
Suite 308, 586 Eglinton Avenue East,
Toronto, ON M4P 1P2
Tel: (416)488-3260
Fax: (416)488-3864
Toll free: 1-800-END-SIDS
Web: www.sidscanada.org

Candlelighter's Association—Childhood Cancer Foundation Canada
Suite 401, 55 Eglinton Avenue East,
Toronto, ON M4P 1G8
Tel: 1-800-363-1062 or (416) 489-6440
Fax: (416) 489-9812
Toll free: 1-800-700-4437
Web: www.candlelighters.ca

Caring for Kids—Canadian Paediatric Society
Web: www.caringforkids.cps.ca

Children's Wish Foundation
Suite 404, 95 Bayly Street,
Ajax, ON L1S 7K8
Tel: (905) 426-5656
Fax: (905) 426-4111
Web: www.childrenswish.ca

Family Support—Health Canada
Web: www.hc-sc.gc.ca/hppb/childhood-
youth/cyfh/family_support

Multiple Births Canada
PO Box 432,
Wasaga Beach, ON L0L 2P0
Tel: (705) 429-0901
Fax: (705) 429-9809
Toll free: 1-866-228-8824
Web: www.multiplebirthscanada.org

Parent Help Line
Kids Help Phone National Office
Suite 300, 439 University Avenue,
Toronto, ON M5G 1Y8
Tel: 1-888-603-9100
Web: www.parentsinfo.sympatico.ca

Parents Without Partners
Suite 510, 1650 South Dixie Highway,
Boca Raton, FL 33432
Tel: (561) 391-8833
Fax: (561) 395-8557
Web: www.parentswithoutpartners.org

Sudden Infant Death Syndrome Alliance
Suite 210, 1314 Bedford Avenue,
Baltimore, MD 21208
Tel: (410) 653-8226
Fax: (410) 653-8709
Web: www.sidsalliance.org

CARE AND EDUCATION

Canadian Child Care Federation
Suite 201, 383 Parkdale Avenue,
Ottawa, ON K1Y 4R4
Tel: 1-800-858-1412 or (613) 729-5289
Fax: (613) 729-3159
Web: www.cccf-fcsge.ca

FIRST AID AND SAFETY

Canadian Red Cross
170 Metcalfe Street,
Ottawa, ON K2P 2P2
Tel: (613) 740-1900
Fax: (613) 740-1911
Web: www.redcross.ca

Product Safety Division—Health Canada
MacDonald Bldg.,
4th Floor, 123 Slater Street,
Address Locator: 3504D
Ottawa, ON K1A 0K9
Tel: (613) 957-4467
Fax: (613) 952-3039
Web: www.hc-sc.gc.ca/ehp/ehd/psb

Canada Safety Council
1020 Thomas Spratt Place,
Ottawa, ON K1G 5L5
Tel: (613) 739-1535
Fax: (613) 739-1566
Web: www.safety-council.org

Children's Safety Association of Canada
Suite 250, 385 The West Mall,
Etobicoke, ON M9C 1E7
Tel: (416) 620-1584
Fax: (416) 620-0048
Web: www.safekid.org

Safe Kids Canada
180 Dundas Street West,
Toronto, ON M5G 1Z8
Tel: 1-888-SAFE TIPS (723-3847) or
416-813-6766
Fax: 416-813-4986
Web: www.safekidscanada.ca

St. John Ambulance Canada
312 Laurier Avenue East,
Ottawa, ON K1N 6P6
Tel: (613) 236-7461
Fax: (613) 236-2425
Web: www.sja.ca

CHILDREN WITH SPECIAL NEEDS

Autism Society Canada
PO Box 65,
Orangeville, ON
Tel: (519) 942-8720
Fax: (519) 942-3566
Toll free: 1-866-874-3334
Web: www.autismsocietycanada.ca

Canadian Directory of Genetic Support Groups
London Health Sciences Center
Web: www.lhsc.on.ca/programs/
medgenet

Canadian Down Syndrome Society
811 – 14 Street N.W.
Calgary, AB T2N 2A4
Tel: (403) 270-8500
Fax: (403) 270-8291
Toll free: 1-800-883-5608
Web: www.cdss.ca

Canadian Cystic Fibrosis Foundation
Suite 601, 2221 Yonge Street,
Toronto, ON M4S 2B4
Tel: (416) 485-9149
Fax: (416) 485-0960
Toll free: 1-800-378-2233
Web: www.cysticfibrosis.ca

Learning Disabilities Association of Canada
323 Chapel Street,
Ottawa, ON K1N 7Z2
Tel: (613) 238-5721
Fax: (613) 235-5391
Web: www.ldac-taac.ca

Muscular Dystrophy Association of Canada
Suite 900, 2345 Yonge Street,
Toronto, ON M4P 2E5
Tel: (416) 488-0030
Fax: (416) 488-7523
Toll free: 1-800-567-2873
Web: www.mdac.ca

Spina Bifida and Hydrocephalus Association of Canada
#977 – 167 Lombard Avenue
Winnipeg, MN R3B 0T6
Tel: (204) 925-3650
Fax: (204) 925-3654
Toll free: 1-800-565-9488
Web: www.sbhac.ca

INFANT/CHILD HEALTH

Canadian Immunization Awareness Program
Canadian Public Health Association
400 – 1565 Carling Avenue
Ottawa, ON K1Z 8R1
Tel: (613) 725-3769
Fax: (613) 725-9826
Web: www.immunize.cpha.ca

Canadian Institute of Child Health
Suite 300, 384 Bank Street
Ottawa, ON K2P 1Y4
Tel: (613) 230-8838
Fax: (613) 230-6654
Web: www.cich.ca

National Institute of Child Health and Human Development (U.S.)
Bldg 31, Room 2A32, MSC 2425,
31 Center Drive,
Bethesda, MD 20892-2425
Web: www.nichd.nih.gov

INDEX

ACKNOWLEDGMENTS

Dorling Kindersley would like to thank **Elizabeth Fenwick**, the author of the English edition, for all the work she put into writing and revising the book.

Original edition
Senior Art Editor Carole Ash
Project Editors Sarah Pearce, Tanya Hines (Pregnancy and Birth), Claire Le Bas (Your Child's Health)
Art Editors Rowena Alsey (Pregnancy and Birth), Tina Hill (Your Child's Health)
Production Manager Michel Blake
Editorial Direction Daphne Razazan
Main photographers Antonia Deutsch, Dave King, Susannah Price

This revised edition
Produced for Dorling Kindersley Limited by Design Revolution, Queens Park Villa, 30 West Drive, Brighton, BN2 2GE
Senior Art Editor Becky Willis
Project Editor Julie Whitaker
Index Milla Hills, Indexing Specialists

This Canadian edition
Dorling Kindersley would like thank the following for their design and editorial work on this edition: Corinne Asghar, Liz Brown, Caroline Buckingham, Liz Coghill, Karen Constanti, Anne Esden, Kathy Fahey, Emma Forge, Edward Kinsey, and Nicola Rodway.
Index Dorothy Frame

Canadian Medical Association
President Dana W. Hanson MD, FRCPC
Secretary General and CEO
William G. Tholl
Executive Director, Publications
Pat Rich
Editor-in-chief, Publications
John Hoey MD
Medical Editor
Catherine Younger-Lewis MD, MJ
Program Manager, Books
Christine Pollock
Assistant Nunzia Parent
Information Services Elizabeth Czanyo

Special photography
(Abbreviations key: t=top, b=bottom, r=right, l=left, c=center)
Andy Crawford assisted by Gary Ombler: 192bc, 197tl;
Antonia Deutsch assisted by Pamela Cowan: 6cl, 17, 19t, 21, 27b, 29b, 37–42, 43t, 44–49, 56t and br, 57–61, 64, 67, 71t, 72–73, 90tr and br, 91tl, tc and cr, 92bl

and br, 94, 95tr, tl and cr, 97;
Trish Gant: 55c and b, 82b, 86cl, 95br, 100cr and c, 121br, 123, 160t, 161b, 191cr, 201b, 216t, 243b, 246cl and tr, 247b, 249b, 250c and cl, 251;
Steve Gorton: 145cr;
Dave King: 4: 1st column pictures 2–4, 2nd column pictures 1–4; 6: 2nd column t and lower c, 7: 1st column, 2nd column all except bl, 50–52, 53b, 54 tr and c, 55tl, tr and c, 76–81, 88tl, 95bl, 98, 99t, l, and tc, 100tl, 101, 104, 105 all except bl, 108 all except t, br, bl and cr, 109br, 110–111, 112tl, 114–16, 117t, 2nd row r, 121 all except t and tl, 124bl, 125tr and b, 128–33, 134t, 138–41, 145t and cl, 146t, 149cl, bl and bc, 154, 159, 162–63, 166–73, 175, 180t and l, 182b, 183tr, cr and br, 182–202 all except 197tl, 204r, cr and b, 205tr and br, 206–7, 209br, 210tr and b, 211–12, 213tl, tr and cr, 214t, 216b, 218–23, 225, 226c and r, 227t and bl, 228cl, cr, and b, 229tl, tr and bl, 230tl and cr, 231tl, cr and b, 232c and r, 234t, 237, 254b, 255b, 256–57;
Ray Moller: 6: 2nd column upper cr, 99b, 100t and b, 106cl, cr, bl, and br, 107, 136t, cr, and br, 137 all except br, 142bl and br, 143, 146bl, 181c;
Stephen Oliver: 4: 1st column pictures 1 and 5; 10, 15, 54l and b, 55tr, 56bl, 99bc and br, 103, 105bl, 108t, 120br, 121t and tl, 125tl, 134 all except t, 135, 148, 149tr, box tr, cl and cr, 153, 155, 156;
Susannah Price: 6: 2nd column upper cl and b, 7: 2nd column bl, 68–69, 84, 86 all except cl, 87, 88bl, and br, 90tl and c, 91tr and bl, 92tl and tr, 93, 112tr, c, and br, 117 2nd row l, 3rd row l and r, 4th row l, c, and r, 120t, 124 all except bl, 125c, 127, 136bl and bc, 137br, 142tl, 144bc, and br, 150–52, 158t, 174, 254t, 255t;
Steve Shott: 2: 2nd column picture 5; 157, 158t, 159.

Picture credits
Picture Researcher Anna Grapes
Picture Librarians Melanie Simmonds, Marcus Scott

The publisher would like to thank the following for their kind permission to reproduce their photographs:
(Abbreviations key: t=top, b=bottom, r=right, l=left, c=center)
Sue Ford, Western Ophthalmic Hospital: 181tr, 183bl, 209r; **Genesis Film Productions Ltd/Neil Bromhall:** 23; **Getty Images:** 1 (Dennis

O'Clair), 11 (Neil Harding); **Lesley Howling:** 43b; **Meningitis Research Foundation:** 208; **Mother and Baby Picture Library/Emap Esprit:** 31; 74–75 main picture, 89, 178–179 main picture (Ian Hooton), 2–3 main picture, 8–9 main picture (Paul Mitchell), 12–13, 12t, 16, 18, 20, 22, 24, 26, 28, 30 (Steve Shott); **National Medical Slide Bank:** 181br, 204tr, 209tl, 213bl, 226l, 227cl, 232l; **St. John's Institute of Dermatology:** 228tl, 231tr; **St. Mary's Hospital:** 183tl, 205tl, 205bl; **Science Photo Library:** 70 (Hank Morgan), 206br (Dr. H. C. Robinson); **Tony Stone:** 1 (Dennis O'Clair), 11 (Neil Harding); **Ron Sutherland:** 67c; **Dr. I. Williams:** 180br, 181cr, 182t and cr, 203r, 210l, 214b, 227bl, 229br, 230t, bc and b.

Jacket images
Image Bank/Sandy King; all other images © Dorling Kindersley. For further information see: www.dkimages.com

Loan or supply of props
Baby B's, Fulham, London, England; Diana Dolls Fashions Inc., Stoney Creek, Ontario; The Nursery Collection, Watford, England; Porter Nash Medical, London, England; Seward Ltd., London, England. **Special thanks to:** Mary Snyder at Snugli, Inc.; Gerry Baby Products Company, Denver, Colorado; Judi's Originals, Scottsdale, Arizona.

Illustrators
Coral Mula: all line artwork except 14t; **Nick Hall:** 14t; **Kevin Jones Associates:** 234, 235, 236; **Richard Tibbitts:** 14, 16, 18, 20, 22, 24, 28, 30

Consultants
Dorling Kindersley acknowledges the contribution of the following consultants to the original edition:
Professor R. W. Taylor MD, FRCOG, Head of Department of Gynaecology, The United Medical Schools of Guy's and St. Thomas's Hospitals, London; **Professor Jon Scopes** MB, PhD, FRCP, Department of Paediatrics, St. Thomas's Hospital, London; **Christine Williams** RGN, HV, FWT, Health Visitor and Family Planning Nurse; **Janice Leighton** RGN, RM, Community Midwife; **Alan McLaughlin** RGN, Department of Clinical Neurology, St Thomas's Hospital, London.